GROUP DYNAMICS
in Occupational Therapy

The Theoretical Basis and Practice Application of Group Intervention

THIRD EDITION

GROUP DYNAMICS
in Occupational Therapy

The Theoretical Basis and Practice Application of Group Intervention

THIRD EDITION

Marilyn B. Cole, MS, OTR/L, FAOTA

Associate Professor of Occupational Therapy

Quinnipiac College

Hamden, Connecticut

SLACK
INCORPORATED

An innovative information, education, and management company
6900 Grove Road • Thorofare, NJ 08086

ISBN-13: 978-1-55642-687-2
ISBN-10: 1-55642-687-9

The work SLACK Incorporated publishes is peer reviewed. Prior to publication, recognized leaders in the field, educators, and clinicians provide important feedback on the concept and content that we publish. We welcome feedback on this work.

Printed in the United States of America.

Library of Congress Cataloging-in-Publication Data
Cole, Marilyn B., 1945-
    Group dynamics in occupational therapy : the theoretical basis
and practice application of group intervention / Marilyn B. Cole. --
3rd ed.
        p. ; cm.
    Includes bibliographical references and index.
    ISBN 1-55642-687-9 (alk. paper)
    1. Occupational therapy. 2. Group psychotherapy. 3. Social
groups.   I. Title.
    [DNLM: 1. Occupational Therapy--methods. 2. Psychotherapy,
Group--methods.   WM 430 C689g 2005]
RC487.C65 2005
616.89'165--dc22

                    2004024893

Published by: SLACK Incorporated
               6900 Grove Road
               Thorofare, NJ 08086 USA
               Telephone: 856-848-1000
               Fax: 856-853-5991
               www.slackbooks.com

Last digit is print number: 10   9   8   7   6   5   4

Contents

Acknowledgments

For the Third Edition, I'd like to thank Mary Donohue, Anne Scott, Pat Schaber, Roxie Black, Mildred Ross, and Roseanna Tufano for their feedback, contributions, editing, and helpful suggestions. A special thanks also goes to my husband, Marty, for his support and encouragement as I worked overtime to complete this project while teaching full-time at Quinnipiac University.

About the Author

Marilyn B. (Marli) Cole, MS, OTR/L, FAOTA, is a tenured Associate Professor of Occupational Therapy at Quinnipiac University, Hamden, CT, and an Occupational Therapy Consultant. She holds a Bachelor's degree in English from the University of Connecticut, a graduate certificate in Occupational Therapy from the University of Pennsylvania, and a Master's degree in Clinical Psychology from the University of Bridgeport. She is licensed by the state of Connecticut to practice occupational therapy and is certified by the Center for Study of Sensory Integrative Dysfunction to administer the Southern California Sensory Integration Tests. The author's clinical experience includes 16 years in mental health, 3 years in pediatrics, and 5 years in geriatrics.

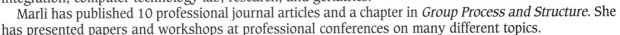

The author has more than 24 years of experience, including Eastern Pennsylvania Psychiatric Institute in Philadelphia; Middlesex Memorial Hospital in Middletown, CT; Lawrence and Memorial Hospitals in New London, CT; and Newington Children's Hospital in Connecticut. She has also served as consultant for the West Haven VA Medical Center, the Portland Public Schools, Fairfield Hills Hospital, the Institute of Living, and St. Joseph's Manor, all in Connecticut.

This is Marli's 21st year of full-time teaching. She has taught courses in psychiatric clinical media, group leadership, group dynamics, frames of reference, fieldwork I and II, psychopathology, sensorimotor integration, computer technology lab, research, and geriatrics.

Marli has published 10 professional journal articles and a chapter in *Group Process and Structure*. She has presented papers and workshops at professional conferences on many different topics.

Marli has also delivered professional presentations to Yale psychiatric residents, the Connecticut Occupational Therapy Association, the New York State Occupational Therapy Association, the American Occupational Therapy Association, and the World Federation of Occupational Therapy.

Currently, she is involved in research investigations of the relationship of group size with cohesiveness and meaningfulness, the status of the therapeutic relationship in occupational therapy, and the development of cultural competence. In recent years she has taken groups of students to England and Costa Rica.

Introduction

Much has changed over the past 5 years, both in the occupational therapy profession and in health care generally. The *Occupational Therapy Practice Framework*, passed by the American Occupational Therapy Association's (AOTA's) Representative Assembly in 2002, has changed the language of our profession and has expanded the scope of our practice (AOTA, 2002). The health care paradigm has shifted away from a reductionistic medical model and toward a holistic community model, which embraces a positive view of health. In it, health is defined as not only the absence of disease, but also life satisfaction and a sense of well-being (World Health Organization [WHO], 2001).

Accordingly, our use of groups for evaluation and intervention is reframed in the third edition of *Group Dynamics in Occupational Therapy*. It reflects the changes in terminology put forth by the new *Occupational Therapy Practice Framework*, as well as elements of the new paradigm, which is holistic, client centered, and systems oriented. The use of group interventions continues to grow in practice, not only because groups are cost-effective, but because of their potential for providing social and emotional support, encouraging client participation, and motivating clients to make therapeutic changes in their occupational choices and performance. When therapeutic groups are skillfully planned, client participation in them parallels their participation in life. There is no better arena for occupational therapists to evaluate and build upon client socialization, communication, and group interaction skills than while enabling their participation in a well-designed and facilitated therapeutic group.

One major change is the inclusion of Chapter 3, Client-Centered Groups, as a part of Section One, Acquiring Group Skills. This chapter formerly defined a "humanistic" approach, which is based in part on the theories of Carl Rogers, the same Carl Rogers whose writings form the underpinnings of the Canadian-founded Client-Centered Model (Law, 1998). In Chapter 1, Cole's seven-step format provides for the highest level of client participation. Using the seven steps, occupational therapist group leaders learn to recognize and encourage expression of each client's unique culture and values to create an atmosphere of nonjudgmental acceptance, and to maximize the group's potential for providing one another emotional and social support. Processing enables emotional self-expression, generalizing allows clients to individualize learning, and application focuses on verbalization of and support for each client's goals. As such, the seven-step format is a good fit with both the *Occupational Therapy Practice Framework* (AOTA, 2002) and with the principles of client-centered practice.

Using frames of reference, or practice theories, will probably always be a part of the reasoning process occupational therapists use to evaluate clients and design interventions. The six frames of reference chapters have also been updated. These chapters illustrate how Cole's seven-step format for groups can adapt to different theoretical perspectives in meeting the needs of a wide range of client populations. While these adaptations take into account different levels of client ability, they do not deviate from the original client-centered focus. *Note: The grand theories, sometimes called overarching theories or occupational performance models, that have recently emerged in the occupational therapy literature are not included (except for MOHO) because their broad nature does not lend itself specifically to the planning of group interventions.

The group protocol, Chapter 11, has been updated to include applications from the *Occupational Therapy Practice Framework* (AOTA, 2002) as well as a wider variety of practice areas, including wellness, prevention, and community-based settings. Another change is greater emphasis on developing a method for measuring outcome. Outcome is presented in the *Occupational Therapy Practice Framework* as an area equal in importance to evaluation and intervention. The two outcomes defined by the framework are "engagement in occupation" and "participation" in life. "Outcomes may be measured by occupational performance, client satisfaction, adaptation, role competence, health and wellness, and quality of life" (AOTA, 2002, p. 619). Setting outcome criteria was an essential step in the planning of group interventions in the first and second editions. However, the third edition includes the discussion of outcomes throughout the group sessions, rather than only at the end. Outcome measures have always addressed the therapeutic goals, but the new process requires that goals be derived from those verbalized by clients during the member selection process. These additions take into account a greater emphasis on collaboration with clients in every aspect of client-therapist interaction.

In addition to these changes, two new chapters have been added. The new Chapter 4, Groups as Social Contexts, explores the design of group interventions for families, work teams, caregiver groups, and community organizations. A six-session protocol for families with dementia, based on Schaber's (2002) application of the family FIRO model, provides an example of how Cole's seven-step format could be adapted for a home care setting. This chapter includes a new measure of social participation designed by Mary Donohue (2003), which is based on Mosey's definition of group interaction skill.

The second new chapter, Chapter 13, presents an additional laboratory experience for students, entitled "Developing Cultural Competence." This group protocol incorporates current research on culture from a variety of sources and presents 6 original structured group activities, based primarily on the cultural competence model published by Shirley Wells and Roxie Black (2000). In the facilitation of client-centered groups, occupational therapists need cultural competence to create an atmosphere of nonjudgmental acceptance, to recognize and encourage the expression of cultural differences among members, and to maximize the value of diversity. Teaching students about culture prepares them to interact effectively with clients and others in the ever-changing multicultural world of the 21st century.

Bibliography

American Occupational Therapy Association. (2002). Occupational therapy practice framework: Domain and process. *American Journal of Occupational Therapy, 56,* 609-639.

Donohue, M. (2003) Group profile: Studies with children: Validity measures and item analysis. *Occupational Therapy in Mental Health, 19,* 1-23.

Law, M. (Ed.). (1998). *Client-centered occupational therapy.* Thorofare, NJ: SLACK Incorporated.

Schaber, P. (2002). FIRO model: A framework for family-centered care. *Physical & Occupational Therapy in Geriatrics, 20*(4), 1-18.

Wells, S., & Black, R. (2000). *Cultural competency for health professionals.* Bethesda, MD: American Occupational Therapy Association.

World Health Organization. (2001). *International classification of functioning, disability, and health.* Geneva, Switzerland: Author.

Section One

Acquiring Group Skills

Introduction

This section begins with experiential learning. Chapter 1, Group Leadership: Cole's Seven Steps, shows the beginning occupational therapy student how to lead an occupational therapy group. This format reflects a client-centered approach that facilitates client participation at every level of the process. The chapter includes many examples, learning activities, and opportunities for practice. Three occupational therapy leadership styles--director, facilitator, and adviser--are outlined, followed by guidelines for co-leadership of groups.

Chapter 2, Understanding Group Dynamics, selects from the vast body of knowledge about group dynamics those elements of groups that have the most impact for occupational therapy. An understanding of the process of groups, group development, and group norms and roles plays an integral part in the design and leadership of group activities. Guidelines on how to approach common member problem behaviors are also helpful to the beginning therapist. Learning exercises in this chapter are intended to increase awareness of the more abstract aspects of group process. This is best accomplished concurrently with experience, such as the series of six group sessions described in Chapter 12, A Group Laboratory Experience. In this way, as students absorb the content of Chapter 2, they can apply the principles directly to their own experience.

Chapter 3, Client-Centered Groups, reviews the basic concepts of client-centered practice as they apply to occupational therapy group leadership. Concepts such as respect, genuineness, and non-judgmental acceptance form a central core for group facilitation using Cole's seven-step format. Many of the basic assumptions are similar to the humanistic approach described in previous editions. This chapter includes skill-building exercises for the therapeutic use of self during group leadership. An outline of Cole's seven steps discusses ways in which each step applies client-centered principles.

Chapter 4, Groups as Social Contexts, is new. Its content discusses the design and leadership of occupational therapy groups in family, work, school, and social group contexts. This chapter's inclusion in Section One demonstrates the expanded role of occupational therapy groups in community and nontraditional settings. A series of six family group interventions is given as an example. Donohue's Group Profile (2003) provides an evaluation tool for the observation of both therapeutic groups and naturally occurring groups in the community.

Bibliography

Donohue, M. (2003). Group profile: Studies with children: Validity measures and item analysis. *Occupational Therapy in Mental Health, 19*, 1-23.

Chapter 1

Group Leadership: Cole's Seven Steps

It has been my observation that students learn best by experience. They are anxious to know how to "do" occupational therapy. They are both eager and afraid to begin working with clients. To the beginning student, occupational therapy is just a label. Only when students are put in the role of a professional do they become aware of what needs to be learned.

Acting like a professional is often difficult for students, whose only experience in group leadership is often with groups of their peers. Part of making the transition to a professional role is learning that it is different from a social role. Professionalism carries with it an authority and a directness of purpose that will need to be practiced by students before they begin interacting with clients.

This book begins with a technique that is a concrete form of group leadership training. This allows students to practice the role of a professional. It is as generic as any technique can be and is intended as a beginning experience for students entering the profession. As the educational process continues, it is expected that the technique will be modified many times over to match the needs of each unique group. It is changed in content to meet new goals and address different age groups and health conditions. It is changed in process and structure to align with different frames of reference. But learning has to begin somewhere. Just as motor development precedes cognitive awareness in the infant, a concrete experience in group leadership becomes the forerunner of the knowledge and understanding of its purpose and application in intervention.

These seven steps incorporate the basic concepts of the *Occupational Therapy Practice Framework*, which "is client centered and facilitates engagement in occupation to support participation in life" (American Occupational Therapy Association [AOTA], 2002, p. 609).

Seven-Step Format for Group Leadership (Cole's Seven-Step Groups)

These seven steps can meet the needs of the highest level groups and so are very appropriate for student groups. They are chosen for maximum integration of learning by the members. Clearly this format will not fit every need, goal, or client population. However, the format is easily adapted to meet the goals of any group. How and why it will be modified will be described later. The steps in group leadership are:

1. Introduction
2. Activity
3. Sharing
4. Processing
5. Generalizing
6. Application
7. Summary

The original idea for this format comes from Pfeiffer and Jones' *Reference Guide to Handbooks and Annuals* (1977), which presents a five-step format that is expanded and adapted for occupational therapy here.

Step 1: Introduction

Let us assume the occupational therapist is leading the initial session of a group. The therapist does not know the members well, although it is presumed he or she knows who they are and something about their disability and the reasons they have been assigned to the group. (In many settings, the occupational therapist would select the members him- or herself.) The members may not know one another. Once the group is gathered, the occupational therapist introduces him- or herself to the group. This introduction includes the therapist's name, title, and the name of the group that is about to begin. Then, even if people know one another, the therapist asks the members to greet the group by saying their names in turn. This procedure does more than just help the members learn one another's names; it acknowledges their membership in the group and invites them to be a part of it. In subsequent groups, it may not be necessary to say names around the room, but acknowledgment of each member's presence should still be done. A friendly "hello" or "welcome back" from the therapist may accomplish this.

Warm-Up

The next thing the leader should be concerned with is the receptivity of the members. How alert are they? How preoccupied are they? How are they feeling? Are members ready to begin a new experience, or do they need to be "warmed up?" A warm-up is an exercise that captures the group's attention, relaxes them, and prepares them for the experience to follow. Warm-ups can be structured or casual and impromptu. A nice collection of structured warm-up activities can be found in Rider and Ridrer's *The Activity Card Book for Mental Health* (2000). An example of a structured warm-up is "Grandma's Trunk." Each member says, "Grandma has an old trunk up in the attic and in it I found ____." Members fill in the blank by saying the name of something that begins with each letter of the alphabet in order. All items must be repeated each time. For example, the first person says she found an Acorn, the second found an Acorn and a Bonnet, etc. If there are eight members to the group, the eighth one must remember the seven items preceding his or her contribution.

This warm-up obviously requires members to have a good short-term memory. The occupational therapist should choose a warm-up that challenges members enough to hold their interest but is not beyond their capabilities. Warm-up activities accomplish several important goals. The game creates an atmosphere of spontaneity and fun. It also refocuses members' thoughts from whatever they came to the group thinking about to this group right here, right now. If a warm-up works properly, it gets the members listening for what will come next and encourages their cooperation in the group experience to follow.

All groups do not need a formal warm-up. Sometimes the best warm-up is a casual conversation about how members are feeling today. If the group is to engage in a discussion, just getting the members talking may prepare them adequately. If the agenda is more creative in nature, an imaginative warm-up may be in order. Remembering what happened last week may be an appropriate warm-up to an activity that will be the next step in a sequence. It is important to make the warm-up relevant to the activity to follow. One does not set a mood of fun and games when the agenda for the group is a serious issue like coping with loss or finding new employment.

Setting the Mood

Setting an appropriate mood is an important objective in choosing the most appropriate warm-up. However, setting the mood for a group is not only accomplished with a warm-up. The environment, the therapist's facial expression and manner of speaking, and the media used all contribute to the mood. Care should be taken before the group begins to set up the environment accordingly; this includes proper lighting; getting rid of clutter; setting out equipment, supplies, and the correct number of chairs; and avoiding distractions as much as possible.

Expectation of the Group

The therapist's manner and expression should generally reflect his or her expectation of the group. A therapist cannot expect group members to take an activity seriously if the therapist does not appear to do so. The therapist will always be a role model to members, whether or not it is his or her intention. If the therapist begins by saying, "Okay you guys, listen up!" the members will be expecting a pep talk before a football game, rather than a serious discussion about managing their time. A direct and authoritative presentation of the group is one of those skills students must learn that make up the role of the professional.

Explaining the Purpose Clearly

Clearly explaining the purpose of the group is a primary task in the introduction phase. How this is done depends on the type of group and the clients' level of understanding. This is a step that should never be left out. The intent of the group has undoubtedly been explained individually to each member why he or she was assigned to this particular group. But it should not be taken for granted that the clients remember, or even fully understand, the purpose of a group from a previous explanation. The purpose should be reiterated by the occupational therapist in a way the clients are likely to understand. A higher level group of clients will want to know why they are being asked to do a particular activity. If they are asked to do calisthenics, it will be helpful to tell them that physical exercise has been known to change brain chemistry, to relieve stress, to elevate their mood, and to energize their muscles. Clients who understand and believe this will be much more motivated to participate.

Clients with mild to moderate cognitive disability are unlikely to understand such abstract explanations of purpose. For them, a modified explanation, such as "These exercises will make you feel better so you can do more for yourself," may suffice. For clients with severe cognitive disability, a friendly expression and a gentle touch that says, "Trust me, this will help you" may be all it takes to engage them in the group activity (Allen, 1999; Allen, Earhart, & Blue, 1992).

We started out assuming that the occupational therapist is introducing a new group experience to a new set of clients. In an initial session, more time is taken in explaining the purpose than in subsequent sessions. In describing the purpose of the group, the goals of the whole series of group sessions should be outlined in the initial session. If possible, the goals should be spelled out in concrete terms. For example, money management is an activity of daily living that occupational therapists often help clients work on improving. In a money management group, members may be expected to plan and carry out a realistic budget for 1 month and keep accurate records in a notebook. Therapists often use behavior change as a measure of progress in their clients. When clients are informed about the behavior that is expected to change, they can keep track of their own progress. This becomes motivating when clients in groups start measuring each other's behavior change (or lack thereof). Peer pressure is a powerful motivator of change in human behavior.

Describing the purpose of each session will not take as much time as the initial explanation. However, the goals for each activity should always be stated clearly at the beginning of each session. Clients need to be reminded of how the group is expected to help them. As the therapist gets to know the members better, explanations can be more individualized and related to the problems each member presents. For example, in introducing a stress management session, the therapist might mention that: "In the previous sessions, you've been complaining about how difficult it is to carry out daily activities when you're feeling so much stress. Today's activity will give you some new strategies for reducing the stress in your lives." Generally, when clients understand exactly how an activity will help them, they are much more interested in doing it.

Brief Outline of the Session

Finally, the introduction ends with a brief outline of the session to immediately follow. The time frame, the media, and the procedures are included. For example, if the activity for a 1-hour session is "Draw Yourself," the therapist might say: "We will be using the paper and markers provided to do a drawing for the next 20 minutes. After we are finished, I will ask each of you to explain your drawing to the group, and we will discuss the activity for the last half of the session." This explanation serves several purposes. It tells the client how long he or she has to complete the activity. A complex artistic drawing cannot be done in 20 minutes, so if he or she is to finish, he or she knows he or she must keep it simple. The explanation also warns him or her that he or she probably should not draw anything he or she does not wish to discuss. Although this may be seen as inhibiting the client's creativity, it also allows him or her to control the image of him- or herself he or she projects to the group. How the therapist handles this will depend on the goal of the activity. If self-awareness is more important than social awareness, the clients may be given the option not to explain everything about their drawing. They need only say as much as they are comfortable sharing.

As well as understanding the purpose of the drawing activity, clients will want to know what is to be done with it afterward. When they know they will be expected to talk about their work, their drawing may be more focused, and they will be more prepared to speak when it is their turn. It may be helpful to tell clients ahead of time whether their drawings will be kept by the therapist or if they can keep them. The disposition of drawings produced will differ depending on the goals and the frame of reference used. However, stating the procedures ahead of time is most respectful to the client and may also prevent difficulties later in the session.

The brief outline of the session also gives members a clue to the session's focus. The example given tells clients that the activity portion is relatively short (20 minutes) compared with the discussion portion (at least 30 minutes). Members will see that the focus is on the discussion rather than the drawing and on learning and interaction rather than artistic talent. The outline helps clients and therapist get the whole session in perspective.

The introduction is one of the steps that is consistently kept in every frame of reference and every type of group. The structure may become less formal, with practice, but the essential elements must remain. An introduction can make or break a group, and each element plays a part in the effectiveness of group outcome.

Step 2: Activity

Many factors should be considered when planning the activity. In a professional setting, this is, in fact, a tremendously complex process. It incorporates all we know about clients; health conditions; and their corresponding dysfunctions, assessment, intervention planning, activity analysis, and synthesis and group dynamics. Selecting a therapeutic activity involves the entire process of clinical reasoning that occupational therapists take 2 or 3 years of academic training to learn. One of the problems in learning group technique before the theory is that the process will seem oversimplified and incomplete. However, students should have a positive experience in trying out the role of an occupational therapist, even though there is much more to be learned before they can adequately do it in the clinic.

Designing the group experience is a very complex process and many issues should be considered. All of them cannot be addressed here. For the purposes of simplification, the following issues will be presented for consideration in selecting a therapeutic activity: timing, therapeutic goals, physical and mental capacities of the members, knowledge and skill of the leader, and adaptation of an activity.

Timing

With five more steps to go (sharing, processing, generalizing, application, and summary), it should be evident that the activity to be experienced should be kept fairly simple and short. This will vary, of course, but for our purposes in learning to plan and lead groups, the activity portion should last no longer than one-third of the total session. For example, in this seven-step process for a 1-hour group, the activity used must be adapted to fit a time frame of 15 to 20 minutes and to meet a preset therapeutic goal.

Therapeutic Goals

It is impossible to plan an activity without first planning and structuring the goals. Goals are desired outcomes, something clients and therapists strive together to accomplish. Setting therapeutic goals for clients involves assessing their needs and applying our knowledge of their abilities and disabilities. The referral source, such as the hospital treatment team, the doctor, or the nursing home staff, may have already defined the problem (e.g., "This client needs to develop adequate social skills" or "Help client to learn joint protection and energy conservation techniques"). In planning our practice groups for peers, the student might first think about what goals might be useful for him- or herself. Perhaps coping with stress, setting priorities, clarifying values, managing money, managing time, and asserting one's self in social situations may be troublesome areas for students. The group goals should be chosen to meet the needs of most of the members. Once the goal is defined, an activity is designed or selected to help members achieve that goal. For example, when goals have to do with personal growth, for example, creative activities such as drawing, sculpture, dramatics, and storytelling can be helpful. Through the creative process, many parts of the self can be revealed and explored. If goals are more socially oriented, structured group tasks involving interaction of the members are appropriate (e.g., communication exercises or group decision making and problem solving).

Physical and Mental Capacities of the Members

Selection of the activity or experience is further determined by the physical and mental capacities of

Table 1-1	Activity Analysis	

Playing Bingo

Activity Components	Skills Needed
A letter and number are called	Client must hear the call and associate it with written letters and numbers
The bingo card is scanned	Client must read and understand written letters and numbers
A marker is placed on the number called	Client must have eye-hand coordination, fine motor skills, and grasp release
When a row of five is marked, patient calls out "Bingo"	Client must have good visual perception and must be able to speak loudly

the members. If members are college students around age 20, without physical or mental disabilities, the possibilities are almost unlimited. The challenge would be to find an activity that holds their interest and from which they can learn something new and meaningful. When members of the group are geriatric clients, the physical and fine motor components of the activity may be limited. A game of balloon volleyball or a lively discussion about a topic of interest might be suitable. When cognitive limitations must be taken into account, the activity will need to be more physical and concrete (not abstract) in nature. Cooking and simple crafts and games are often useful activities with adult clients who have developmental delays. Assessment of the physical and mental functioning of an individual is the subject of other textbooks in occupational therapy, and so will not be covered here. In the clinical setting, assessment would be done on each member prior to starting the group.

Knowledge and Skill of the Leader

Another factor in the activity selection process is the knowledge and skill of the leader. What activities that are familiar to the leader can be adapted to this group experience? Student leaders usually choose activities for the group that they themselves are comfortable with or have done before. A student who has had dance lessons may feel very comfortable introducing a movement activity; a leader with artistic talent may choose a drawing activity. Crafts, games, and educational or social experiences may be sources of familiar activities to be adapted. There are a wealth of resource books available offering ideas for structured experiences

in human relations. An example is Rider and Rider's *The Activity Card Book for Mental Health* (2000), which is updated every few years. When using these references, it should be kept in mind that most of the exercises cannot be done as written but will have to be adapted to the specific goals set by the occupational therapist.

Adaptation of an Activity

Adaptation of an activity requires some knowledge of activity analysis and synthesis. Activity analysis is the "process of examining an activity to distinguish its component parts. Activity synthesis is the process of combining component parts of the human and non-human environment so as to design an activity suitable for evaluation or intervention relative to performance" (Mosey, 1981, p. 114). The analysis of activities is the subject of other textbooks and will not be fully described here. This is yet another example of the complex process of clinical reasoning in occupational therapy, in bringing together concepts from many bodies of knowledge to influence our intervention choices.

Activity analysis is the breaking down of an activity into its component parts and matching each part with the human functions required to accomplish it. Playing bingo, for example, may be analyzed as shown in Table 1-1.

In this oversimplified illustration, the therapist must know 1) how to play Bingo and 2) what physical and mental skills are required to play. Knowing this, the client's skill is matched with what is required to do the activity. Modifications can then be made in the activity to suit the client's abilities. This is activity synthesis. For example, a group of clients with poor vision may need Bingo cards with larger letters and numbers and bright-colored markers. A hearing impaired group will need to have the calls written on a blackboard or flashed on a screen. Clients with poor motor control may need a Bingo card with magnetic markers that will stay in place even if the card is moved. Higher functioning groups may need more challenging requirements to win, such as markers all around the edge or in the shape of an "H" or an "S." Additional motivation may be built in by offering appealing prizes.

Once selected, the therapeutic activity should be presented in a systematic way. First, the activity should be explained as directly and simply as possible. Procedures and instructions are given in language appropriate to the level and background of the group.

The therapist should get feedback from the group as to whether they understood the directions and should answer any questions before proceeding. Materials and supplies, if needed, should be hidden from view until they are actually needed. As the activity is in progress, the therapist may choose to participate in order to avoid making members feel self-conscious or watched. However, a leader should not allow his or her participation to detract from making relevant observations of the group to be discussed later.

When the activity portion of the group is finished, any materials used such as pencils or paints should be collected and placed out of sight before moving to the discussion stages. This will avoid having some members continue working after time is up or be distracted by the extraneous items. It may be necessary to stop some individuals before they are finished in order to keep the group moving along. The leader needs to be prepared to continually adapt and structure the group.

Step 3: Sharing

After completing the activity, each member is invited to share his or her own work or experience with the group. The structure and process for sharing will vary with each activity. If the activity involves drawing or writing something individually, members will show the drawing and explain it to the group or read to the group what was written. In activities involving interaction, members share what the experience was like for them or what it meant to them. In either case, the therapist is responsible for making sure each member has a chance to do this.

Another important responsibility in this phase is to make sure each member's contribution is acknowledged. Acknowledgment may be done verbally or nonverbally. Sometimes just a smile and a nod may be all that is necessary. Members often want to respond to one another's sharing, but the therapist may need to model this to be sure the responses show caring and concern. Empathy is an important factor here. This means the therapist responds to the client in a way that communicates understanding of how the client feels. Empathy will be discussed in more depth in a later chapter.

Some members may be reluctant to share for various reasons. The therapist may need to support and encourage clients to share or to reassure them that they can do it without negative consequence. However, if a client refuses to share, this must be accepted; clients should not be unduly pressured to disclose anything about themselves that they do not feel comfortable sharing.

It does not matter in what order the members share, but often it is easier to keep track if members go in order around the circle. It is usually best to ask for a volunteer to start the process, so that clients feel some control over the group. However, the therapist can start to role model for the group what is expected to be shared. For example, in the "Best Friend" exercise from Pfeiffer and Jones (1973) (Worksheet 1-1), the therapist might begin by getting up and standing behind a chair and saying, "This is my best friend Beth (indicating an invisible self in the empty chair). She's a person who likes cooking healthy food, doing creative projects, and helping other people. Her pet peeve is people who smoke. She has always wanted to write a book... etc." The therapist models the format the members will use in sharing.

There are a few activities for which sharing is not a separate step but is incorporated into a discussion activity. For example, "The Doctor's Dilemma" (see p. 223) is a group decision-making task that involves extensive discussion as part of the activity. Expressing one's opinion on a given issue is built into the actual task. In this case, the therapist may be more involved during the activity to make sure all of the members participate and express their views and that their responses to one another are respectful and courteous.

Step 4: Processing

This is the most difficult step for students to learn. Inexperienced group leaders often skip this step entirely. Processing involves members expressing how they feel about the experience, the

Worksheet 1-1
Best Friend Introduction Sheet

Directions: Answer the questions as you would expect your best friend to describe you.

This is my best friend _____ (your name).

He or she is the kind of person who likes:
1.

2.

3.

He or she greatly appreciates and values:
1.

2.

3.

Some of his or her dislikes or pet peeves are:
1.

2.

3.

Someday he or she would like to:
1.

2.

3.

From Cole, M. B. *Group dynamics in occupational therapy: The theoretical basis and practice application of group intervention* (3rd ed.). Thorofare, NJ: SLACK Incorporated. © 2005 SLACK Incorporated.

(Adapted from Pfeiffer, J., & Jones, J. (1973). *Reference guide to handbooks and annuals*. La Jolla, CA: University Associates.)

leader, and each other. Feelings guide our behavior more than we know, and they certainly influence clients' behavior in occupational therapy groups. If these emotions remain unexpressed, the outcome of the group can never be fully understood. Expressing feelings is not so difficult when the experience has been positive. But if there are negative feelings, people often wish to avoid expressing them, and this includes both the group members and the leader.

Done correctly, processing can reveal some important and relevant information. If members felt anxious, embarrassed, or belittled while doing an activity, this will help to explain some of their responses when sharing and discussing it. Perhaps they felt intimidated by the leader or angry with some of the other members. Feelings like this can override any possible benefit the activity may have, if they are not expressed before the group ends. When they are expressed, the therapist has the opportunity to incorporate them into the subsequent discussion and to help the clients understand the significance of the feelings related to the group experience. From the *Occupational Therapy Practice Framework* perspective, this process helps to identify issues that encourage or discourage "engagement in occupation" or emotions that facilitate or present "barriers to participation" (AOTA, 2002).

Processing also includes a discussion of the nonverbal aspects of group. Underlying issues, such as struggles for power and control, subgrouping, scapegoating, conflict, attraction, and avoidance, are dynamics that may never be verbalized but will have a powerful influence on the group. These issues are highly complex for the beginning student; however, they should be well-understood by the beginning therapist. Underlying dynamics such as those mentioned can and do occur naturally in all groups. They will strongly influence the outcome of our occupational therapy groups, both positively and negatively, and must be handled openly and skillfully. More will be discussed about the underlying process of groups in a later chapter.

Step 5: Generalizing

This step addresses the cognitive learning aspects of the group. Here the therapist mentally reviews the group's responses to the activity and tries to sum them up with a few general principles. If the activity has gone as expected, some of the general principles derived from the group should closely resemble the original goals. However, few groups go exactly as planned. The general principles discussed in the group should not be preplanned but should come directly from the response of the members.

For example, an occupational therapist did an activity called "Incomplete Sentences" with a group of emotionally disturbed adolescents. The goal of the group was to clarify their values, and, in fact, the group did accomplish this. However, some additional principles were brought up during the processing phase, which are important to note. Principles of the "Incomplete Sentences" group were:

- The members generally value making decisions independent of their parents.
- The most valued activities were those the members chose to do themselves, such as sleeping late on Saturdays or buying their own clothes.
- Although wishing to be independent, members generally needed and wanted to be accepted by their parents as autonomous adults.

The third principle is the one not planned. During the processing phase, a member pointed out how good it was to be able to ask the leader to complete the sentences too. The group felt positive toward this leader, who, unlike their parents, seemed to accept them as equals. The comment brought forth many spontaneous stories of parental nonacceptance and it was evident that this was the important issue for the group.

General principles may be arrived at in several ways. The leader can look at the patterns of response among members. What opinions do they have in common? What were the common elements of their drawings or stories? For example, persons with alcohol abuse may see their drinking as the obstacle to reaching their vocational ambitions; bottles or glasses may appear in their drawings, or they may talk about highly unrealistic vocational ambitions. These common elements are easily seen as general principles.

Another way to distinguish general principles is to look at areas of disagreement. What are the conflicted areas in the group? Some members, for example, may see stress as a motivator to get moving, while others may find it overwhelming and the cause of their inaction.

A third important clue to the general principles is the group's energy. The therapist should follow up on issues that seem to energize the group and stimulate spontaneous conversation. An example is the third principle in the "Incomplete Sentences" activity mentioned earlier. This is one of those unpredictable aspects of groups that makes them continually exciting and interesting.

Step 6: Application

The application phase closely follows the generalizing phase, but takes it one step further. The therapist helps the group to understand how the principles learned during the group can be applied to everyday life. The goal is for each member to understand how he or she will apply the results of this group experience to help make his or her own life more functional outside the group.

To begin this process, the therapist should attempt to verbalize the meaning or significance of the experience—"Now that we know how important it is to have our parents' respect and acceptance, each of us needs to find a way to communicate this need to our parents." Application answers the question, "Now that you know how things are, what are you going to do about it?"

The answer to this question will be different for each individual. Knowledge of the client's background is helpful. The therapist discusses with each member how the principles learned in the group relate to problems or issues each has expressed earlier. For example, Sue will have a hard time explaining to her father, who thinks of her as a child, that she needs for him to trust her judgment about whom she dates and where she goes on Saturday nights. Laura, whose mother travels extensively on business, will have difficulty just getting her mom's attention long enough to talk about it. She sometimes wonders if her mother cares about her enough to take the time. Both girls will have difficulty in communicating with their parents, but in very different ways. Application may sometimes resemble a kind of group problem solving as members help each other find ways to apply the newly learned information. In client-centered terms, this part of the group's session encourages collaboration. In the *Occupational Therapy Practice Framework*, application addresses how the group learning will facilitate "participation in life."

One way the therapist can help the group with application is through limited self-disclosure. The therapist can role model application by saying, "When I need to discuss something with my mother and there never seems to be a good time, sometimes I suggest we make a date to go out to dinner together. She has to eat anyway and so do I, so

that plan works well for both of us. How do you see that?" The self-disclosure is not so personal as to be distracting, but offers a possible method of getting parents' attention for the group to consider. It gives group members a concrete example and opens the door for them to make their own suggestions.

Step 7: Summary

The final phase of the seven-step group is the summary. The purpose of the summary is to verbally emphasize the most important aspects of the group so that they will be understood correctly and remembered. Like generalizing, there is really no way to preplan a summary. The points to emphasize should come directly from the group's responses. A good summary may take 4 or 5 minutes. It reviews the goals, the content, and the process of the group. Sometimes the therapist asks the group members to help summarize by remembering the activity and giving their ideas about what was learned. The general principles are almost always included in the summary. Having members explain their own views of the group and how it can be applied often reinforces the learning that took place.

The emotional content of the group is also important to summarize. Especially when the group feels positive or the mood has changed for the better, verbal recognition of the good feelings by the therapist will help members remember the group as a positive experience.

One way for the therapist to acknowledge feelings is to thank the members for their participation in the group. While this is not a formula, addressing and thanking individuals for their openness, honesty, and willingness to share or trust in the group is always welcomed.

A final responsibility of the therapist is to end the group on time. If the group is well-planned and led, this will mark the completion of all seven steps. If, for some reason, all the steps have not been completed by the end of the session, the missing parts and the reasons for this can also be dealt within the summary.

Before leaving the "how to" section, three additional factors of leadership need to be explored:

1. Group motivation
2. Setting limits
3. Leadership styles

All are the responsibility of the leader and should occur throughout the seven steps as they are needed.

Group Motivation

Ideally, the therapist will have a group that comes to meetings with enthusiasm and interest to participate. Such a group will be eager to listen to the therapist and take direction. A group that is motivated will interact freely with one another, will share with one another easily, and will spontaneously seek to know the meaning of the group activity and how it can be applied. Such a group is probably too healthy to need therapy. Therefore, the leader needs to develop skills in how to motivate groups that may not be so eager.

Confidence in the Leader

An important factor in the group's motivation is its confidence in the leader. If the leader takes charge of the group with some authority and sounds like he or she knows what to do, the leader will inspire the group's confidence and trust. This confidence is further enhanced by the support and encouragement offered to the members. If clients feel that the therapist empathizes with them and understands their situation, they will tend to be more cooperative in accepting leadership. Trust is the important issue here. Clients need to feel that the leader is sensitive to them and that he or she can and will respond to their needs. They also need to know the leader is in control in order to feel safe.

Encouraging Enthusiasm

A leader also motivates the group members by encouraging their enthusiasm. This can be done in a number of ways. First, the leader can show enthusiasm for the group both verbally and nonverbally. A leader who smiles and speaks in a lively tone, makes frequent eye contact, and demonstrates energetic movements often passes on enthusiasm to the group. Talking to members individually and encouraging them to participate may be effective. The approach to clients has to be adapted to the cognitive level of the clients. An explanation of how the group will make a difference in their lives will work for higher level clients. A more immediate benefit may need to be offered to lower functioning clients (e.g., "Doing this activity will make you feel more relaxed"). Activities such as games or creative efforts chosen for the group may stimulate enthusiasm. Some activities will have built-in rewards (e.g., cooking groups and craft groups).

Encouraging Interaction

A final motivating factor is encouraging group interaction. It has been said that people get as much out of a group activity as they put into it. When group members are interacting with one another, they are not only participating, but also taking over some of the responsibility for the group. Interaction should be encouraged, especially in the sharing, processing, generalizing, and application phases of the group. A good leader allows the group members to share the leadership to the extent that they are capable. If they can support one another during sharing, express how they feel about one another during processing, notice similarities and differences during generalizing, and offer ideas to each other about application, they will then learn a lot more than if the leader does all these things for them. The leader can get the group to interact by indirectly encouraging them or by asking them to do so directly; the leader might ask, "Susan, what do you think of Peter's drawing?" or "Peter, what do you think the group had in common?" Often, the leader only needs to ask questions a few times in order for the group to understand what is expected.

A leader who does all the talking in the seven-step group is working too hard. It benefits both the leader and the group by getting the group to talk more. Members who interact, respond, and ask questions are showing their enthusiasm and helping others to become enthusiastic also. With the leader's guidance, the group can help accomplish many of its goals through interaction.

Setting Limits

This has to do with how the leader exerts authority over the group. The goal is to achieve a balance between control and leniency.

Assuming Appropriate Authority

The leader should assume appropriate authority, guiding the group through all its stages, while giving members the freedom to express their thoughts, feelings, and opinions. A good leader will guide the group assuredly but will not dominate or intimidate its members. Neither does a good leader allow him- or herself to be dominated by the group. If the group goes its own way unguided, the members will not learn and make therapeutic change, and the group may never reach its goals.

Equal Time

Another part of setting limits is allowing sufficient time for each member to contribute. There are always a few members of a group who seem to take up more time and attention than the others. It is up to the therapist to see that all the members have a chance to participate. The leader controls the pace of the group and lets members know when they are taking more than their share of the time available. In this way, the group can be guided through each stage and can end on time.

Limiting Inappropriate Behavior

Limiting inappropriate behavior is perhaps the most difficult for students to learn. It generally requires that the leader interrupt the process going on in order to request that it be changed. If Joe has embarked on a lengthy discussion about a staff member who has treated him unfairly, but the issue has nothing to do with the goals of the group, it may be necessary for the leader to stop him and redirect the group back to the task at hand.

Respectful Limit Setting

Limits are best set with respect, and without anger, so that the group members will not become defensive. The therapist should develop skill in empathizing with the offending client. When the leader asks Joe to stop his tirade about the staff member, it is more likely to be heard if he or she first acknowledges his anger: "Joe, it sounds like you're very angry at ____, and I'd be happy to listen to you tell me about it after the group. But for now, I'd like to hear what all the members have to say about leisure planning." Other types of inappropriate behavior might be members showing disrespect for or disinterest in one another or physical expressions of emotion.

One important principle to keep in mind is always put the good of the group first. When individuals behave in ways that distract the group from benefiting in an occupational therapy activity, the leader is obligated to intervene on behalf of the group. Techniques for dealing with specific client behaviors that are difficult will be discussed in the next chapter.

Leadership Styles

The leadership style a therapist uses will profoundly affect the outcome of the group. Furthermore, different frames of reference require very different leadership approaches. Knowing the characteristics of several approaches and their likely effects on the group allows us to be flexible and use our skills more effectively to achieve desired outcomes.

According to Lewin and colleagues (1938, 1939), there are three fundamental leadership styles: autocratic, democratic, and laissez-faire.

Autocratic leadership implies complete control of the group with little or no input from the members. Democratic leadership allows members to make choices and to have a say in what the group does and becomes. Laissez-faire is a French expression meaning literally "to let do" or to let the people do as they choose. Laissez-faire leadership implies a minimum of control and a deliberate noninterference in the natural forces of a group or the freedom of individuals within it. Lewin studied the effects of these three styles of leadership at a boys' summer camp. He found that autocratic leadership resulted in the greatest productivity, but created hostility and resentment, poor quality of work, and dependency on the leader. Laissez-faire leadership produced independence in the members, but morale was not very high. It was democratic leadership that resulted in the highest morale and the most group cohesiveness. However, Lewin's study should be understood in the context of the boys' camp. The democratic style that worked best for campers may not work for other populations, and other styles may be more appropriate. Posthuma (2002) suggests that characteristics from all the above styles become a part of each leader's repertoire.

Three types of occupational therapy group leaderships will be presented in this text: director, facilitator, and advisor. All may be defined democratic in spirit, but with varying amounts of member input. Each is appropriate in different situations and for different levels of client functioning.

Directive Leadership

In politics, an autocratic leader rules a dictatorship; he or she fashions the nation according to his or her own vision, setting up the structures of government and making all the decisions. In therapy, it would not be ethical or desirable to hold this much control over a group of clients. However, as a director, the occupational therapist defines a group, selects activities, and structures the group in ways that he or she knows to be therapeutically appropriate for a specific group of clients. The director uses authority sparingly, only as necessary to make the group therapeutic for its members. Used inappropriately, too much direction can cause members to feel infantilized, treated like children who cannot think for themselves; it can stunt the growth and development of a group by crushing attempts to question or challenge the leader.

However, directive leadership is absolutely necessary for lower functioning clients who do not have the cognitive capabilities to make decisions or solve problems. These clients do not feel safe when the therapist is not in control. In a sense, the therapist is always in control, even in the more democratic approaches. The leader sets the goals, the level of structure, the media used, and the extent to which leadership responsibilities are shared with the group. The therapist's decisions about how to lead are, hopefully, based not only on his or her own preference or style, but on the therapist's expert assessment of the needs of the group. For example, Allen suggests that the therapist structure the environment and the task demand, but within that context, allow clients to do as much as they can for themselves (Allen et al., 1992). If the therapist is knowledgeable about Allen's theory, he or she will be able to predict fairly accurately how much assistance the clients will need to accomplish a task and will plan the structure of the group accordingly.

Frames of reference for which a directive leadership style is most appropriate are cognitive behavioral, sensorimotor, and cognitive disabilities. (Note: The term "directive" as used here does not relate to Kaplan's "Directive Group," which is discussed in Chapter 10.)

Facilitative Leadership

The next style of leadership on the control vs. freedom continuum is democratic. Just as the democratic leader is voted into power by the citizens, a facilitator gathers support from constituents. The facilitative leader must convince the members of the group that he or she is on their side and represents their best interests. The facilitator earns the support of the members by allowing them to make choices and showing care and concern. Decisions are made by the group with the facilitator's guidance. The therapist is a resource person, providing the group with needed information, needed structure, and needed equipment and supplies. The occupational therapist facilitator openly discusses the purpose and goals of the group. Just as a democratic government presumes and requires a certain level of education in its citizens in order to work effectively, democratic leadership in therapy requires that the members have a certain level of knowledge and skill. Without the required knowledge, members cannot make good decisions or share the leadership effectively. So the role of a facilitator is also that of an educator. The therapist explains the therapeutic aspects of activity so that the group can choose tasks that are likely to be of benefit to them.

Lewin said that democratic leadership is the most likely to lead to group cohesiveness. This is confirmed in reviewing the group developmental process (further described in Chapter 2). As a group reaches the "control" phase, members must challenge the leadership, the structure, and/or the group task. A facilitator can allow him- or herself to be challenged, use reason and logic to explain the way things have been, and give the group choices about changing them in ways that are not destructive to the group's integrity.

Group facilitation also has its limitations. It is not suitable for clients functioning at a low cognitive level. It presumes a certain level of self-awareness, intelligence, insight, and self-understanding. It is most useful in frames of reference that make personal direction and choice a priority. The developmental, psychodynamic, and model of human occupation approaches depend on a facilitative leadership style to promote a certain level of independent functioning and decision making in client group members. However, when the goals of intervention are to develop specific skills and abilities or to promote neurophysiological or cognitive development, a democratic approach may not be appropriate.

Facilitation is the most useful in motivating clients and getting them involved. It is a widely recognized phenomenon that people tend to be more committed to pursuing goals that they have a part in choosing. The more cognitively aware they are, the more they resent goals that are imposed on them. Therefore, discussions that precede a group may use a facilitative approach as a motivator, even when the group itself is more directive.

Group Leader as Advisor

The advisor is the most passive of leadership styles. Occupational therapy consultants use advisory leadership when working with groups of professionals or community groups. Its use in therapy is limited to the most highly functioning groups working on goals like problem solving or attitude change. An occupational therapy consultant/advisor may be appropriate in emerging practice areas like prevention or health maintenance. Clients who seek assistance with specific problems may need an occupational therapist to advise them on issues such as coping with stress on the job, conserving energy in the home, or eliminating architectural and social barriers. The advisor offers expertise as needed or requested, but does not provide structure or goals. Motivation comes from the group itself, and change is produced intrinsically as a

Table 1-2	Leadership Style Guidelines		
Member Characteristics	*Directive Leadership*	*Facilitative Leadership*	*Advisory Leadership*
Cognitive level	Low	Medium-high	High
Insight capacity	Minimal	Fair-good	Very good
Group maturity	Immature	Medium-high	Mature
Verbal skills	Poor	Average	High
Motivation	Low	Medium	High
Activity Characteristics	*Directive Leadership*	*Facilitative Leadership*	*Advisory Leadership*
Structure	Therapist selects activity	Therapist and members select activity	Members select activity
Goals	Accomplish task	Learn skill from experience	Understand process
Instruction	Therapist demonstrates/ teaches	Therapist and members teach process	Members seek advice as needed
Group maintenance roles	Mostly done by therapist	Members share in leadership	Members lead themselves
Feedback	Given mostly by therapist	Members encouraged to give to each other	Natural consequences from environment

result of the internal processes of each member or extrinsically as a result of social action. This type of leadership is most appropriate when working with families, caregivers, self-help groups, or community organizations.

General Principles of Group Leadership

Leaders of therapy groups, whatever their particular style, have certain obligations to the group. Designing the group is the most obvious of these. This planning phase involves choosing the members, setting or acknowledging the goals, setting the time and place, organizing the environment, and choosing the activity or media (sometimes with help from members). The group protocol described in Chapter 11 serves as a guide for how to design a therapy group. Decisions about the best leadership style to use within a given client setting are often complex. Table 1-2 may be helpful in choosing the best leadership style for certain member and activity characteristics.

The ongoing functions of the leader are to help the group achieve its goals (task function) and to maintain the group's integrity (maintenance function). The therapist may need to focus the group on the task to prevent it from getting sidetracked. He or she may have to adapt the activity or task along the way. Maintaining the group can involve the use of many leader skills. Setting group norms, like confidentiality and mutual respect, can be important. Modeling behaviors to be learned or effective interaction skills can help the group communicate and resolve its conflicts. The counseling skills Egan (1986) writes about are all useful in leading a therapeutic group; accurate empathy, concreteness, genuineness, confrontation, and self-disclosure are examples. These are elaborated in Chapter 3. Giving members feedback and helping members to give and receive feedback is an important function of the leader. Keeping the communication channels open is vital to the survival and growth of groups. These norms and roles are elaborated in Chapter 2.

A Leadership Experience for Students

To practice the seven-step group leadership, students may be divided into groups of eight members. Each student should plan and lead a group of his or her peers for 45 minutes, followed by a 15-minute feedback session from the instructor (and members). Students who are beginning their professional training should not attempt to play the roles of clients. There are plenty of goals students will find useful to work on for themselves in these groups.

To help the student plan a group, the Practice Group Plan (Worksheet 1-2) is suggested. The student's leadership skills may be evaluated by using Worksheets 1-3 and 1-4.

Co-Leadership

While leadership skills are best learned individually for practice purposes, students may feel more comfortable facing client groups in the company of a co-leader. Having a co-leader in an occupational therapy group with six to eight clients has a number of advantages. Some of these are mutual support, increased objectivity, collective knowledge, modeling for each other, and taking different roles.

Advantages of Co-Leadership

- Mutual support. Even if your co-leader is an inexperienced peer, you will be able to encourage one another and cover for each other's weaknesses. One of you is bound to remember what the other one forgets. Overcoming one's fear of coping with difficult clients and situations in the group will be easier when you have a partner to fall back on.

- Increased objectivity. Much more can be learned by the group when there are two leaders who can compare observations and give each other feedback. An objective understanding of the process of the group will be easier to achieve using both leaders' points of view. This is especially advantageous during supervision.

- Collective knowledge. Two leaders means twice as much knowledge and experience available for the group. Both leaders will be able to contribute ideas in the planning stage, as well as providing skilled interventions and leadership during the group itself. A discussion between co-leaders after the group is over is an important learning tool for novice leaders. Yalom (1995) writes discussion is an "essential ingredient" of a good co-therapy team. He suggests at least 5 minutes before each meeting and 15 to 20 minutes after each meeting be reserved for planning strategy and sharing reflections about each other's behavior during the group. If there are differences of opinion about how to handle difficult clients or interactional problems, this postgroup discussion would be the time to work them out. Co-leaders who cannot come to terms with their differences would be well-advised to seek out supervision before they re-enter the group arena for another session.

- Models for each other. Peer co-leaders have much to learn from each other. Every leader has different strengths and weaknesses, as well as different styles of intervention. Co-leader teams can help each other best by taking turns being active or directive and being attentive listeners and observers. In the clinic, students may have practicing therapist as co-leaders; beginning therapists may have experienced co-leaders as models. Each has its obvious advantages. However, ongoing co-leadership teams should eventually equalize their roles so that both are contributing and sharing the responsibility.

- Different roles. Good co-leadership teams learn to take advantage of each other's strengths by taking on different leadership roles. Some leaders are especially effective in setting limits when group members lose control. Other leaders are better at giving empathetic support. Co-leaders should take turns doing the confronting and rescuing so that no one has to play the "bad guy" all the time.

A much discussed issue in co-leadership is whether or not the group leaders should air their disagreements openly during the group or save them for the postgroup discussion. Yalom (1995) points out that timing is the deciding factor here. Newly formed groups should not be exposed to disagreement among the leadership. However, more stable and cohesive groups have much to

Worksheet 1-2
Practice Group Plan

1.   Title of group:

2.   Purpose of the group:

3.   Brief description of activity:

4.   Supplies and equipment needed:

5.   Goals of the group:

6.   Questions for discussion in:
     • Processing

     • Generalizing

     • Application

7.   Points for summary:

From Cole, M. B. *Group dynamics in occupational therapy: The theoretical basis and practice application of group intervention* (3rd ed.).
Thorofare, NJ: SLACK Incorporated. © 2005 SLACK Incorporated.

Worksheet 1-3
Leadership Evaluation

Student Name: _____ Date: _____ Time: _____

Group Title: _____

_____ Written Group Plan (10 points)

_____ Introduction (10 points)
Explains purpose clearly
Uses warm-up to relax/prepare group
Communicates expectations
Outlines timeframe/structure of group

_____ Activity (10 points)
Adequately prepared
Asks for feedback from the group
Directions clearly given
Timing appropriate
Materials appropriate
Environment appropriate

_____ Sharing (10 points)
Invites each member to share
Uses appropriate verbal and nonverbal communication
Empathizes and acknowledges feelings of members

_____ Processing (10 points)
Elicits members' feelings about the experience
Elicits members' feelings about each other
Elicits members' feelings about the leader (when appropriate)
Helps group understand its own processes

_____ Generalizing (10 points)
Points out like or similar responses
Points out contrasts or differences
Develops one or two principles learned

_____ Group Motivation (10 points)
Inspires confidence of group
Encourages enthusiasm
Encourages group interaction

From Cole, M. B. *Group dynamics in occupational therapy: The theoretical basis and practice application of group intervention* (3rd ed.). Thorofare, NJ: SLACK Incorporated. © 2005 SLACK Incorporated.

Leadership Evaluation (Continued)

_____ Limit Setting (10 points)
 Allows sufficient time to each member
 Limits inappropriate behavior
 Assumes appropriate authority (but not too controlling)

_____ Application (10 points)
 Verbalizes meaning of this experience (significance)
 Shows how this experience can relate to everyday life
 Relates this experience to issues/problems of members
 Uses concrete examples and/or self-disclosure

_____ Summary (10 points)
 Chooses most important points to emphasize
 Verbally reinforces group learning
 Acknowledges contributions of members
 Ends group on time

_____ Total Leadership Score

Member Evaluation Summary (from Worksheet 1-4)
 Average leadership score: _____

 Summary of strengths:

 Summary of suggestions for improvement:

Worksheet 1-4
Member Evaluation of Leader

Directions: This form may be used to obtain reactions of student members prior to discussion of student leader's performance in practice groups. The forms are then collected by the instructor and are considered when rating the student leader. Member evaluations are anonymous.

Date and Time: _____ Title of Activity: _____

How satisfied were you with the way the group was planned and led? (Please check one of the following.)
- ❑ 1 Not at all satisfied
- ❑ 2 Somewhat satisfied
- ❑ 3 Satisfied
- ❑ 4 Very satisfied
- ❑ 5 Extremely satisfied

Please comment on how you found this group experience.

What did you see as the leader's strengths?

What did you see as the leader's weaknesses? (Must state at least one.)

From Cole, M. B. *Group dynamics in occupational therapy: The theoretical basis and practice application of group intervention* (3rd ed.). Thorofare, NJ: SLACK Incorporated. © 2005 SLACK Incorporated.

learn from observing two mature leaders model the open discussion and respectful consideration of their differences of opinion.

Male/female co-leadership can be particularly enlightening to group members when they model different roles. Their interaction during the group generally brings up issues relating to the primary family. They are also prone to the stereotyping of gender roles. That is, typically the female leader is expected to take on supportive and nurturing roles, while the male leader is perceived as critical and judgmental. Male/female co-therapy teams are well-advised to share a variety of confrontive and harmonizing roles, so that both are perceived as capable leaders with mutual respect for one another's professional strengths.

Occupational therapists in the clinic may be asked to co-lead groups with professionals from other disciplines. Physicians, psychologists, social workers, nurses, recreation therapists, and dietitians are some of the many possibilities. An occupational therapist and a registered nurse may co-lead a medication education group. An occupational therapy assistant may co-lead a sensory awareness group with a recreation therapist. Each profession brings a different knowledge base and a different point of view. Teams such as these require careful planning to be sure the goals and leadership roles are clear and that their attitudes are compatible. Interdisciplinary collaboration has many potential advantages, but also pitfalls for the inexperienced occupational therapist. A well-established professional identity should be in place before attempting to co-lead a group with a person from another discipline. It is not recommended for students.

Disadvantages of Co-Leadership

Although there are many advantages to co-leading groups, there are a few common difficulties to be wary of. These difficulties must be overcome, if the co-leadership is to be effective.

- Splitting. When there are two leaders, group members have a tendency to favor one over the other. Clients often put pressure on one co-leader to take sides against the other. Like children who, when they are criticized by one parent, turn to the other for refuge, so clients in groups will try to get the co-leaders to disagree or to form alliances with subgroups. Co-leaders should be watchful for such

attempts and openly discuss them in the group. Not doing so can divide the group and create power struggles, which usually have nontherapeutic consequences.

- Competition. A certain amount of competition in co-leading a group is normal. Leaders seek to establish themselves as competent therapists, and the approval of others does much to enhance their self-esteem. Student leaders or beginning therapists may be looking for high marks from a supervisor as well. While all competition is not a bad thing, open communication about the feelings it evokes between co-leaders is necessary in order to avoid destructive consequences.

- Unequal contribution. This disadvantage occurs when one leader does most of the work, while the other sits back and watches. Resentment is bound to develop on both sides. Students have often complained of this problem during supervision of fieldwork experiences. In resolving this dilemma, it must first be acknowledged that both parties are to blame. Once again, the problem must be openly discussed and supervision sought as needed. The partner who is more active may not see the situation as problematic. It is usually the silent partner who feels uncomfortable and increasingly afraid to speak up. Often the passive leader feels dominated by his or her partner, prevented from doing his or her part in leading the group, and deprived of the opportunity for needed experience. This problem does not resolve itself and only grows worse as time goes on. Considerable effort and determination on both sides must be given, to set aside the blame and to equalize the balance of leadership, in fairness to the group members.

Stages of Co-Leadership

Lessler, Dick, and Whiteside (1979) studied the development of the co-therapy relationship. They identified four developmental stages, which parallel the group's development (described in Chapter 2).

1. Formative stage. In this stage, co-leaders are preoccupied with their feelings of self-worth as a leader and plagued by fears of inadequacy. These feelings naturally lead co-leaders to compete with one another. By trying too hard

to be "good" leaders, they could end up in a power struggle with one another or a popularity contest with the group members.

2. Development stage. This stage requires much interpersonal discussion and the recognition of differences. This stage must be resolved if the co-therapy team is to work effectively together.

3. Stabilization. After having their fights and talking it out, co-therapists view each other as individuals and recognize each other's strengths and weaknesses as well as their own. They are able to capitalize on their differences by taking on different leadership roles and discussing their perceptions openly during the group as well as afterwards.

4. Refreshment. From the process of the first three stages, a relationship between co-leaders forms that allows each to grow in his or her role as leader. Their interaction results in renewed enthusiasm for the group experience and its potential to help others. They may experiment with new ideas, do research together, or present their group experiences at professional meetings. They take pride and enjoyment from working with each other, and this energizes the group members with a sense of hope and anticipation.

The lesson from this classic research outcome is that competition in co-leadership can lead to a positive outcome when it is openly discussed and dealt with constructively. However, some leaders may find that after a few sessions, they are incompatible as partners. If mutual respect cannot be achieved through discussion of differences, it is best to find another co-leader. The focus of the group should be therapy for its members, not training for the co-leaders.

Co-leadership has many advantages in practice. However, co-leaders should be chosen carefully and matched for compatibility. Students are advised to master individual leadership first before attempting co-leadership of groups. Those who take on the co-leadership should be prepared to work hard, be open to feedback, and take time to discuss the issues of working together on a regular basis.

Conclusion

Section Two will review six frames of reference occupational therapists have used to guide them in planning and leading groups. However, students often understand theory best when it relates to their experience. Therefore, it is suggested that students learn to lead groups first. They can practice their skills by leading groups of their peers.

Although the seven steps of group leadership are described without reference to theory, it should be noted that no approach is entirely atheoretical. The theoretical basis for this approach is client centered and has some elements of the cognitive behavioral frame of reference as well. It has a sequence of steps that may be seen as developmental in their hierarchical order. These approaches and their application to occupational therapy groups will be discussed in later chapters. Cole's seven-step approach is not intended to meet all needs for all clients. It can be adapted in many ways to reflect differing clients, goals, and frames of reference.

Bibliography

Allen, C. (1999). *Structures of the cognitive performance modes.* Ormond Beach, FL: Allen Conferences, Inc.

Allen, C., Earhart, C., & Blue, T. (1992). *Occupational therapy treatment goals for the physically and cognitively disabled.* Bethesda, MD: American Occupational Therapy Association.

American Occupational Therapy Association. (2002). Occupational therapy practice framework: Domain and process. *American Journal of Occupational Therapy, 56,* 609-629.

Egan, G. (1986). *The skilled helper* (3rd ed.). Monterey, CA: Brooks/Cole.

Lessler, K., Dick, R., & Whiteside, J. (1979). Stages of cooperation: Co-therapy viewed developmentally. *Transactional Analysis Journal, 9*(1), 67-73.

Lewin, K., & Lippitt, R. (1938). An experimental approach to the study of autocracy and democracy: A preliminary note. *Sociometry, I,* 292-300.

Lewin, K., Lippitt, R., & White, R. (1939). Patterns of aggressive behavior in experimentally created social climates. *Journal of Social Psychology, 10,* 271-299.

Mosey, A. (1981). *Occupational therapy: Configuration of a profession.* New York: Raven Press.

Pfeiffer, J., & Jones, J. (1973). *Reference guide to handbooks and annuals.* La Jolla, CA: University Associates.

Pfeiffer, J., & Jones, J. (1977). *Reference guide to handbooks and annuals* (2nd ed.). La Jolla, CA: University Associates.

Posthuma, B. (2002). *Small groups in therapy settings: Process and leadership.* Toronto: Little, Brown & Co.

Rider, B., & Rider, J. (2000). *The activity card book for mental health.* Kalamazoo, MI: Author.

Stevens, J. (1971). *Awareness.* Moab, UT: Real People Press.

Yalom, I. (1995). *Theory and practice of group psychotherapy* (4th ed.). New York: Basic Books.

Chapter 2

Understanding Group Dynamics

The large body of knowledge regarding group dynamics developed by behavioral scientists over the past 60 years offers a great deal of help in our understanding of how groups work. This body of knowledge comes from a variety of theoretical bases: psychoanalytic, existential, behavioral, cognitive behavioral, and, more recently, systems theory. Around the mid 1970s a paradigm shift occurred in group dynamics research. Older theories were challenged, and new theories and models have come into focus since then. This chapter retains the best of traditional research while presenting an overview of representative updated theories.

Because of the verbal nature of the groups being researched, some assumptions have been made about the populations upon which these theories are based. Although even the most dysfunctional groups achieve some level of social organization, members of a group who have verbal skills and are capable of interaction can more easily demonstrate the dynamics described. Another assumption is that when there is enough freedom within the group structure for members to initiate and make choices, the dynamics will be more obvious. A third assumption is that the members are intrinsically motivated to self-improve through self-understanding and by increasing their interaction skills. All of these assumptions are consistent with the client-centered approach described in Chapter 3.

Group dynamics may be defined as the forces that influence the interrelationships of members and ultimately affect group outcome. It is important for occupational therapists to understand these forces when planning and implementing group interventions. Groups have predictable stages of development and will respond best to different activities at different stages. As leaders, our recognition of our group's stage of development should influence our selection of activities. How we design and lead groups also depends on our recognition and understanding of the various dynamics. Some of the dynamics that will be included in this chapter are group process, group development, group norms and roles, client problem behaviors, and termination of groups.

Group membership experiences are emphasized in this chapter so that students can gain an appreciation for what clients might be experiencing under different group conditions. It is hoped that membership experiences will help occupational therapy students to be more observant and empathetic group leaders.

Group Process

We have already discussed processing as one step in group leadership. An awareness of the underlying process of groups is essential to our approach as therapists. It gives us many clues as to the feelings and motives of members and helps the therapist to make clients aware of these and their impact on wellness and on group function. Irvin Yalom (1995) has written a great deal about the process of psychotherapy groups. Process is often first understood by what it is not. It is not content. The content of a group is what is done and what is said. For example, the group did pencil drawings, and topics discussed were the jobs members had and how they liked them. Bob said he likes being a carpenter, but Sarah hates being a teacher. Process does not include past history or even recent history of the members. Its thrust is what is happening in the group, between and among members, right now. Process concerns the interpersonal relationships among the participants.

There are two parts to process in groups, according to Yalom: "If the powerful therapeutic factor of interpersonal learning is to be set into motion, the group must recognize, examine, and understand process. It must study itself; it must study its own transactions; it must transcend pure experience and apply itself to the integration of that experience" (Yalom, 1995, p. 129). So the process is experienced first, and then it "performs a self-reflective loop," examining what just occurred. The "processing" step in the preceding chapter represents a simplified self-reflective loop (Figure 2-1). Members are asked to reveal how they felt about the activity they just experienced, as well as how they felt about the leader and each other. So the process commentary begins. Its emphasis is often on emotion, and its purpose is to establish a cognitive framework that permits members to retain the group experience so that it can be generalized and applied.

The process comments are largely the responsibility of the therapist. The leader can and should request member participation, but he or she chooses the direction of intervention according to the needs of the group.

Example

In a task-oriented group, the occupational therapist had taken considerable time in helping the group plan their next activity. They were going to construct kites. The plan for Monday was to walk to a craft store (about four blocks from the hospital) to buy paper, string, sticks, and paint. The kites would be constructed during the next two sessions. The seven members of the group assembled, wearing jackets and sneakers and ready for the walk. Hannah, age 63, the eldest member of the group, was not feeling well and refused to go. Dave, a 23-year-old member, bluntly asked the therapist if Hannah was too sick to walk. The reply was that she was fine medically. So Dave proceeded to call Hannah a "lazy, do-nothing complainer." The other members verbally attacked Dave for his rudeness and insensitivity to the elder member, and a heated argument ensued until it was too late to carry out the plan.

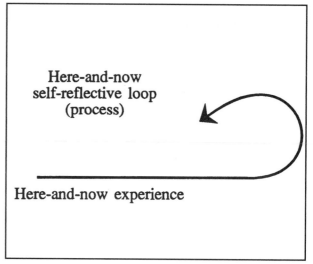

Figure 2-1. Yalom's self-reflective loop.

Content

As an occupational therapy leader, how would you process this group? First, it is helpful to identify content. What was the overt experience? The group came prepared to walk to the craft store as planned. The plan was not carried out because Hannah refused to go. What was verbalized? Dave was verbally abusive to Hannah. The other members verbally attacked Dave for being abusive, and he defended himself with counter attacks, shouting loudly at the group. The virtues of courtesy to one's elders was discussed.

Process

The process involves what is implied by the content. The therapist might consider the following possibilities:

- Hannah wanted some attention and chose to pursue it by her passivity. Perhaps her refusal was her way of exerting control over the group, or perhaps illness is her usual way of getting attention.
- The other group members were frustrated at not being able to carry out their plan and were looking for someone to blame.
- Hannah was to blame, but she seemed too frail and vulnerable to be verbally accused.
- Dave was impatient and expressed his frustration aggressively. Perhaps aggressiveness is his usual way of coping with frustration, a habit that often gets him into trouble, or perhaps he feels guilt and is looking for a way to be punished.

- The group's frustration, diverted from Hannah by her vulnerability, was vented onto Dave instead. Dave was made the scapegoat of the group. A *scapegoat* is something that symbolizes all the badness of the group or someone who is blamed for its problems. The scapegoat generally serves the purpose of allowing the group to avoid its own responsibility for what has occurred.

- Perhaps the group wanted to avoid either the walk or the activity. Dave and Hannah gave them an excuse to avoid doing any task-oriented problem solving.

Needs to Be Addressed

Which hypothesis is correct? Any or all of them are. How, then, should the therapist intervene to help the group understand its process? The first thing a leader should ask him- or herself is "What does this group really need?" Here are some possible needs to be addressed:

- The foremost need is to get Dave off the "hot seat." He may have been rude and aggressive, making him an easy target for the group, but he is certainly not the direct cause of their frustration. If Dave is not rescued, he will probably be forced out of the group and will be left feeling angry and hurt. Being scapegoated is not a therapeutic experience. For Dave, the therapist might point out how his behavior tends to elicit this kind of response from others, and how he set himself up to be the scapegoat. For the members of the group, the therapist might discuss their feelings about Hannah. They need to understand why they avoided blaming her, how they ended up in a struggle with Dave, and what they themselves were avoiding by pursuing the argument.

- The therapist might then want to examine the issue of Hannah's control. What are her real needs (attention, respect) and how might they be pursued more appropriately? An awareness of her pattern of controlling others with her illness, real or otherwise, might be very helpful as a beginning step toward therapeutic change. The group's collusion with her in achieving her goal to keep the group from acting is another important issue. Why did they allow her to exert such control? What purpose did it serve for them? Why did they not exclude her instead of Dave?

- The final issue of importance is the group's relationship to the task. How did they feel about the activity they chose? Were they really that invested? Or were they looking for an excuse not to pursue it? What were the group's choices? Could they have found an alternative way to get their supplies? Could they have reorganized their roles so that Hannah would not have to go on the walk, without excluding her from the group as a whole? If walking is important to them in getting out of the hospital to enjoy the spring weather, perhaps Hannah could have been wheeled in a wheelchair, or she could have walked part of the way and then waited with another member.

If the group is to learn from this rather frustrating and upsetting experience, it is evident that they need the occupational therapist's guidance in problem solving. Finding alternative solutions and compromising are essential if the group is to accomplish its task. Learning depends on the effectiveness of the group's reflection about the reasons for the unfortunate outcome. The occupational therapist guides the group to discover what steps should be taken before the end of this group to avoid a reoccurrence of frustration in the next session.

Discovering the Process of Groups

The best way for students to learn about group process is to experience it. Therefore, a real example taken from a student group experience is best used for this exercise. However, if that is not available, the student may use the following example. Use Worksheet 2-1 to evaluate the experience.

The group was engaged in doing an assertiveness exercise. All the members had anonymously written down situations on a card and put them in a basket in the center of the table. Members had to draw a card, read it, and tell what they would do to assertively handle the situation described on the card. Mary drew a card and read it to the group. It said, "On my fieldwork experience, I was working with two clients and one of them started to cry. I didn't know why she was crying so I ran down the hall to find a nurse, leaving the two clients alone in the clinic. I couldn't believe that my supervisor, Miss Hunt, failed me for leaving the clients alone." Mary looked bewildered. "How could the supervisor expect you to know what to do? You're just a

Worksheet 2-1
Content-Process Reaction

Directions: Write the answers to these questions after you have participated in the group session.

I. Content
   A. Give a brief description of the activity.

   B. Identify three major participants and what topics they discussed. If there were more than three, choose the three you think were most important.
      1. Person:
         Topic:
         Others offering feedback:
         Approximate length of time:
      2. Person:
         Topic:
         Others offering feedback:
         Approximate length of time:
      3. Person:
         Topic:
         Others offering feedback:
         Approximate length of time:

II. Process
   A. Name three feelings you personally experienced during the group. To whom or what were the feelings directed?
      1.
      2.
      3.

   B. Based on your observations of verbal and nonverbal behavior, what are some hypotheses (possible explanations or interpretations) about the process of the group?
      1.
      2.
      3.
      4.
      5.

   C. Based on the above hypotheses, what therapeutic intervention(s) would you make as a leader and why?

From Cole, M. B. *Group dynamics in occupational therapy: The theoretical basis and practice application of group intervention* (3rd ed.). Thorofare, NJ: SLACK Incorporated. © 2005 SLACK Incorporated.

Table 2-1		Comparison of Various Theories of Group Development				
Theorist	Year*	Beginning of the Group				End of the Group
Bion	1961	Flight		Fight		Unite
Schutz	1958	Inclusion		Control		Affection
Tuckman	1977	Forming	Norming	Storming		Performing
Yalom	1985	Orientation		Conflict	Cohesiveness	Maturity
Poole	1983	Multiple sequences, cycles, and breakpoints; multiple activity tracks				
Gersick	1984	First meeting	Phase 1	Midpoint transition	Phase 2	Conclusion

* Years represent earliest introduction of group development theory.

student." Maureen, another member said, "How could the student be so stupid? If she doesn't know what to do, she shouldn't be in occupational therapy." Susan added, "But I had Miss Hunt, too. She's really a hard nose." Several others commented on Miss Hunt's inadequacy as a supervisor. Laurie agreed with Maureen, "Yes, but the student should have known better." Roberta listened silently to this debate, looking more and more distressed as the end of the session approached.

Group Development

Group development refers to the stages groups go through as they progress from initiation to termination. Several theorists have contributed to this aspect of groups, including Tuckman, Bion, Schutz, Yalom, Poole, and Gersick (Table 2-1). Knowing the characteristics of each stage helps the therapist to anticipate problems. It helps him or her predict how the group will respond to certain activities, and therefore plan appropriately.

Traditional researchers (Bion, Schutz, Tuckman, Yalom, and many others) suggest that all groups progress through a series of predictable stages. Many theories have been suggested as to what these stages are, and, in fact, all seem to have similar characteristics. There is an initial stage of orientation, with its search for structure, goals, and dependency on the leader. Next, there is a stage of conflict with its struggle for dominance and rebellion against the leader. Following resolution of conflicts, interpersonal harmony and intimacy emerge, sometimes called cohesiveness.

Newer theorists (Poole, Gersick) challenge traditional phase theories and tend to use systems theory to study the process of small group communication, behaviors, and decision making. Our knowledge of group development comes from a collection of studies including observations of therapy groups, training groups (educational), natural groups, laboratory groups, and work teams. The final outcome of development is a mature working group characterized by high cohesiveness and commitment to the goals of the group. This outcome is agreed upon by older and newer theorists. Cohesiveness is the ideal to which we will aspire as occupational therapy group leaders.

Tuckman

Tuckman (1965) published the first major review of these studies from which he abstracted a theory of four stages of group development:
1. Forming
2. Storming
3. Norming
4. Performing

Tuckman believed that all the stages occur in some way regardless of the duration of the group (e.g., shorter length groups impose the requirement of the problem-solving stages to be reached quickly); therefore, the rate of development tends to adjust to the time available.

Tuckman's initial stage, forming, involves orientation and testing regarding the group task and a dependence on the leader for guidance. Storming involves conflict among group members as they challenge the task, the rules, and the leader. In the norming stage, harmony prevails and members accept and trust one another while conflicts are avoided. The last stage, performing, goes beyond cohesiveness to a point where conflict can be openly discussed and resolved. A performing group can effectively work together in a supportive emotional environment that encourages growth and therapeutic change.

Bion

Bion's work is also frequently quoted, especially with the easy-to-remember titles of the three stages:

1. Flight
2. Fight
3. Unite

Bion (1961) looked at the behavior of groups at conferences, having a task rather than a therapeutic focus. Flight represents an avoidance of some problem or threat. Members tend to turn to each other in pairs for more intimate emotional response in this stage. The fight stage represents the challenge of the leader (and possibly scapegoating a rival member-leader). Uniting follows these two emotional states; it settles down the members to a stable working group with relatively little emotionality. Bion's work, although emerging from the corporate and industrial arena, has many parallels in the therapeutic group. This may be especially applicable to the occupational therapy group, which, although therapeutic in its goal, tends to be more task focused.

Schutz

Schutz's (1958) theory, while similar to those previously described, tends to have the clearest interpersonal focus. He says that every individual has three interpersonal needs:

1. Inclusion
2. Control
3. Affection

These needs parallel those of a child in the family and are generalized to any interpersonal relationship among two or more individuals. In other words, groups follow the same sequence of interpersonal concerns as individuals do. Schutz's stages are shown to have both individual and group characteristics.

Inclusion Stage

In the inclusion stage, the individual is concerned with being accepted: "Where do I fit in? Will I be important, respected? Can I be myself? How will the leader respond to me?" The group behaviors observed are overtalking, attention seeking, territoriality, and individual self-centeredness. Members listen but do not really hear what others say. They tend to look to the leader when they speak rather than each other. In this initial phase, the rational approach is dominant; emotions do not flow freely. The group explores the goals, rationale, and structure. The leader is looked to for the answers. There are multiple attempts at sizing each other up. Members look for similarities and tend to downplay differences. There is concern over those who have not made a contribution, and rightly so. If members are continually passive, they can become blockers to the progress of the group as a whole.

Control Stage

Schutz's control stage also has individual and group concerns. The individual now questions: "Where do I stand in relation to power and authority? How much influence do I have? Will I have too much responsibility?" The group is generally, at some point, engaged in a leadership struggle. The once all-powerful and all-knowing leader (therapist) is now viewed with skepticism and mistrust.

If the leader abdicates (i.e., gives up the leadership), a struggle among members ensues to fill the void. Scapegoating of a would-be leader is common, and attempts to lead are often met with severe criticism or are ignored. Members often disagree about how much structure is needed or how the group should be led, and subgroups may arise. There is ambivalence about the leader; like a 2-year-old child, the group at once wants to be autonomous but needs the leader's support and protection.

The importance of all this for occupational therapists is in knowing that rebellion and challenge among group members is normal and necessary to the healthy development of the group. Be prepared to be challenged, and do not take it as a personal affront. How then should we as occupational therapists handle the challenge? There are three choices:

1. An advisor as leader would tend to back down, to abdicate leadership. To do so invites intragroup conflict that could be more stressful than clients can handle.

2. A director would subdue the rebellion. In this case, the therapist remains the leader and encourages further dependency of the group. Such an approach has been known to stifle group development.

3. The democratic leader would not abdicate all the control, but would encourage the group to share the leadership. This is Yalom's approach. He states that the group needs to experience the freedom and the responsibility for the group outcome. He suggests the leader not abdicate, but allow expression of dissension and acknowledge it. The therapist should "take the blows" and not allow any group members to become a scapegoat. Ideally, the therapist will make some changes in response to the group to allow the conflict to resolve while preserving the integrity of the group.

Affection Stage

If the conflict in leadership is resolved successfully, the group progresses to the affection stage. This is the stage of group cohesiveness when attention focuses on "How do others feel about me?" and then "How do we feel about each other?" The group is characterized by expression of positive feeling and emotional investment in the group. Members are able to really listen to each other and even direct hostility may be expressed without devastating consequences.

The affection stage is the goal for any therapy group. Here is where members feel safe, cherished, and trusting in one another. This allows members to explore new behaviors and to grow. They value one another, and therefore, they value themselves. There is real altruism and real consensual validation; members want to help each other and accept feedback from each other to validate their own self-perceptions. It is part of our role, as occupational therapists, to help our groups to reach this stage.

Nevertheless, there are some real barriers to achieving the affection stage. Schutz (1958) tells us that groups tend to regress easily, even after they have reached this stage. Events such as the arrival of a new member, leaving of an old member, leadership changes, and long holidays will all cause a group to regress. Furthermore, clients who are lacking in social and interpersonal skills and/or who are unable to trust others may be incapable of reaching the affection stage. Anticipation of termination of the group inevitably causes the development to reverse. A cohesive group may sink, once

again, into conflict in preparation for breaking the ties and moving on.

Yalom incorporates characteristics of Schutz's theoretical group phases in his theory. He dubs Schutz's Stage 1, In or out, Stage 2, Top or bottom, and Stage 3, Near or far.

Yalom

In the most recent update of his classic textbook on group psychotherapy, Yalom synthesizes much of the previous research regarding group development. He concedes that the issues of each phase may, in fact, be revisited in later phases. That being said, the "crude schema of developmental phases" he describes are:

- Orientation (hesitant participation, search for meaning, dependency)
- Conflict (dominance, rebellion)
- Development of cohesiveness (early phase and late phase) (Yalom, 1995, pp. 293-307)

Orientation

Yalom points out that the group therapist's preparation of members regarding the purpose for joining the group will affect its early development. In occupational therapy groups, pre-group interviews with potential clients might serve a dual purpose of determining collaborative goals and discussing group membership as an intervention strategy. According to Yalom, a client's hesitant participation in the initial stage of the group stems from his or her need to understand how group membership will help meet individual goals. Socialization is also inherent in the process of a therapeutic group. Accordingly, members size each other up in order to determine whether or not they belong as they search for acceptance and approval.

Dependency, another characteristic of the initial stage, stems from the members' wish to be rescued from the dilemma that brings them to therapy in the first place. Yalom suggests that group leaders take advantage of this early need for structure and answers to shape therapeutic norms in the orientation stage.

Conflict

In the second stage, members are preoccupied with issues of power and control. As social conventions are abandoned, members feel free to make personal comments and criticism. Yalom states that "the struggle for control is present in every group" (p. 298). However, the urge to rebel might not be a conscious process. For example, latent conflict may create group stagnation or boredom. Or, rebellion might take the form of complaining about the structure, such as the time or place of group meetings, or some other aspect of group content. In this case, the leader's role will be to promote awareness of the conflict through processing. Hostility toward the leader, as mentioned earlier, might be the most overt expression of conflict. How the therapist handles the hostility or criticism has a powerful effect upon group development.

Cohesiveness

The earliest phase of cohesiveness occurs when the group successfully resolves the conflicts of the previous stage. It is characterized by the emergence of a group spirit, high morale, and heightened mutual support. Competition among members is replaced by intimacy and trust, and an emotional atmosphere of nonjudgmental acceptance is created. As members feel free to self-disclose, "long past transgressions are publicly unearthed" (Yalom, 1995, p. 302), and previously unexpressed emotions from past sessions may surface. However, the early stage does not represent true cohesiveness because negative affect remains suppressed.

Maturity

Not until both negative and positive can be freely expressed does the group reach true cohesiveness or maturity. The mature working group will demonstrate "true teamwork in which tension emerges not out of a struggle for dominance but out of each member's struggle with his or her own resistances" (Yalom, 1995, p. 303). This is the more advanced stage of group cohesiveness.

Yalom, in his review of criticisms of group development theory, states that the boundaries between phases are not clearly demarcated. As such, the above stages may be more accurately named developmental tasks, not phases. Research shows that the same themes are repeatedly revisited, and that some group events have an unpredictable effect on group development.

Poole's Multiple Sequence Model

This model is included as representative of an updated approach that challenges the validity of previous group development phase theory. Poole focused on decision making in work groups for his

research. He suggests that group decision making generates multiple clusters of associated behaviors along at least three activity tracks:

1. Task process activities, which the group enacts to manage its task
2. Relational activities, which reflect or manage relationships among the members (process)
3. Topical focus, which includes issues and arguments of concern to the group (discussion, conflict resolution)

Central to Poole's developmental theory is the concept of breakpoints. Breakpoints are points of change or transition, and Poole acknowledges three types:

1. Normal (changes in discussion topic, different parts of the task)
2. Delays (setbacks due to emerging problems, group problem solving)
3. Disruptions (major conflicts, major changes required for the group to proceed) (Poole, 2003)

Poole suggests that no distinct phases occur in all groups, but that different tasks, goals, and group member characteristics produce unique patterns of content and process.

Gersick's Time and Transition Model of Group Development

Gersick (2003) studied eight diverse work teams to discover how their function changed over time. Her findings also contradict prior stage theories, but she replaces them with an alternate structure. Gersick points out that most organizations consist of permanent and temporary groups, which function as teams to carry out the work of the organization. She changes the focus of group development from one of typical behaviors, to one that attempts to explain the mechanisms of change and considers environmental contingencies. In a broad-based research study, Gersick observed that while groups use a wide variety of behaviors, "the way they worked was highly congruent" (p. 62). Her model consists of a first meeting, phase 1, midpoint transition, phase 2, and completion. The theory Gersick identifies is called "punctuated equilibrium" (Eldridge & Gould, 1972), which theorizes that systems progress through an alternation of stasis (inertia) "punctuated by concentrated revolutionary periods of quantum change" (Gersick, 2003, p. 62).

Phase 1

The first half of the group's calendar time is an inertial movement whose direction is set by the end of the group's first meeting. This places great importance on the first meeting as a time that the group's process and content may be easily shaped. During the first meeting, Gersick speculates, member behaviors may be influenced by prior expectations, contexts relating to the sponsoring organization (social, cultural contexts), and preferred behaviors or strategies characteristic of their personalities (client factors).

Midpoint Transition

At the midpoint of the allotted calendar time, groups undergo a transition during which the direction of the group is revised for phase 2. Gersick calls this a "problemistic search and pacing," which stems from the group's awareness of problems with initial norms and the pressure exerted by external deadlines. The group transition is compared to Levinson's "midlife crisis" in which around age 40 to 45, an adult reappraises his or her life so far and redefines his or her remaining life as "time left to live" (see Chapter 8). At the midpoint transition, the group faces the reality of limited time left to complete its task and picks up the pace accordingly. The ideal outcome gives way to a more realistic one, and both content and process change to accommodate this altered goal.

Phase 2

The second period of inertia focuses on carrying out the plan formulated during the transition. Progress may spurt ahead in order to reach a markedly accelerated conclusion, in which the group finishes off the work generated during phase 2.

Role of Context

The environmental influences on groups, not addressed by phase theorists, play a significant role in Gersick's model. Context impacts the group's development at three critical periods:

1. Design of the group
2. The first meeting
3. The midpoint transition

Translated into occupational therapy terms, the occupational therapist's selection of members for the group, structuring of the task, and support for the group from outside sources greatly influences the initial group functions. During the group's first meeting, both content (the task and its purpose) and process (the norms for interaction and reflection) have a lasting impact on subsequent groups. During the phases of inertia, groups are less responsive to environmental influence. The next and final time the group opens itself to outside influence is the midpoint transition. At this time in the life of the group, members are familiar enough with the task to realize that outside resources, requirements, and guidance are needed as a basis for recharting their work, and the stress of a rapidly approaching deadline motivates them to pick up the pace while there's still time to produce a reasonably successful outcome.

Relevance for Occupational Therapy

The importance of Gersick's study for occupational therapy group leaders is to acknowledge the importance of initial planning and to establish therapeutic norms aggressively during the first meeting. Secondly, occupational therapy group leaders should anticipate the midpoint transition in ongoing task groups and use it as a second chance to redirect and refine goals, correct nontherapeutic norms, and provide needed resources to increase the likelihood of a positive outcome.

How Groups Reach Maturity

Why should occupational therapists study group development? There are several reasons. First, understanding the progression to maturity in groups gives us something to strive for; it shows us what is the true capacity of a mature, cohesive group. We as therapists should do whatever we can to help the group reach a mature, working stage. Corey, Corey, Callanan, & Russel (1988) suggest one way to speed up the process is to prepare members to get the most from a group. Corey's guidelines are helpful to students participating in a group lab and may be kept in mind as suggestions for our higher functioning clients. Some of the suggestions are summarized as follows.

Have a Focus

Think about what you would like to get from the group, what issues you would like to explore, and changes you would like to make. Writing down your goals prior to each group is often helpful.

Pay Attention to Feelings

Groups are an opportunity to explore personal issues that are often heavily laden with emotion. It is often the emotions that emerge that offer important insights and an opportunity for personal growth. The group is not a place to censor expression of emotions, but rather to let them flow. Feelings that are bottled up session after session will eventually "dam up the flow of the group" (Corey et al., 1988, p. 48).

Be an Active Participant

You will help yourself most if you take an active role in the group. Silent observers are not as likely to get as much from their participation in the group, and others may believe their silence means they are being judgmental. (Corey et al., 1988, p. 48)

Give Feedback

Whether positive or negative, your honest and direct response to others will move the group toward a deeper level of trust. Occupational therapists look forward to a long career of giving constructive feedback to clients. It is essential for occupational therapy students to develop the skill of giving honest feedback in ways that are empathetic and respectful of the other member.

Be Open to Feedback

Others in the group may not have perfected the art of giving constructive feedback. When someone responds honestly but bluntly, it is natural to get defensive in justifying your own standard and therefore to reject his or her feedback. Instead of letting defenses sabotage your work in the group, use the group as an opportunity to discover your defenses, which might include "rationalizing, withdrawing, denying, or turning a specific criticism into a global 'I'm no good'" (Corey et al., 1988, p. 51). Try to get beyond your defenses and learn to use feedback constructively.

Take Responsibility for What You Accomplish

It is easy to blame others when you are bored, annoyed, or unable to self-disclose in the group. Take a look at your own contribution to this state of affairs and instead of blaming the group, think about what you could do to make things better. You have a great deal of control and choice about how you interact with others in the group, and in the final analysis, what you accomplish is up to you. Corey's suggestions are some individual behaviors and beliefs that can help groups move toward cohesiveness. We as occupational therapists have many activities at our disposal that

encourage the group to move in the direction of cohesiveness. An example is the structured group activity called "Giving and Receiving Feedback" (Session 3 in Chapter 12).

Secondly, because the stages are predictable, knowledge of group development prepares us for what is coming next. It makes us better able to plan occupational therapy activities that are appropriate at each stage of development. For example, a "Trust Circle" exercise, requiring members to intentionally fall into the arms of other group members and trust that they will be protected, may not be a good activity to introduce in the control stage of a group. Even the best laid plans might have to be changed because of changes in the stage of the group's development. For example, in a student training group, I had planned a structured exercise in setting priorities for the sixth session of the group. The group had developed beyond the control stage to a level of intimacy that made them almost cohesive. Sharing their priorities seemed too superficial, so they rejected it and modified the activity to a discussion of how to rescue their troubled relationships. The group let me know very quickly that they needed to deal with something on a deeper level.

Another reason for studying group development is that the role of the leader changes with each stage. As occupational therapy leaders, we need to know what to expect. Imagine if you were a student leading a group and one week the clients all decided to rebel against you. Suppose you did not know that this is a normal process for groups? How would you feel? One student leading time management group for substance abusers was faced with a client uprising. Quite unexpectedly, several members of the group refused to do the prescribed activity. Rather than forcing them to do it, she changed the agenda to a discussion of what they did and did not like about the group. This student did not get defensive (fortunately) but listened intently to the clients' complaints and wrote down their suggestions. Group development theory had given this student some guidelines about how to handle the conflict. She knew she could not give up her leadership role, but neither was there any way she was going to force six grown men to do an activity they did not want to do. By listening to them and taking them seriously, she allowed them to challenge her in a way that did not threaten her and did not threaten the integrity of the group either. The following week they were able to approach the activity (one they themselves had suggested) with renewed interest and enthusiasm.

Table 2-2	Schutz's Stages of Development of Groups

I. Inclusion—behaviors
  1. Depend on leader to structure
  2. Look to leader for answers
  3. Rational approach dominates
    discuss topics/opinions/thoughts
    avoid feelings
    look for purpose/goals for group
  4. Individual behaviors predominate
    attention-getting or withdrawal
    humor/laughter
    territoriality/pairing
    talking but not listening
    referring back to prior experiences
  5. Search for similarities
    energy is in keeping harmony
    find "what we agree on"
    avoid conflicts
  6. Concern over belonging/approval
    only say what will be accepted
    eye contact, verbalize mostly with leader
    seating changes frequently

II. Control—behaviors
  1. Ambivalence toward leader
    challenge structure/purpose
    challenge leader style
    challenge authority of leader
    test limits/rules
    need for leader protection/approval
  2. Disenchantment with group
    subgroups struggle among selves
    leader viewed with mistrust
    members critical and discounting group
  3. Sharing group responsibility
    dependence-independence struggle
    members share leadership functions
    suggestions for change in structure and task emerge
    members-leaders emerge
    competition, not cooperation, predominates
    leader bends toward will of group

III. Affection—behaviors
  1. Focus on feeling
    express feelings about each other
    express feelings about the leader
    consensual validation occurs
    direct hostility expressed constructively
  2. Delight in company of others
    identify with group
    feel one is lovable and loved
    concern that one is not lovable and not loved
    altruistic desire to help others
    separation anxiety
    new behaviors are explored

Identifying Group Stages

A good way to learn about the stages of group development is to reflect on a group one has participated in for several sessions. If the group meets for 10 weeks, the self-reflection about the stage of development should not start until at least the fifth session. If the stages are discussed too soon, before the conflicts begin, the discussion will not be meaningful.

Furthermore, too close a scrutiny will make the group self-conscious and, therefore, inhibit its flow. The leader takes his or her cue from the group itself in the timing of a discussion of developmental stages.

As a self-learning tool, the student group member might look at the characteristics of each stage and see if these behaviors can be found in his or her group. Table 2-2 may be useful in assisting with this process. As behaviors are recognized, examples of these in one's own group may be cited. Generally, if three or four of the behaviors

are present for a given stage, that one is likely to be correct. As an example, my student group lab was scheduled to do the "Giving and Receiving Feedback" exercise. Some of them questioned if they were ready for it. They claimed they did not know each other well enough to say anything critical. They asked me to allow them to modify the activity so they would not have to say anything negative. A few said, with hostility, they would just have to "make something up." A few others counterattacked with the rationale that they would soon have to give constructive feedback to clients and this would give them some practice. I did not allow them to modify the activity but did allow them to vent their frustrations and fears and make their suggestions. Clarification and examples were given on how to give constructive feedback. The activity was carried out with a great deal of anxiety, but ended in relief when it was "not as hard as we thought."

Considering the above example, try Worksheet 2-2.

Worksheet 2-2
Group Development Evaluation

Directions: List six different behaviors or events in the group in the first column. Then in the second column, identify the stage of development in which this behavior would best be categorized.

Group Behaviors	Stage
1.	
2.	
3.	
4.	
5.	
6.	

Stage of development for this group is _____.

From Cole, M. B. *Group dynamics in occupational therapy: The theoretical basis and practice application of group intervention* (3rd ed.). Thorofare, NJ: SLACK Incorporated. © 2005 SLACK Incorporated.

Group Norms and Roles

Norms

Norms are present in every group; they incorporate certain attitudes and standards of behavior that are acceptable to the group. Norms may be specified and verbalized by the leader, or they may not be verbalized but only implied by the behavior and interactions of members. The norms of a group may change as it develops or as members come and go. The therapist's awareness of the norms and their acceptance by the group helps him or her understand better the behaviors observed in the members.

The leader is responsible for establishing explicit ground rules for the group, like being on time and respecting the opinions of others. These are expectations the leader will announce at the outset and enforce as the group continues. Confidentiality has been mentioned earlier as a common explicit norm of groups. This means that what members say and do during group sessions should not be revealed or discussed with nonmembers. The agreement to keep group work confidential is an extension of the client-therapist relationship: what clients say and do is considered privileged information. Knowing this, the clients can trust one another and are more likely to open up to the group.

Nonexplicit norms are more elusive because they are seldom verbalized. These may even be beyond the group's awareness. They may be understood in terms of behaviors that are acceptable or nonacceptable in the group. For example, the avoidance of conflict may be a norm in the beginning stages of groups. Certain topics may be considered taboo, to be discouraged or avoided. Norms develop in all groups, therapeutic or otherwise.

Yalom points out that the norms of a therapy group are radically different from the rules of etiquette in social groups. In therapy, not only must members interact freely, they must also feel free to comment spontaneously on their immediate feelings about each other and the leader. Yalom describes the desirable norms of a therapy group as "active involvement in the group, non-judgmental acceptance of others, extensive self-disclosure, desire for self-understanding, dissatisfaction with present modes of behavior, and eagerness for change" (Yalom, 1995, p. 117). These norms do not develop automatically. The leader uses considerable influence to shape the norms of a therapy group, with necessary help from its members.

Furthermore, the leader should closely monitor the nonexplicit norms of the group. The adoption of nontherapeutic norms must be avoided at all costs because once norms are established, they are very difficult to change. The therapist is the key influence in shaping norms. Yalom suggests that therapists do this in two ways: as a technical expert and as the model-setting participant.

As technical expert, the therapist relies on his or her experience and knowledge to introduce therapeutic norms and the reasons for them. Then, as the group goes on, the therapist may use social reinforcement to encourage the enactment of therapeutic norms, while discouraging antitherapeutic norms. For example, one pattern that should be discouraged is the group members speaking only to the leader. We have already learned that dependence on the leader is a characteristic of the early stages of groups. A typical picture of this interaction is shown in Figure 2-2.

In the earliest stages, the leader establishes a norm of group interaction in several ways. He or she can refuse to answer the questions of members and reflect these to other members. For example, Mary asks the leader, "What are we supposed to talk about?" The leader does not answer, but responds with a question, "What might be some meaningful issues to talk about today?" As members begin to give their ideas, the therapist might ask, "Mary, what do you think about Sally's idea?" or "Sally, why don't you give Bill some feedback about his suggestion?" In this way, the leader tactfully establishes a communication pattern that looks more like Figure 2-3.

Members are speaking not only to the leader, but addressing each other as well. This is an important norm to set in an interactive occupational therapy group, where members are expected to give each other feedback and learn from each other. This norm also helps the group to progress beyond the initial stage of development.

In this example, the therapist has used his or her role as both technical expert and model-setting participant. The therapist has guided the group by telling them that they should interact with one another and demonstrated the behaviors by asking specific group members to respond to one another.

Self-disclosure might be another way to model expected behaviors. When asking members to share their feelings, the leader may begin by sharing his or her own. Referring to the situation described earlier, the therapist might say: "When

Figure 2-2. Leader-centered interaction.

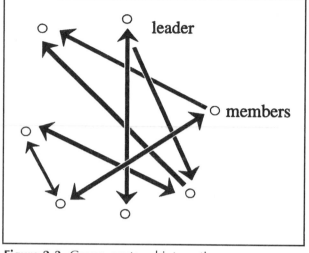

Figure 2-3. Group-centered interaction.

Maureen criticized the student for not knowing what to do with a client who cried, I felt very concerned about how that student was feeling. Yet I was frustrated, because the situation was presented anonymously and I didn't know who wrote it. I didn't want to force this student to reveal herself, but I was afraid she would really be hurt and I wanted to protect her from the attack. I wonder if other members had some of these feelings also." This example demonstrates several expectations. The norm of free expression of emotion in the group is demonstrated by the leader's expression of both concern (fear) and frustration. The focus on "here and now" is demonstrated in the leader's encouragement of responses to one another within the group about what just occurred. The therapist's encouragement of concern for one another and not allowing members to criticize one another in a hurtful way helps establish a norm of safety and trust. Finally, this self-disclosing comment invites the group to reflect on its own process, encouraging a norm of self-reflection in the group.

The norms in this example are some of what Yalom considers to be therapeutic norms. Some therapeutic norms Yalom refers to are:

- Self-reflection of the group
- Encouraging self-disclosure
- Encouraging free interaction among members
- Reinforcing the importance of the group
- Regarding members as agents of change and setting an atmosphere of safety and support

Norms will necessarily change in different groups. In occupational therapy groups, norms will vary with the client populations with which we deal and our frame of reference. Norms also change as the group moves through the stages of development. A comment that is unacceptable in Stage 1 may be right on target in Stage 2 or 3. For example, the avoidance of conflict may be normal in Stage 1, but gives way to open criticism of the leader and the group structure in Stage 2. The norm of open conflict in turn gives way to a norm of acceptance of constructive feedback in Stage 3.

If a group is to progress in its development, norms must, from time to time, be challenged. Members who do so are considered to be taking a risk. Risks involve revealing yourself to the group in a way that makes you vulnerable and taking the chance that you will be accepted and supported. In risks, there is always the chance that you may not get the response you are looking for. For example, after a very tense session in "Giving and Receiving Feedback," Roberta shared with the group that she was rather hurt that someone in the group considered her to be aggressive and intimidating. Another member, Jennifer, took Roberta's cue and shared that she was confused by someone's comment that she was a snob and "looked down her nose" at peers who were not as smart as she was. The comments of Roberta and Jennifer were met with silence. Shortly afterward, the group ended.

What risks did Jennifer and Roberta take? How did the group respond? How do you think the group changed (or should change) as a result of their risk-taking behaviors? What norms did these two students challenge? Use Worksheet 2-3 to evaluate a group experience.

In considering the example of Roberta and Jennifer, it is clear that neither left the group

Worksheet 2-3
Monitoring Norms

Directions: As a learning exercise, complete the following after each group experience. Your comments can address many individual and group behaviors, but here are some suggestions: seating pattern, structure and format of the group, timing, silence, topics discussed, communication pattern, expression of emotion, discussion of process, and leader intervention.

List three behaviors that were accepted by the group.
1.

2.

3.

List three behaviors that were not (or would not be) accepted by the group.
1.

2.

3.

List three expectations established by the leader.
1.

2.

3.

List three of your own expectations for this group.
1.

2.

3.

What norms have changed from the last group? Which norms would you like to see changed?
1.

2.

3.

From Cole, M. B. *Group dynamics in occupational therapy: The theoretical basis and practice application of group intervention* (3rd ed.). Thorofare, NJ: SLACK Incorporated. © 2005 SLACK Incorporated.

happy. They were both angry and silent during the next group session. The group, left on its own, perhaps would have continued to ignore the behavior, which in some way threatened the group's status quo. In this case, the therapist has to make some judgment calls. Are Jennifer and Roberta mature and stable enough to handle the group's response, or do they need support in continuing to take risks? Is the group ready to change its norms and open up to challenge and conflict? In the group exercise "Giving and Receiving Feedback" (Chapter 12, Session 3), the members' feedback to one another is anonymous. At what point are members ready to accept responsibility for their comments and give up the safety of anonymity? The leader's intervention should be protective of Roberta and Jennifer and supportive of their vulnerability, while being sensitive to the level of trust within the group. The best intervention, considering these factors, would be to use these members' risk-taking behaviors as a way of encouraging the silent members to take risks also. Only when the writers of the seemingly hurtful comments take the risk of revealing themselves can the issues be discussed and resolved. Members can learn a great deal from this process, not the least of which is learning to give critical feedback in a caring and helpful way and learning to accept critical feedback as an opportunity to grow and make therapeutic change.

Roles

Roles are the result of the members dividing the work of the group among themselves. Members play roles, such as follower, initiator, energizer, and blocker, spontaneously as the group progresses, or roles may be assigned by the leader. Researchers have identified the more frequent roles played in groups and have organized these according to their functions. Some roles tend to help the group accomplish a task, while others help maintain the group's lines of communication. Still other roles tend to interfere with group function, such as an attention seeker or a monopolist. The therapist not only needs to recognize these roles, he or she should help members take on a variety of roles and to change those roles that are detrimental to the group. It is often through taking on different roles that much of the therapeutic learning takes place in the group setting.

The concept of group roles was introduced in 1948 by two researchers, Kenneth Benne and Paul Sheats. Their idea was to look at leadership of the group not as solely present in the identified leader or therapist, but as a shared responsibility of all the members. These writers suggest that "the quality and amount of group production is the 'responsibility' of the group ...(and) the setting of goals and the marshalling of resources to move toward these goals is a group responsibility in which all members of a mature group come variously to share" (Cathcart & Samovar, 1974, p. 180). Benne and Sheats (1948) developed from their research at the National Training Lab in Group Development in 1947, their now-classic breakdown of member roles into the following:

- Group task roles
- Group building and maintenance roles
- Individual roles

A group role is a behavior pattern or structured way of behaving within the group. Group roles tend to remain stable regardless of who is in them. Thus, a single group member can take on a variety of roles within the group, and members can change their roles as often as they wish. Since there is a relationship between personality and the roles one typically plays with others, the roles members find themselves taking on can, in itself, be revealing. However, the roles themselves are interchangeable. Maturity has been measured by the ability to take on a variety of group roles.

Group Task Roles

These are the 12 roles that help the group to get its work done:

1. **Initiator-contributor:** Suggests new ideas, innovative solutions to problems, unique procedures, and new ways to organize.
2. **Information seeker:** Asks for clarification of suggestions, focuses on facts.
3. **Opinion seeker:** Seeks clarification of values and attitudes presented.
4. **Information giver:** Offers facts or generalizations "automatically."
5. **Opinion giver:** States beliefs or opinions.
6. **Elaborator:** Spells out suggestions and gives examples.
7. **Coordinator:** Clarifies relationships among various ideas.
8. **Orienter:** Defines position of group with respect to its goals.
9. **Evaluator-critic:** Subjects accomplishments of group to some standard of group functioning.
10. **Energizer:** Prods the group into action or decision.

11. Procedural technician: Expedites group's movement by doing things for the group such as distributing materials, arranging seating.
12. Recorder: Writes down suggestions and group decisions, acts as the "group memory."

Group Building and Maintenance Roles

These are seven supportive roles that keep the group functioning together:

1. Encourager: Praises, agrees with, and accepts the contributions of others.
2. Harmonizer: Mediates the differences between other members.
3. Compromiser: Modifies his or her own position in the interest of group harmony.
4. Gatekeeper and expediter: Keeps communication channels open by regulating its flow and facilitating participation of others.
5. Standard-setter: Expresses ideal standards for the group to aspire to.
6. Group observer and commentator: Comments on and interprets the process of the group.
7. Follower: Passively accepts ideas of others and goes along with the movement of the group.

Individual Roles

These are opposed to group roles and indicate the use of the group to serve one's individual needs. These roles tend to interfere with group functioning. Benne and Sheats (1948) suggest that a high incidence of individual behaviors is symptomatic of various group malfunctions such as inadequate group skills of members (including the leader), low level of group maturity, discipline and morale, or an inappropriately chosen and inadequately defined group task. There are eight individual roles defined by these authors:

1. Aggressor: Deflates the status of others; expresses disapproval of the values, acts, or feelings of others; attacks the group or group task, etc.
2. Blocker: Tends to be negativistic or stubbornly resistant, opposing beyond reason or maintaining issues the group has rejected.
3. Recognition-seeker: Calls attention to self through boasting, acting in unusual ways, or struggling to remain in the limelight.
4. Self-confessor: Uses group as an audience for expressing nongroup-oriented feelings, insights, or ideologies.

5. Playboy: Displays lack of involvement through joking, cynicism, or nonchalance.
6. Dominator: Monopolizes group through manipulation, flattery, giving directions authoritatively, or interrupting the contributions of others.
7. Help-seeker: Looks for sympathy from the group through unreasonable insecurity, personal confusion, or self-depreciation.
8. Special interest pleader: Cloaks his or her own biases in the stereotypes of social causes, such as the laborer, the housewife, the homeless, or the small businessman.

Admittedly, the group roles are, in part, a function of the group's stage of development. More of the task and maintenance roles can be observed in a mature group than one that is less mature. No statements are made as to the relative value of the various roles. It can be assumed that all roles are equally valuable and necessary to the group's positive outcome. Too many opinion givers and not enough compromisers are likely to create chaos rather than productivity. A well-functioning group needs a balance of roles, and this requires members to take on a mixture of roles that are compatible.

As a learning experience, it is helpful to analyze member roles (Worksheet 2-4). This gives members some feedback about what roles they tend to take on in groups and how they are contributing to the group outcome. It is easiest to see roles in groups that require extensive interaction, problem solving, and decision making. Remember, a single member can take on several roles. After everyone has written down their ideas, group members should compare notes and discuss their answers and the reasons for them. See if the group can reach a consensus about who played which roles.

For further self-awareness, the questions in the Self Role Analysis (Worksheet 2-5) can be answered concerning your own role in the group. Since flexibility in roles is considered a sign of maturity, it may be set as a goal in groups to have each member try a few new roles over the course of group meetings.

Client Problem Behaviors

It is evident from our discussion of individual roles that certain member behaviors can interfere with or severely constrict the functioning of groups. Knowledge of group dynamics also helps

Worksheet 2-4
Role Analysis Exercise

Directions: After your group ends, take a few minutes to identify which members played the various identified roles. Give an example of the behavior that supports your choices.

Group Task Roles

Role	*Member Name*	*Sample Comment or Behavior*
1. Initiator-contributor		
2. Information seeker		
3. Opinion seeker		
4. Information giver		
5. Opinion giver		
6. Elaborator		
7. Coordinator		
8. Orienter		
9. Evaluator-critic		
10. Energizer		
11. Procedural technician		
12. Recorder		

From Cole, M. B. *Group dynamics in occupational therapy: The theoretical basis and practice application of group intervention* (3rd ed.). Thorofare, NJ: SLACK Incorporated. © 2005 SLACK Incorporated.

Role Analysis Exercise (continued)

Group Building and Maintenance Roles

Role	Member Name	Sample Comment or Behavior
1. Encourager		
2. Harmonizer		
3. Compromiser		
4. Gatekeeper/expeditor		
5. Standard-setter		
6. Group observer/commentator		
7. Follower		

Individual Roles

Role	Member Name	Sample Comment or Behavior
1. Aggressor		
2. Blocker		
3. Recognition-seeker		
4. Self-confessor		
5. Playboy		
6. Dominator		
7. Help-seeker		
8. Special interest pleader		

From Cole, M. B. *Group dynamics in occupational therapy: The theoretical basis and practice application of group intervention* (3rd ed.). Thorofare, NJ: SLACK Incorporated. © 2005 SLACK Incorporated.

Self Role Analysis

1. What role(s) did you see yourself playing in the group?

2. Were these the same or different from the role(s) others saw you playing?

3. How does your role in this group compare with the one you usually play in groups?

4. What other roles would you like to try?

5. What comments or behaviors can you use to help you take on a new role?

the leader know how to deal with special problems. For example, if the leader understands why the monopolist needs to monopolize and how his or her behavior affects the other group members, then the type of therapeutic intervention needed can be determined. Sometimes the problems that arise are best dealt with by the leader, while others are handled more effectively by the group itself.

Yalom (1995) points out that all clients are problems. Indeed, clients are often assigned to therapy groups for the purpose of attempting to change problem behaviors. The behaviors to be reviewed here are monopolizing, attention-getting, silence, and psychosis. It is very important for the occupational therapist leading groups to gain an understanding of each member's needs and develop skills in handling problem behaviors.

Members who display these problem behaviors are those who play the individual roles in groups, often blocking the group's progress and frustrating its members. Dealing effectively with these clients in the group involves several challenges for the therapist. First, the therapist should develop an understanding of the individual dynamics of the client: What does this client really need? Second, the therapist needs to develop strategies for preserving the integrity and cohesiveness of the group: What does the group need? How can the leader handle this client so that the group can continue to function therapeutically? Ideally, both the client need and the group need can be satisfied. Realistically, it is not always possible for the leader to do both. If a choice is to be made, the group should be preserved first, even if that means an individual member must leave it. A good group therapist will never sacrifice the whole group for the sake of an individual member.

The Monopolist

Harry came into the group angry. He refused to listen to the purpose of the group or to participate in the activity. "I'm not going to draw like I'm in kindergarten. Excuse me, but you girls (occupational therapy student leaders) don't know anything about alcohol abuse. When I was in County Hospital, they had me doing paintings and sculptures, and what-all, and it never did anything for me..." Five other members listened to this outburst in silence. They had heard Harry's routine before.

How should the leaders handle Harry? First, let us ask two key questions. What does Harry need? Perhaps he needs to control the group, to maintain the group's (or leader's) attention, or perhaps he needs to avoid his own hurtful issues. What do the members of the group need? Probably, they need to get Harry to "shut up." However, when a silent group allows a monopolist to control things, there is always an element of ambivalence. In some ways, Harry may be serving their needs as well, particularly if they, too, wish to avoid revealing hurtful issues or feelings.

In this example, Harry is playing the role of the aggressor, by devaluing both the task and the leaders of the group. The leaders, in this case, are more likely to stop Harry's tirade by appealing to the other group members. Ask them, "Why do you allow Harry to monopolize the group? Why are you silent?" The group might be encouraged to give Harry feedback by completing the sentence, "When you speak like that, it makes me feel _____." If the group is able to express its frustration with Harry, then Harry might be helped by learning to control the behaviors that elicit negative feelings from others.

The Silent Member

Silent behaviors occur frequently in occupational therapy groups. In active groups, silent members may go unnoticed for a session or two, but will eventually block the group's progress. Why? Because, as the group becomes aware of a member's silence, members begin to imagine what the silent member must be thinking. Soon resentment develops over the silent, passive member's "not pulling his or her weight" in the group. In truth, a silent member might feel inadequate, out of tune with the others, and fearful of self-disclosure. What the group wants most is for the silent member to talk and to allay its fears about what he or she may be thinking. For example, in a group of students, Patty usually made two or three non-committal comments in each session, just enough to keep her from being noticed. Patty's greatest fear was becoming the center of attention. But as members got to know one another through mutual participation in group activities, it soon became clear that no one was getting to know Patty. Two group members finally confronted her angrily at the beginning of a group. Once begun, she continued speaking in a very pressured way, hard to interrupt: "I've been listening to you all discussing your life in the dorms and your problems with your boyfriends. But I'm a commuter. I leave right after class and go to my evening job and I don't get home until midnight. On weekends I help my handicapped mother with the housework and help her shop and pay her bills. I don't have time for a boyfriend and homework too. I can't think about having fun when I'm wondering how I'll manage to pay next semester's tuition or how I'll get the money to fix my car. I have nothing in common with this group. I'm not resentful or angry and I learn a lot from listening. But don't ask me to join in when I have nothing say." After allowing the group to respond, the occupational therapist suggested that the group try to find things Patty and they had in common, rather than things that singled her out as being different. Patty was still quiet and had a hard time feeling like part of the group. But after this "event," the group no longer regarded her as an impediment. They empathized with her and collaborated to help involve her as much as she could tolerate.

Attention-Getting Behaviors

There are various forms of attention-getting behavior. Most represent self-centered patterns of interaction that reflect low self-esteem and the need for external evidence of one's worth. The three types we will discuss are self-depreciation, complaining, and narcissism or self-love.

The Self-Depreciator

The self-depreciator is the client whose stories you hear over and over. He's/she's always putting him- or herself down and seems unresponsive to overtures of acceptance from others. Janice loved to do activities, so she participated willingly in occupational therapy group. But whenever she finished a project, she talked on and on about all of its flaws and imperfections. The group used to argue with her and tell her how nice her project looked. But the routine was repeated too often, so they stopped responding to Janice at all. This "fed up" group behavior made Janice feel all the more rejected. Getting the group to help Janice to see her self-defeating behavior was a key intervention here. Through group feedback, Janice learned how she made her expectation of rejection a self-fulfilling prophecy. The leader encouraged Janice to accept the group's support and stop devaluing herself before the group gave up on her.

The Help-Rejecting Complainer

The help-rejecting complainer, referred to by Yalom as the "HRC" (1995, p. 379), chronically rejects the very help he or she asks for from the group. Yalom explains this behavior as unresolved dependency: the HRC is dependent on authoritative others, but at the same time, is unable to trust others. After the fifth or sixth "yes, but..." response, the group usually becomes frustrated and angry at having all its advice rejected. The HRC is seen as using up a lot of time and energy and getting nowhere. Marge, for example, had chronic headaches and was addicted to several medications, which, in turn, caused a barrage of other symptoms from constipation to irrational anger. An unknowing doctor tried to help Marge by lowering her pain medication prescription. Predictably, the doctor's well-meaning action not only did not help Marge, it made him the target of all her irrational anger. She complained incessantly in group and would not be consoled. Marge had once again painted herself into a corner. Not only had the group rejected her, but she had rejected the only one (the doctor) who had the credentials to help her with her addiction problem. Why does this happen? Because the client is stuck in a self-defeating cycle (Figure 2-4).

What to do? Do not give the client the help requested. Why? Because he or she will reject the help and therefore reinforce the self-defeating cycle. The only hope for the HRC is to break the cycle. The therapist can help the group to empathize with Marge, to understand and acknowledge her feelings of defeat and frustration. As a bond with the group forms, the client might be helped to see how her own behavior invites rejection.

The Narcissistic Member

These attention-seekers seem to demand the constant and undivided attention of the group. I have known doctors to come across this way in team meetings. Narcissistic clients have an exaggerated self-love; they feel they deserve concern, compliments, gifts, and surprises, although they give none of these to others. For example, Franklin, a small, clever, and attractive man, seemed to have a natural talent for comedy. He held the group's attention with his humor, but rarely listened to the other members. Franklin did a lot of talking about the women he had affairs with; he could not understand why these relationships never lasted. The group's need was to have Franklin contribute to the group by listening to and empathizing with others.

Groups can be very useful to clients like this, who need to alter their perception of themselves

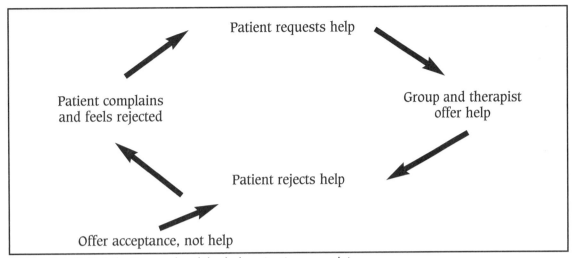

Figure 2-4. Self-defeating cycle of the help-rejecting complainer.

and others. It is important, however, for the therapist to protect them because of their high degree of vulnerability. The group's feedback can be accepted if it is presented in a gentle and caring way. Franklin, for all his humorous overconfidence about his sex appeal to women, had a very fragile sense of self-worth. He was highly dependent on the acceptance or rejection of others. The group, in their anger, could easily burst his bubble and their rejection would sink him to the depths of depression. Franklin needed the group's high regard to sustain him through their feedback about how his lack of caring makes them feel. The therapist might look for an opportunity to ask the group to comment about Franklin's rejection of them in ways that are not likely to evoke defensiveness.

Psychotic Client Behavior

The client who becomes psychotic and is out of touch with reality does not benefit from group intervention, according to Yalom (1983, 1995). Irrational and illogical clients take up vast amounts of group energy and may bring the group process to a halt. Such clients should be removed from the group until their psychosis comes under control through medical treatment. Posthuma (2002), however, suggests that psychotic clients may benefit from occupational therapy group intervention in which the activity is the focus, rather than discussion and social interaction.

Additionally, psychosis may not always be easy to identify. Some clients continue to interact in a seemingly rational manner and may deceive the group by creating distractions or personal crises to cover their breaks with reality. Clients with borderline personality disorder provide good examples of this problem behavior. Borderline clients have been identified as exceedingly difficult to treat. Yalom describes them as having an "outward veneer of integration" that "conceals a chaotic, primitive personality structure" (Yalom, 1995, p. 399). Borderline clients often thrive in occupational therapy groups because they have developed a great deal of skill. Often they are excellent artists, craftsmen, and writers, as well as convincing talkers. In groups (as in life), they seem to go from crisis to crisis. Self-destructive acts can be an everyday occurrence, although often unpredictable. Group members and therapists alike are taken in by the borderline client's great potential to achieve and disappointed again and again by his or her impulsive self-destructiveness.

Group intervention can be valuable to the borderline client because of the many opportunities to test reality. Feedback from the group can keep his or her numerous perceptual distortions and primitive needs and fears in check. However, the therapist needs to be constantly in touch with the amount of the group's time and energy taken in meeting the needs of the borderline client. Sometimes these clients leave little time for the other group members.

Termination of Groups

Finally, as the time for ending a group approaches, the leader will need to help the group through the process of termination. Some groups prepare for termination from the day they begin, while others avoid dealing with issues of termination altogether. The therapeutic learning that takes place in the group can be greatly enhanced by a good termination, or it can be destroyed by an inadequate termination. The leader should be keenly aware of the issues groups need to deal with in terminating so that he or she can help the group face them in a healthy and effective way.

This rather gruesome word *termination* is used here simply to mean the end of something. In the case of groups, it refers to the point at which groups cease to meet together as a group. Whether or not members expect to encounter one another as individuals in another context, termination of a group usually means the end of relationships as they exist within the group. The end of a group is a real loss, and involves some of the same feelings associated with other losses.

Termination, when faced directly, usually involves pain and anxiety. Group members tend to avoid these feelings in a number of ways: withdrawal, devaluing the importance of the group, anger toward the leader or other members, silence and inactivity, or leaving the group prematurely. It was mentioned in the section on group development that some research shows group regression as the end approaches. A group that has reached maturity may go backwards and re-enter a state of conflict prior to termination. Some groups just ignore the impending termination by bringing up new issues as if the group would continue as usual.

A healthy termination is never easy. However, leaders can help group members to go through the process, which involves several steps:

- Review the group experience, the goals, and the learning that took place over the life of the group. Even though members may wish to devalue the group, the leader can encourage members to verbalize the goals they have accomplished or can help them recall positive learning experiences.
- Review concerns and feelings regarding separation and loss. A good therapist will encourage the expression of painful, sad, angry, or anxious feelings to prepare the members for separation. Often the leader will experience these feelings and can share them with the group as an example.
- Use counseling skills. Empathy and confrontation (detailed in Chapter 3) are often useful in this process to help members acknowledge their feelings instead of avoiding them.

- Finish unfinished business. This seems obvious, but there may be various reasons why members wish to avoid doing it. A therapist should encourage members to bring up issues that are pending and follow up on past conflicts to bring closure.
- Give feedback on skills learned. Group members may be engaged in giving one another feedback about changes they have made or learning what has been gained from the group's activities.
- Help generalize learning. As a way to help members accept separation, an emphasis can be placed on how what was learned in the group can be practiced and applied elsewhere. When members understand how they can apply their skills to their lives outside of the group, they can move on without diminishing the importance of their group experience.

Summary

Students learn best about group dynamics through experience. So it is recommended that students meet in a series of six to 10 group sessions. These can be led by peers or can follow the format of Chapter 12 or 13, led by an instructor.

As a way to enhance an awareness of group dynamics, it is suggested that the Personal Group Reaction Paper Outline (Worksheet 2-6) be used to record student reactions after each group session.

The Group Leadership Analysis Assignment (Worksheet 2-7) is a new addition for the more advanced student. Students in a group lab sign up to lead one of the groups described in Chapter 12 or 13 and videotape the group. The analysis assignment serves as a guide to more in-depth observation of group process from an occupational therapy leadership perspective.

Bibliography

Benne, K., & Sheats, P. (1948). Functional roles of group members. *Journal of Social Issues, 2*(4), 123-135.

Bion, W. (1961). *Experiences in groups and other papers.* New York: Basic Books.

Cathcart, R., & Samovar, L. (1974). *Small group communication: A reader* (2nd ed.). Dubuque, IA: W. C. Brown Co.

Corey, G., Corey, M. S., Callanan, P., & Russel, J. (1988). *Group techniques* (Rev ed.). Pacific Grove, CA: Brooks/Cole.

Eldridge, N., & Gould, S. J. (1972). Punctuated equilibria: An alternative to phyletic gradualism. In Schopf (Ed.), *Models in paleobioloby*. San Francisco: Freeman, Cooper & Co.

Gersick, C. J. (2003). Time and transition in work teams. In R. Hirokawa, R. Cathcart, L. Samovar, & L. Henman (Eds.), *Small group communication: Theory and practice: An anthology* (8th ed.). Los Angeles: Roxbury Publishing.

Hirokawa, R., Cathcart, R., Samovar, L., & Henman, L. (Eds.). (2003). *Small group communication: Theory and practice: An anthology* (8th ed.). Los Angeles: Roxbury Publishing.

Poole, M. S. (2003). A multiple sequence model of group decision development. In R. Hirokawa, R. Cathcart, L. Samovar, & L. Henman (Eds.), *Small group communication: Theory and practice: An anthology* (8th ed.). Los Angeles: Roxbury Publishing.

Posthuma, B. (2002). *Small groups in counseling and therapy: Process and leadership* (4th ed.). Boston: Little Brown.

Schutz, W. (1958). The interpersonal underworld. *Harvard Business Review, 36,* 123-135.

Tuckman, B. (1965). Developmental sequence in small groups. *Psychological Bulletin, 63,* 384-399.

Yalom, I. (1983). *Inpatient group psychotherapy.* New York: Basic Books.

Yalom, I. (1995). *The theory and practice of group psychotherapy* (4th ed.). New York: Basic Books.

Worksheet 2-6
Personal Group Reaction Paper Outline

Title (a few words expressing theme): _____

Date of Session: _____

Seating Pattern Diagram:

1. Draw a diagram of the seating arrangement, listing names of each member present and his or her position within the group.

2. Discuss significance of seating pattern, positions near leader, opposite leader, pairing, subgroups.

3. Note absences and impact of these.

Norms: Identify "rules" of the group (confidentiality, respect, etc.).

1. Which are verbalized (explicit)?

2. What norms are not verbalized (implicit) (e.g., What behaviors are acceptable to the group? Not acceptable?)?

3. Each week note any changes in group norms from previous weeks.

Content: Identify the major discussion topics of the group.

Process:

1. Theme—Based on the topics discussed, identify the predominant theme of the session in a few words or a phrase (this becomes the "title" of your paper). The theme should have both a content and a process (or feeling) component. Then explain how you arrived at this theme. How do the topics reflect the theme and why were they verbalized (or not verbalized) in this manner?

```
┌─────────────────────────────────┐
│         Seating Diagram         │
│                                 │
│                                 │
│                                 │
│                                 │
│                                 │
│                                 │
│                                 │
│                                 │
│                                 │
│                                 │
└─────────────────────────────────┘
```

From Cole, M. B. *Group dynamics in occupational therapy: The theoretical basis and practice application of group intervention* (3rd ed.). Thorofare, NJ: SLACK Incorporated. © 2005 SLACK Incorporated.

Worksheet 2-6
Personal Group Reaction Paper Outline (continued)

3. Verbal communication—What significant interpersonal interactions took place between group members? Be sure to name names. Vagueness is not helpful to the understanding of process. Interpret what was implied or hidden in the group discussion. What subjects were avoided and why?

4. Nonverbal communication—What was the general mood of the group? What was communicated by nonverbal behaviors of members, especially feelings of members? Interpret significance. How did nonverbal behaviors affect group functioning?

Personal Reaction: Identify your role and impact you had on the group. Describe your personal feelings.
1. How did you respond to this group?

2. How do you feel about your relationship to individual group members (give names)?

3. How did you react to the leader (honesty counts)?

Self-Evaluation: What did you learn about yourself today in group (strengths, weaknesses, values, interactive style)?

Goal: What are your personal goals for the next session?

From Cole, M. B. *Group dynamics in occupational therapy: The theoretical basis and practice application of group intervention* (3rd ed.). Thorofare, NJ: SLACK Incorporated. © 2005 SLACK Incorporated.

Group Leadership Analysis Assignment
(Due 2 Weeks After You Lead Group)

Video and Preparation

You must videotape your group. As a group leader, you are responsible for arranging to borrow a camera and tripod from AV for your assigned date. (Plan ahead!) Please purchase a good quality videotape as you will need to keep it for use in a graduate course next year. You are responsible for the quality of the finished video. Position the tripod so that you are facing the camera and all group members are visible and away from distracting noises (vents) so that voices may be clearly heard. No adjustment of taping should be necessary after you start your group, so that you will be able to give the group your full attention as a leader. Also, prepare copies of worksheets and written group plan.

Analysis Guidelines (four pages or more, double spaced, 1-inch margins)

1. *Steps:* Watch the videotape and summarize what occurred during each of the seven steps.
2. *Goals:* What were the therapeutic goals and how well were they achieved? Be specific.
3. *Process:* Discuss the process of the group. What was the prevailing theme? What feelings were expressed verbally/nonverbally? What was the level of self-disclosure (Stage of group development)? What barriers or conflicts became evident (must name at least one)?
4. *Member Roles:* What roles did each member play? What emotional issues were expressed by each member? (Should list names individually and answer for each.)
5. *Meaningful Interactions:* Choose three significant interactions that occurred between members in this group; describe and discuss why they were significant.

Self-Analysis

1. *Leadership Role:* Discuss your leadership role in this group. Compare your own expectations with the group experience. What challenges did the group members represent for you as leader? What could you have improved or done differently and how?
2. *Highlights:* Identify three highlights of your leadership skills during this group (list videotape positions for these). These should represent group reactions or interactions that challenged you as a leader and for which you demonstrated effective group leadership. Write a short paragraph describing each, including what was stated, what interventions you used, and why.
3. *Transference/Countertransference:* What emotional responses did members evoke for you and what prior relationships or experiences help explain these responses (either positive or negative)?
4. *Personal Reaction:* How did you feel about leading this group? What was most personally meaningful about it and why?

** *Videotapes of group sessions must be kept confidential. As a precaution, after you hand it in, your instructor will keep your videotape until the end of the semester.*

Chapter 3

Client-Centered Groups

First and foremost, all seven-step group interventions described in this text are client centered. The primary purpose for which this method of group facilitation was designed is to enable the participation of members in doing a shared task or activity and to reflect upon its meaning for each of them. Every step in the process calls for the group leader's therapeutic use of self to enact the principles of client-centered practice. While the seven steps can be adapted for use with different frames of reference, their basic approach remains client centered. This chapter reviews some basic principles of client-centered occupational therapy practice as they relate to group interventions.

Client-centered practice as an approach in occupational therapy was developed by the Canadian Occupational Therapy Association (1991, 1997) in the 1980s and earlier. Only recently have these principles been incorporated into the American Occupational Therapy Association's (AOTA's) core values (AOTA, 2004; Law, 1998). Client-centered principles are based, in part, on the theories of Carl Rogers, Abraham Maslow, and Robert White. This set of compatible concepts has also been called the humanistic approach. In addition, the writings of Irvin Yalom and Rollo May enlighten us on how many of these principles can be enacted in groups. Irvin Yalom has long been recognized as an existential group psychotherapist, and Rollo May is credited with translating existential ideas from many sources for use in mainstream American psychotherapy (Corey, 1996). Many of the concepts reviewed here are also reflected in AOTA's core values, ethics, and philosophy of occupational therapy (Crepeau, Cohn, & Schell, 2003). People

are seen as equally valuable, regardless of their race, religion, sex, level of intellectual ability, socioeconomic position, or state of health. The "Philosophical Base of Occupational Therapy," adopted by the AOTA in April 1979, states that "human beings are able to influence their physical and mental health and their social and physical environment through purposeful activity" and "adaptation is a change in function that promotes survival and self-actualization" (AOTA, 2004, p. 403). Client-centered groups using the seven steps outlined in Chapter 1 will bring our group interventions into harmony with the fundamental philosophy and values of our profession (see The Philosophical Base of Occupational Therapy on p. 56).

Person-centered therapy provides guidelines that help us develop skills for forming and maintaining therapeutic relationships. Matheson (1998) calls this therapeutic engagement. He makes a distinction between client centered and person centered "because being a person is more basic and encompassing than being a client" (p. 108). A therapeutic relationship has been defined as "a trusting connection established between therapist and client through collaboration, communication, therapist empathy, and mutual understanding" (Cole & McLean, 2003). A group therapist forms this connection with group members through the therapeutic use of self. The counseling skills contributed by Gerard Egan (2001) are useful for students in the helping professions when learning to communicate empathy, understanding, concern, and guidance to clients, both as individuals and in groups.

The Philosophical Base of Occupational Therapy

Man is an active being whose development is influenced by the use of purposeful activity. Using their capacity for intrinsic motivation, human beings are able to influence their physical and mental health and their social and physical environment through purposeful activity. Human life includes a process of continuous adaptation. Adaptation is a change in function that promotes survival and self-actualization. Biological, psychological, and environmental factors may interrupt the adaptation process at any time throughout the life cycle. Dysfunction may occur when adaptation is impaired. Purposeful activity facilitates the adaptive process.

Occupational therapy is based on the belief that purposeful activity (occupation), including its interpersonal and environmental components, may be used to prevent and mediate dysfunction, and to elicit maximum adaptation. Activity as used by the occupational therapist includes both an intrinsic and a therapeutic purpose.

This statement was adopted by the April 1979 Representative Assembly of The American Occupational Therapy Association, Inc. as Resolution C #53-79. The text can be found as noted below:

American Occupational Therapy Association. (1979). The philosophical base of occupational therapy. *American Journal of Occupational Therapy, 33,* 785.

American Occupational Therapy Association. (1979). Policy 1.11. The philosophical base of occupational therapy. In *Policy manual of The American Occupational Therapy Association, Inc.* Bethesda, MD: Author.

Contributing Concepts

Existential Concepts

Existential theory can be seen as the forerunner of humanism and person-centered therapy. Existentialism focuses on understanding the person's subjective view of the world. "Therapy is a journey taken by the therapist and client into the world as perceived and experienced by the client" (Corey, 1996, p. 237). The major contributions of the existentialists lie in three key concepts:

1. Freedom and responsibility
2. Aloneness and relatedness
3. Existential anxiety and search for meaning

Freedom and Responsibility

Freedom implies that an individual has a capacity for self-awareness and awareness of his or her environment that allows him or her to make choices. An individual who is aware need not allow his or her present behavior to be determined by others, his or her situation, or his or her past experiences. He or she alone is responsible for his or her own life dilemmas. Therapy that utilizes this approach is aimed at getting clients to see that they have choices, have always had choices, and helps them take responsibility for the choices that have made them who they are now. Adults can stop blaming their parents for their shortcomings, and instead, take on the responsibility of correcting them. The concept of freedom to choose is what allows clients to take charge of their own lives, to leave the past behind, and to make positive changes for the future (Corey, 1986).

Aloneness and Relatedness

Existentialists believe that we are social beings who depend on interpersonal relationships for our humanness. Awareness of our aloneness can be frightening. Some people attempt to hide their fears in superficial relationships or projects and activities. Existential therapists encourage individuals to find their own identity and inner direction before attempting to connect with others. Group interventions necessitate interactions among members and afford opportunities to practice forming meaningful connections. The work of groups in occupational therapy involves reflecting on the experience of interaction with other members and how that experience relates to social participation in the world outside the group. Additionally, occupational therapy group interventions are ideal for evaluating and learning socialization skills and for exploring and problem solving barriers to social participation.

Existential Anxiety and Search for Meaning

Anxiety, in the existentialist view, is a necessary condition of living. Rollo May defines anxiety as "the threat to our existence or to values we identify with our existence" (1977, p. 205). The concept is based on the idea that our existence or "being" (May & Yalom, 1989) has no intrinsic predetermined meaning. The meaning of life is developed by each individual for him- or herself. Thus in therapy, there is an emphasis on one's individual values and in finding or defining what activities are meaningful to the individual. While too much anxiety can immobilize a person, a certain amount of anxiety is normal and positive. Anxiety alerts us that all is not well and that a change is needed. In this case, anxiety is seen as a motivator to make necessary changes in behavior, values, or life structure in order to maintain or promote healthy functioning.

Humanistic and Client-Centered Concepts

The humanistic approach is overwhelmingly positive and is appealing to most therapists. Carl Rogers was perhaps its major spokesman. Rogers developed what is known as nondirective counseling, based on the assumption that the client really knows what is best for him or her. Rogers viewed his clients with "unconditional positive regard" and allowed them to choose the direction of therapy, to set their own goals, and to provide their own solutions to problems (Rogers, 1967). Abraham Maslow added significantly to humanistic thinking through his hierarchy of needs leading to self-actualization. Robert White's theory of occupational competence helps us understand human motivation and the role of occupation. The key concepts of the humanistic (client-centered) approach are:

- Respect
- Genuineness
- Nonjudgmental acceptance
- Deep understanding
- Self-actualization
- Occupational competence and motivation
- Spirituality

Respect

Respect in therapy is not a technique, but an attitude toward the client. In the client-centered approach, the therapist sees the client as the only real expert on his or her own life. Therefore, the therapist makes no predetermined assumptions about the client, but seeks to learn all about him or her by asking open-ended questions and getting him or her to talk about him- or herself as much as possible. Yalom translates this idea in his approach to group intervention by encouraging group members to respect each other and to talk to each other as much as possible. Respect also includes a belief

that when people are realistically aware of their problems, they are capable of creating their own solutions. Therefore, suggestions and advice giving are discouraged and replaced by responses that show empathy. Empathy is expressed by both therapist and group members by statements that not only reflect what the client has said, but also acknowledge how the client is feeling. For example, a client presents the problem that his wife does not understand his need to grieve the death of his mother. The therapist would encourage the group to ask for appropriate details in order to gain a thorough understanding of how this client feels. Then empathy would be expressed with a statement like, "You must be feeling abandoned when your wife cannot share your grief about the loss of your mother." Statements such as this encourage the client to trust the therapist and/or group members and to move ahead to even greater self-disclosure.

Genuineness

Genuineness is also an attitude rather than a technique. It means that the therapist expresses real emotional responses to the client. Clients are keen observers and are quick to sense any dishonesty on the part of therapists. When the therapist tries to cover up anger or frustration, the client usually senses something wrong and the effect is often silence and withdrawal of trust. It is only by expressing negative feelings that honest communication with the client is facilitated. This is not to suggest that the therapist's anger (or other feelings) should be expressed indiscriminately. On the contrary, it takes considerable skill and self-understanding for a therapist to express feelings in a way that is therapeutic (Egan, 2001).

The value of genuineness has a profound effect upon groups. When the therapist encourages the members to be genuine, the responses they give to one another are much more meaningful and helpful. In the initial stages of groups, it is a natural tendency for members to hold back in their responses to one another. Clients are often reluctant to express negative feelings toward other members. Reasons for this have been discussed in the chapter on group dynamics. After members have established a certain degree of trust in one another, they feel much more inclined to share their real feelings. It is one of the therapist's roles to establish an atmosphere of safety and trust, which allows group members to be genuine in their responses to one another.

Nonjudgmental Acceptance

Nonjudgmental acceptance refers to the therapist's relationship with the client as one of caring. In the humanistic approach, the client is accepted for the human being that he or she is, regardless of his or her feelings or his or her behavior. This "unconditional positive regard" allows the client to reveal all his or her inner feelings and secrets without fearing the therapist's rejection. According to Rogers, research indicates that "the greater the degree of caring, prizing, accepting, and valuing the client in a non-possessive way, the greater the chance that therapy will be successful" (Corey, 1991, p. 214). The humanistic therapist needs to be very careful not to allow his or her own values to enter into the therapeutic relationship. Judgments of bad and good feelings or bad and good behavior have no place in the humanistic approach.

Being judged by others is one of the greatest fears clients have in the group setting. For example, when a client speaks in the group, he or she is often uncomfortable with the silence of others. Clients often imagine that silent members are secretly disapproving of what is being said. It is most important for the therapist to establish the norm or expectation early in the group that members not judge one another in this way. All members have a right to have feelings and feelings are neither good nor bad. Likewise, behavior should not be judged for itself, but looked upon in the context of the individual's perceptions of self and environment. If a client got drunk on a weekend pass, this behavior can be seen as one of several responses the client could have to a stressful situation. The object is not to condemn the behavior but to understand it and examine its effect on the client.

Deep Understanding

In the humanistic approach, behavior change is considered to be the by-product of a deep self-understanding. For this reason, considerable time and energy in therapy is devoted to uncovering hidden aspects of the self. In occupational therapy groups, structured activities are often helpful in fostering self-understanding among group members. The therapist should continue to gather information from the clients until he or she can almost see the world through the client's eyes. Only then is the therapist able to assist the client in changing his or her behavior. New therapists have a tendency to push for behavior change too quickly. In their desire to be helpful, new therapists might even make a suggestion in the form of a question (e.g., "Have you tried talking to your wife instead of just getting drunk?"). Such a question reveals a lack of respect as well as understanding. Questions should focus on further defining the problem until it is thoroughly explored. When it is revealed that the client depends on his wife so much that he cannot risk disagreeing with her, then getting drunk to numb the pain is less contemptible. Furthermore, the problem is redefined not as one of drunkenness, but one of dependency. That dependency may be further explained by a lack of trust in one's self. Problems are seldom as simple as they may seem. Rogers believes that "When therapists can grasp the present experience of the client's private world as the client sees and feels it without losing the separateness of their own identity, then constructive change is likely to occur"(Corey, 1991, p. 214).

Self-Actualization

Self-actualization is the innate tendency of all human beings to achieve their potential. This concept assumes that each of us has within us an inherent potential that we can actualize and through which we can find meaning. Maslow, the chief proponent of this concept, places self-actualization at the top of a continuum called the hierarchy of needs (Figure 3-1). Maslow sees at the core of human nature a push to satisfy the needs that ensure physical and psychological survival. The satisfaction of each need is a necessary prerequisite to the search for satisfaction of the next. Thus, in Maslow's hierarchy: 1) physiological needs, 2) safety needs, 3) needs for belonging and love, and 4) esteem needs are all prerequisites to the need for self-actualization. In his book *Toward a Psychology of Being*, Maslow (1968) elaborates the idea of self-actualization in his discussion of "peak experiences." These experiences are difficult to describe, but widely documented, according to Maslow. They are moments of ecstasy, of self-discovery, and brilliant creativity or vision; moments when suddenly one's views of him- or herself and the world change permanently forever. Peak experiences are said to cause symptoms to disappear; they can change self-perception in a healthy direction and can release the person for greater creativity, expressiveness, and growth. "The person [after such experiences] is more apt to feel that life in general is worthwhile, even if it is usually drab, pedestrian, painful, or ungratifying, since beauty, excitement, honesty, play, goodness, truth, and

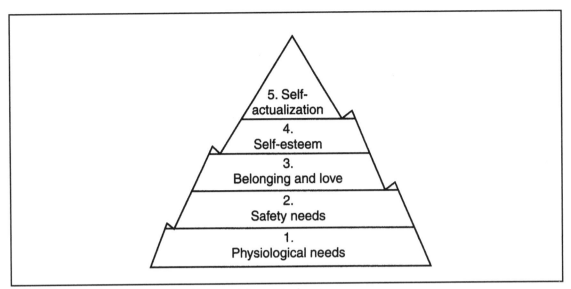

Figure 3-1. Maslow's mountain. (Adapted from Maslow.)

meaningfulness have been demonstrated to him to exist" (Maslow, 1968, p. 101). If only we, as therapists, could make our clients feel that life is worthwhile in this way!

Occupational Competence and Motivation

Robert White (1959) believed that people have an innate motivation toward competence, which translates into an innate drive to explore and master the environment. This idea is certainly compatible with the basic tenets of occupational therapy. Perhaps we would add that occupational therapy interventions improve the quality of client's lives through the engagement in meaningful occupation. Similarly, Maslow views motivation as need satisfaction and a kind of thrust for survival. But this changes from physiological survival to psychological survival as it approaches the top of the needs hierarchy. Self-actualization is seen not as a search for what is missing, but an innate drive toward self-fulfillment. This differs somewhat from the existentialist view that anxiety is the major motivator, that the search for structure and meaning is largely motivated by the desire to escape the anxiety of meaninglessness and nothingness. In client-centered theory, there is an assumption that people have a natural tendency to improve the quality of their lives.

We as therapists need to find out where the dysfunction lies where our client is stuck, and the obstacles preventing him or her from pursuing self-actualization. Perhaps the client is not aware of the freedom to make choices. Many clients I have worked with have felt so defeated by the "system," by the bureaucracy of governments and organizations or by the prejudices of society, that they no longer exercise their ability to choose. Many have had negative life experiences rather than "peak" experiences. Perhaps their more basic needs are not being satisfied; they feel unsafe, unloved, or like they do not belong. People with disabilities, both mental and physical, often feel they are misfits, controlled by others, victims of circumstance, incapacitated by anxiety, and prevented from enjoying the fulfillments of life that "normal" people enjoy. As group therapists, we sometimes facilitate the outward expression of our clients' pain before we can help them begin to find the more positive aspects of themselves.

Spirituality: The Experience of Meaning

One of the unique aspects of the Canadian Occupational Performance Model is the place of the human spirit at the center of the person. Client-centered theory views the human spirit as the unifying force that binds the other parts (physical, psychological, social) together. Spirituality had been defined as "the experience of meaning in everyday activities" (Urbanowski & Vargo, 1994, p. 89). Its scope encompasses religious beliefs but transcends the divisiveness of organized religions. As occupational therapists, we are concerned with the meaning of daily activities for our clients. An activity cannot be separated from its meaning. Through our various roles, it is the routines and activities of everyday life that define us. When clients' lives are disrupted by illness or injury, our first priority might be to find out how to best restore this sense of "ordinary existence," however the client might define it.

Hasselkus (2002) discusses everyday routines as rituals. Unlike other habits, rituals have a meaning not only for the individual, but also attributed by one's culture. For example, baking cookies can have meaning beyond following a recipe; it becomes a ritual when the activity symbolizes motherhood for the individual.

Dixon (1987) states that each (life) crisis has a nucleus, a nuclear problem that threatens something the person considers essential for a meaningful life (Rosenfeld, 1997). Rosenfeld suggests that occupational therapists seek to understand this "nuclear" problem and find "nuclear tasks, that is, the things that need doing to resolve the crisis... The functions of nuclear tasks are to express and manage feelings, sustain occupational patterns and involvements, learn vital new skills, and remotivate by demonstrating self-reliance, and symbolize recovery" (p. 26).

Using the client-centered approach, group interventions with clients might focus on some of the steps Rosenfeld defines in identifying nuclear problems and tasks. The occupational goals clients set for themselves with our help probably relate in some way to this kind of spiritual meaning.

Applications

Practical application of the contributing concepts of client-centered theory will be discussed in four sections:

1. The client-centered nature of groups
2. Selecting group members using the client-centered model
3. Skills of the client-centered leader: therapeutic use of self
4. Benefits of the seven-step format

The Client-Centered Nature of Groups

Ideally, clients come to us with an understanding of what occupational therapy can do for them and already knowing their goals and priorities regarding occupational participation. In reality, that level of awareness rarely exists. Care must be taken during the initial occupational therapy interview to connect with the person who is the client, to evaluate that person's status regarding self-awareness, and to facilitate further client self-

understanding. Only when the occupational therapist has developed an appreciation for the client's own feelings and perceptions regarding his or her occupational status can therapist and client collaborate about what possible occupational therapy interventions might be helpful.

There are many reasons why a client may not have a good understanding of his or her own occupational issues. Psychological barriers such as denial, repression, projection, or reaction formation might prevent client insight. Cognitive disabilities often interfere with the ability to define and communicate problems or to anticipate the consequences of impaired occupational performance. Even the most cognitively able clients may lack an understanding of the barriers to occupational engagement caused by illness or by social and cultural contexts. When the occupational therapist encounters several such clients, designing structured group activities or exercises to enable self-awareness and self-understanding may be the ideal format for initial intervention. Client-centered groups offer a structured way to facilitate client self-expression, awareness of choices, and empowerment for self-direction.

Selecting Group Members Using the Client-Centered Model

In the process of occupational therapy practice, member selection becomes a part of the initial evaluation. In client-centered occupational performance process model, clients identify problem areas during an informal or semistructured interview such as the Canadian Occupational Performance Measure (Fearing, Clark, & Stanton, 1998). While evaluation of clients is beyond the scope of this text, a general description is necessary in order to appreciate how groups can play a part.

The client-centered interview has several purposes:

- To develop a therapeutic relationship (engagement)
- To identify and prioritize problem areas in occupational functioning
- To identify potential interventions
- To discuss the effects of contexts in enabling or creating barriers to occupational performance
- To identify strengths and weaknesses
- To identify targeted outcomes and collaborative action plans

Table 3-1	The Potential Benefits of Groups

- Provide a context of social support
- Enhance communication and self-expression
- Provide an atmosphere of nonjudgmental acceptance
- Allow expression of the unique cultural values of each member
- Offer multiple opportunities to share learning and application of therapeutic strategies
- Impart information in a cost-effective way
- Facilitate client participation
- Promote all levels of client group interaction skill
- Provide ideal context for problem-solving relationships with others

Not all clients are self-aware, and many have not given much thought to their priorities or the effects of the various contexts in which they perform occupations. After collaboratively prioritizing problem areas to address, the occupational therapist may suggest a therapeutic group as a potential intervention. However, to limit the use of groups to interventions would not take advantage of their potential for helping clients with earlier parts of the process. Structured group activities can help clients clarify and prioritize problem areas, explore the enabling and disabling aspects of context, identify strengths and weaknesses through group discussion and mutual feedback, and identify targeted outcomes through group problem solving.

In the client-centered evaluation and intervention process, occupational therapists should consider the advantages of groups listed in Table 3-1. These potential group benefits should be shared with the client during the evaluation.

During the initial evaluation, clients who are good candidates for groups can be identified using an interpersonal relationships interview focus. Yalom (1995) suggests exploring the client's relationships with others, including spouse, family, friendships, and community groups. This can be useful in two ways. It can assist the client in identifying problems with interpersonal relationships that might be preventing meaningful social participation, and it can also help the therapist to evaluate the client's appropriateness for different types of groups.

After a client has agreed that a group intervention would be helpful, the next step is to prepare the client for group participation. The therapist should discuss the goals, benefits, and expectations of group membership. Potential members should have a clear understanding of the targeted outcomes to be worked on during the session before joining the group.

Skills of the Client-Centered Group Leader: Therapeutic Use of Self

The humanists say that we cannot change our clients, that they must desire to change themselves. The function of the therapist is to create an atmosphere of safety and to help the client build the kind of self-image and self-understanding that increases the likelihood of positive change. The client-centered therapist does this through the therapeutic relationship and through the facilitation of therapeutic groups. Rogers (1961, 1975) said that behavior change is really a by-product of a deep self-understanding. To change their lives in a positive way, clients must first feel and believe that they have the strength and the power to make changes. This requires a feeling of self-worth and self-esteem as well as a belief that one has the needed skills and capacities required. A prerequisite for change is the belief that change is possible. All of these are appropriate issues to be addressed in occupational therapy groups.

The occupational therapy group leader focuses on skills that help develop the therapeutic relationship. These skills will be used extensively in planning and leading occupational therapy groups. Leader use of skills in therapeutic use of self gives group members an active part in the direction and process of therapy, while allowing the leader to guide them through the establishment of therapeutic norms.

Knowledge of the stages of groups is important, as well as what skills are appropriate for each stage. The reader is referred to Gerard Egan's *The Skilled Helper* (2001) for a more thorough discussion of these skills. Egan's text is intended for teaching basic counseling skills to those who will be doing individual psychotherapy. However, the stages of counseling that parallel the development of groups and the use of specific skills in group intervention will be the emphasis here.

Egan describes three stages of counseling, that parallel the occupational therapy process:

1. Problem definition (OT, evaluation)
2. Self-understanding (OT, goal setting)
3. Behavior change (OT, intervention)

Stage I is concerned with problem definition. This stage is parallel to the beginning stage of a group, in which members get to know one another and begin to lay the ground rules for how they will interact. The skills Egan suggests for this stage are *attending*, *concreteness*, and *primary accurate empathy* (PAE).

Attending

Attending is something most of us do without even thinking about it. The leader of the group needs to be especially alert and observant since he or she is attending to not one but several people at one time. Attending refers to the attentive physical presence the therapist focuses on the client. It is evident even before anyone begins to speak. Taking note of appearance, body language, posture, seating position, eye contact, and facial expression are all part of attending. The therapist gets from these factors important clues as to how members are feeling and how the group is likely to respond to various activities or interventions.

Skill Practice in Attending

To help you become aware of how powerful these first impressions really are, try sitting in a group for the first few minutes without speaking and do the following:

- Draw a diagram of where people are seated in the room.
- Write a one- or two-word phrase describing the appearance of each member. For example:

  Glenn—Sloppy, poor hygiene

  Mary—Dressed up, neat

  Sue—Provocative, overly made up

  Joe—Preppie, well-groomed

- Write one or two adjectives to describe the posture of each member. For example:

  Glenn—Relaxed, slouching

  Mary—Watchful, tense

  Sue—Uncomfortable, fidgety

  Joe—Alert, open

- Note with whom each member has eye contact. For example:

  Glenn—Looks at no one, looks down

  Mary—Looks at everyone

  Sue—Looks only at Joe

  Joe—Looks at leader primarily

- Write a word of feeling describing the emotional message given by the facial expression of each. For example:

  Glenn—Defiant

  Mary—Anxious, fearful

  Sue—Distracted, blunted

  Joe—Eager, anticipating

It is most helpful to put the descriptions of each individual together so you can begin to get a more complete picture of each (Worksheet 3-1).

Knowing these impressions before starting the group, the leader can predict some responses that can be expected from the four clients. Even if the therapist does not know anything about the clients except their names and ages, an observant leader will begin to adapt his or her approach to the group to accommodate the different expectations.

Which of these clients is most likely to be cooperative? Uncooperative? Which client is most likely to disrupt the group? Which member might be expected to leave prematurely? Attending and forming impressions of members becomes second nature to the skilled therapist, but the beginning therapist perhaps needs some practice. Worksheet 3-1 may be used to practice these observations on your own group.

Concreteness

Concreteness refers to the ability to elicit specific information about a client/problem. If the humanistic therapist's goal is to obtain a thorough understanding of the client, many clarifying questions must ultimately be asked. The most basic skill in concreteness is to ask open-ended questions. These are questions that cannot be answered with a simple "yes" or "no." Open-ended questions encourage the client to clarify his or her perceptions, elaborate on important points, and give specific personal examples. A therapist may use open-ended questions to get the client to discover concrete solutions to problems, but that often happens in a later stage of intervention.

Constructing open-ended questions is not always as easy as it seems. Some beginning therapists are in the bad habit of asking closed questions one after the other, and this kind of habit is

Worksheet 3-1
First Impressions

Directions: List names of group members in the first column. Then use one or two descriptive words to denote appearance, posture, and facial expression. Before beginning to speak, note the person with which each member makes eye contact. This information will make up your first impressions of group members.

Member Name	Appearance	Posture	Eye Contact	Facial Expression
1.				
2.				
3.				
4.				
5.				
6.				
7.				
8.				

From Cole, M. B. *Group dynamics in occupational therapy: The theoretical basis and practice application of group intervention* (3rd ed.). Thorofare, NJ: SLACK Incorporated. © 2005 SLACK Incorporated.

hard to break. Consider the following opening of an occupational therapy session:

OT: Would you like to do some drawing today?

Joe: No.

OT: Are you too tired?

Joe: Yes.

OT: Can you just talk to me for a while?

Joe: I'd rather not.

OT: Do you find it hard to talk?

Joe: Yes.

OT: Why?

Joe: I don't know.

Now consider the following alternative opening:

OT: To begin our session, I'd like to learn how well you express your feelings. What can you tell me about how you're feeling right now?

Joe: Nothing.

OT: What makes it difficult to talk about feelings with me?

Joe: It's nothing against you, I'm just in a bad mood.

OT: What put you in a bad mood?

Joe: My doctor just told me I can't go home this weekend.

In leading occupational therapy groups, open-ended questions are more effective because they encourage communication and interaction among members. Closed-ended questions tend to cut off communication. This is an important point to remember when planning questions for discussion when processing an activity group. In asking open-ended questions, it seems most useful to begin with the words "what" or "how." Using the word "why" is not advisable because it tends to elicit vague answers and because it may sound judgmental, reminding some clients of their angry parents' interrogations. Also, avoid beginning a question with "do you, can you, would you, are you, have you" because these can easily be answered with "yes" or "no," as observed in the above example. Now try Worksheet 3-2.

Primary Accurate Empathy

PAE is discussed by several humanistic theorists, particularly Carl Rogers. The importance of its use early in therapy cannot be overemphasized. PAE is the reflection of the feeling and content expressed by the client. If composed and delivered effectively, an empathetic comment from either the therapist or another group member will convince the client that he or she is being listened to and understood. The effect of empathy is to encourage this client to open up even more. PAE, used often in groups, will help build an atmosphere of safety and trust and will help the group progress toward a state of cohesiveness.

PAE is considered "primary" because it does not reach far below the surface. It reflects, but does not repeat, what the client has actually said. Empathy requires that the feeling of the client be recognized, and that may require careful observation of nonverbal cues as well as what the client actually says. (In the practice exercise, you'll just have to read between the lines.) The "accurate" part of empathy requires that the emotion be identified accurately. Emotions vary in both kind and intensity. Some psychologists have divided feelings into the categories of sad, mad, bad, and glad. It isn't enough to just say "you feel angry." Anger varies from low intensity, like annoyed or perturbed, to very high intensity, like rage. Clients often do not have a very wide "feeling" vocabulary; many are not used to expressing their feelings in words. Often clients need the help of the therapist to find right words to describe their feelings accurately. Worksheets 3-3 and 3-4 will help you to develop a better "feeling" vocabulary.

After expanding our knowledge of "feeling" words, we will apply them to the skill of PAE. When practicing PAE, we will use a sentence completion to facilitate finding the right feeling words. We will complete the sentence, "You feel _____ because _____." "You feel" refers to the feeling word that best reflects how the client is feeling. "Because" refers to the thoughts or behaviors that are seen to have caused the feeling. When leading a group, you will learn to use your own words to show empathy. Now try Worksheet 3-5.

According to Egan (2001), the goal of *Stage II* in counseling is self-understanding. The middle stage of group development is more complex than this, with its subgroups, leadership struggles, and questioning of purpose/value, but the outcome is still a greater self-understanding. It is helpful to groups if the leader uses and teaches the skills of Stage II to get through this vital phase of group development. The skills of Stage II are *immediacy, advanced accurate empathy* (AAE), and *confrontation*.

Immediacy

Immediacy is the direct mutual communication between therapist and client. It enables the therapist to discuss openly and directly what is happening in the here and now of their interpersonal relationship. It is an invitation to process the relationship, and this is how it is best used in groups. When a group bogs down, and nothing seems to

Worksheet 3-2
Open-Ended Questions

Directions: In each of the following examples, respond to the client with an open-ended question that can:
- Elicit more specific information
- Focus the discussion on a specific problem
- Help define the problem

1. "I'm always so unlucky!"
   Therapist response:

2. "No matter what I do, I can't win."
   Therapist response:

3. "I'm not thinking right today."
   Therapist response:

4. "Boy, did I have a boring weekend!"
   Therapist response:

5. "My doctor gave me new medication, and I'm just not myself."
   Therapist response:

6. "Life is so unfair. Do you think there's any justice in the world?"
   Therapist response:

7. "What good does it do to write down a schedule? When I go home, it's all for nothing."
   Therapist response:

8. "I'm really afraid to talk about how I feel."
   Therapist response:

9. "Just let well enough alone. I feel great today."
   Therapist response:

10. "Why should I care what my mother thinks?"
    Therapist response:

From Cole, M. B. *Group dynamics in occupational therapy: The theoretical basis and practice application of group intervention* (3rd ed.). Thorofare, NJ: SLACK Incorporated. © 2005 SLACK Incorporated.

Worksheet 3-3
Developing Your Empathy Vocabulary, Part I

Directions: This exercise may be done as a group or individually. Take 10 or 15 minutes to list as many feeling words you can think of in each category listed at the top of the first four columns. A fifth column is provided for those words that seem to defy categorization but are nevertheless expressive of feelings. You may use a thesaurus to form a more complete list (at least 20 words per column). When you are finished, go to Worksheet 3-4.

Mad	Sad	Bad (fearful)	Glad	Other Emotions

From Cole, M. B. *Group dynamics in occupational therapy: The theoretical basis and practice application of group intervention* (3rd ed.). Thorofare, NJ: SLACK Incorporated. © 2005 SLACK Incorporated.

Worksheet 3-4
Developing Your Empathy Vocabulary, Part II

Directions: From the list you made in Worksheet 3-3, sort the words in each column into the three levels of intensity described to the left: mild, moderate, or severe. For example, in the "Bad" column, a mild emotion might be "worried," a moderate emotion might be "fearful," and a severe one might be "petrified." Refer to your completed list when completing the Primary Accurate Empathy worksheet (Worksheet 3-5).

Mad	Sad	Bad (fearful)	Glad	Other Emotions
Mild				
Moderate				
Severe				

Worksheet 3-5
Primary Accurate Empathy

Directions: After reading each client's comment in group, write a response that completes the sentence: "You feel
_____ because _____" and communicates:
- What emotion that patient is feeling (as accurately as possible)
- A summary of the thoughts or behaviors that are seen to have caused the feeling

1. "I can't draw very well (shows a very faintly drawn picture to the group). This is supposed to be my sofa and my dog."
   "You feel _____ because _____."

2. "He just accused me of being prejudiced! I say he's a moron!"
   "You feel _____ because _____."

3. "Brian is doing so well. He's leaving tomorrow to start a new life, and here I am, still in the hospital."
   "You feel _____ because _____."

4. "Can I leave now? This group is making me very upset, especially when Mark sounds so angry."
   "You feel _____ because _____."

5. "This group just isn't helping me. None of you understand what I'm going through!"
   "You feel _____ because _____."

6. "I didn't want to come to occupational therapy group today. Setting goals is too much work."
   "You feel _____ because _____."

7. "When Laurie tells me I'm being insensitive, I don't know what she means."
   "You feel _____ because _____."

8. "All I know is that I'm restricted to the ward again. They seem to like punishing me."
   "You feel _____ because _____."

9. "My boyfriend always picks on me when he's had a bad day. Now I am too upset to participate in this group."
   "You feel _____ because _____."

10. (Laurie crying) "I don't know why I'm so upset. Just hearing Roy talk about being old and alone. He reminds me of my grandfather who died 2 months ago."
   "You feel _____ because _____."

be happening, a question like "What is happening right now?" or "What do you think the silence means?" will serve to refocus the group on its own process. The group's relationship to its leader is commonly a troubled one in Stage II, with which immediacy can help. For example, the leader can often sense anger, resentment, or rebellion in the members and invite the group to discuss it. He or she could ask, "Are you angry with me for insisting that you give each other constructive feedback?" This direct question encourages the members to examine their own feelings about the leader, an essential task in the "control" stage of groups. Trust is another important issue to help therapist immediacy. A comment like "I can see that you're having a hard time trusting one another in this group today," will invite the group members to examine their relationships with one another. Now try Worksheet 3-6.

Advanced Accurate Empathy

AAE goes a step further than PAE. This skill enables the therapist to bring feelings and thoughts that the client may only be implying to the forefront. Therapists find AAE difficult because it involves forming a hypothesis about the underlying or hidden feelings/topics the client just hints at with his or her statements. Egan (2001) defines AAE as:

> ...sharing hunches about clients and their overt and covert experiences, behaviors, and feelings which the therapist thinks will help clients see their problems and concerns more clearly, and in a context that will enable them to move to goal setting and action.

AAE helps the client in several specific ways. First, it can help him or her become aware of hidden or forbidden feelings. Male clients, for example, often try to hide their sad or hurt feelings because they consider them to be a sign of weakness. Secondly, the therapist can use AAE to help the client see patterns of behavior or general trends. A bad experience with one doctor, for example, may lead a client to mistrust all doctors. A third way that AAE can help a client is to help him or her draw logical conclusions to his or her behaviors or comments. An older teen who feels trapped by his parents' rules and says he is tired of his parents treating him like a child may be expressing a desire to leave home and become more independent. Actually moving out may be very scary to an adolescent who has never been on his own, but that is where his comments seem to be leading.

Since AAE is really the therapist's hypothesis or educated guess about the client's implications, it is best to present these ideas tentatively. Always leave yourself a way out, by using phrases like "could it be that...," "it seems likely that...," or "I could be wrong, but...." The fact is, you could be wrong, and it should always be acceptable for the client to correct you if you are. Even if you are not wrong, if the client really is hiding a seething rage at his or her spouse, he or she may not be ready to face or accept such intense feeling. Tentativeness also leaves the client a way out without damaging the therapeutic relationship.

The easiest way to learn AAE is to begin with PAE. Practice AAE by doing Worksheet 3-7.

Confrontation

Confrontation involves the resolution of possible discrepancies, distortions, games, and smoke screens clients use to avoid self-understanding and/or behavior change. It includes challenging the undeveloped, unused, or misused potentialities, skills, and resources clients may have as well. Confrontation as a technique is actually an extension of AAE or interpretation. However, whereas interpretation involves the therapist's understanding of a client's behavior, confrontation permits the client him- or herself to put his or her own meaning to the behavior. In confrontation, the therapist points out maladaptive behaviors or inconsistent actions and comments and invites the client to explain or make sense of them.

Confrontation has a reputation for being harsh and accusing. However, the skilled confrontation is not harsh, but an act of caring. It should offer genuine feedback to the client about his or her comments or behavior, while leaving the judgment of the behavior up to him or her. The tone of voice used by the therapist is very important here. The correct words, conveyed in an angry or accusing tone, will not achieve the desired result. What is hoped for is self-discovery on the part of the client, using the confrontation as a guide.

For example, when Ben expresses that he's "happy-go-lucky and able to cope with almost anything," the therapist might ask, "If this is true, what are you doing in a psychiatric hospital?" In this confrontation, it is Ben who has to explain the discrepancy between his healthy self-presentation and his psychiatric inpatient status. The therapist might say, "One doesn't get admitted to a psychiatric ward by being healthy and able to cope. How did a healthy person like you end up on a psychiatric ward?" There must be problems Ben is not

Worksheet 3-6
Practice of Immediacy

Directions: In the following examples, respond with a direct question or statement that encourages the group to examine its here-and-now relationships.

1. Group of adolescents hospitalized for drug abuse.
   Tina: "If we discuss our problems in group, you'll just tell our parents. They're the ones who sent us here in the first place."

   Bob: "Yeah, how do we know you won't rat on us?"

   Mikki: "I'm not telling you nothin'. I may have to come to this group, but I don't have to talk."

   Therapist response:

2. Group of eating disorder patients working on vocational readiness. This group has chosen to do one small craft project after another. None of the members have opted to take on anything more challenging, yet three of the members face discharge with only three or four more occupational therapy sessions.

   Therapist response:

3. Group of arthritis patients attending the third session of a leisure planning group.

   Morgan: "What are we in this group for anyway? All I want to do is go back to work. Then I won't have any leisure time."

   Jackie: "I stopped participating in sports back in high school. Sure, it would be good for me, but it's just too much effort."

   Ellie: "Sure, my doctor told me I need to plan time for relaxation and enjoyment, but I'm not sure I need someone telling me how or when to do it."

   Therapist response:

Worksheet 3-7
Advanced Accurate Empathy

Directions: First, respond with a primary accurate empathy statement to the client. Then, respond with some statement of advanced accurate empathy. Freely interpret so as to assist the client in taking a larger view of his or her situation, see the implications, or examine the logical conclusions of what is said or done.

1. Sam, age 54
   Situation: This man has a variety of problems. This time he has just undergone surgery to repair a back injury. His tendency is to ruminate constantly on his defects.
   "To feel bad, all I have to do is review what has happened in my life. This past year I let my drinking get the best of me for 4 months. Over the years, I've messed up my marriage. Now my wife and I are separated. I don't have the kind of income that can support two households, and the job market is really tight. I'm not so sure what skills I have to market anyhow."

   Therapist PAE response:

   Therapist AAE response:

2. Adele, age 44
   Situation: This woman has been admitted for the third time with a bleeding ulcer.
   "I'm completely depressed. I don't feel like working anymore. Actually, I work all the time. I can't think of any day I get up and don't intend to work. I think I begrudge myself the time I take for relaxation. There's been no day for the past 2 years when I said, 'Today's a day off.' I always feel so good about myself after I've worked hard, and after all, it's my choice to spend the time the way I want, isn't it?"

   Therapist PAE response:

   Therapist AAE response:

talking about. However, the point of the confrontation is not to accuse Ben of having problems; the point is to get Ben himself to stop denying or hiding his problems and instead try to solve them.

Use Worksheet 3-8 to practice your skills in confrontation as an act of caring and promoting self-understanding.

Benefits of the Seven-Step Format

The following section of this chapter elaborates upon how the general group format presented in Chapter 1 uses a client-centered approach.

Introduction

In client-centered groups, the purpose should be thoroughly explained, when member self-understanding and insight is possible. Care in this initial explanation will make it possible for the members themselves to strive to accomplish the purpose as they do the activity.

Activity

Selecting activities is guided by the therapeutic goals of the members. Activities will vary widely, depending on the frame of reference used and the interests and preferences clients have expressed. They may involve exploring interests, making choices, or developing new skills. Creative activities like drawing, painting, sculpting, and storytelling or drama often encourage the expression of hidden aspects of the self and are helpful in the goals of self-awareness and insight, as long as these activities are client directed. The therapist selects and structures the activity in collaboration with clients to maximize goal achievement.

For example, when clients express a need to improve their ability to express emotions in their relationships, the occupational therapist might suggest an activity called "Circle of Feelings." This requires each member to draw a circle in the center of a piece of 9 inch x 12 inch white drawing paper. Then they use colored markers to indicate layers of feelings. The outer edge of the circle represents the outer self, the feelings they show to others, while the center of the circle represents the inner core, those feelings kept well-hidden and seldom shown to others. Such an activity serves to focus and guide the group toward a frank discussion of their inner feelings, promoting the goal of greater self-understanding among members.

The time frame for such an activity should adhere to the rule of no more than one-third of the entire group time. Emphasis should always be on discussion and processing.

Sharing

In client-centered groups, feedback is the most vital therapeutic tool available and should be encouraged early in groups, beginning in the sharing stage. The purpose of feedback goes beyond the acknowledgment of member contributions. It is a skill to be taught to all the group members if they are to help one another. Considerable time should be taken with this stage to be sure each member's work is correctly understood and explored by the group. The therapist might ask questions of each member to help clarify and focus their issues. Leader skills in concreteness, PAE, immediacy, confrontation, and AAE can be used effectively in all of the discussion stages of client-centered groups. The occupational therapist can use client issues as examples to demonstrate the techniques of reality testing and consensual validation for the group.

In our example of the "Circle of Feelings" exercise, members may question one another about the meaning of color and about reported feelings. They may agree or disagree about the outer circle a client describes. If Ben draws an outer circle of yellow, and reports feeling that others see him as cheerful and carefree, the statement invites other group members to comment. Some may agree with Ben, that he presents a jovial exterior. Others may see beyond this, to his inner pain and suffering. Ben and the group both benefit from a discussion of how he really comes across to others.

Processing

The potential of members sharing the leadership of groups is maximized in client-centered groups. Thus, the skill of giving and receiving feedback is further defined in the processing stage. As members discuss their feelings about the activity, the leader encourages them to also express feelings about one another. The best that we hope for is a genuine curiosity about one another, leading to concern and caring in the later stages of group development. The focus on feelings in the processing stage leads clients to think about their own subjective experience of engaging in occupation within a social context. The therapist can further maximize benefits of the group context by getting members to use their own experiences and capabilities to help one another.

Worksheet 3-8
Practice in Confrontation

Directions: Respond to each of the following clients first with primary accurate empathy, then with confrontation.

Example: Sheila says "Everything is fine" as she stares at the floor and looks sad.

Therapist confrontation: "You must feel sad, judging from the downcast look on your face. Yet you're telling me everything is fine. How do you see that?"

1. Mike, a spinal cord injured patient, age 25, comments after a visit from his wife. "It really hurts me when I think about what she said to me." He smiles and shrugs his shoulders.

   Therapist confrontation:

2. Anne, age 35, is an arthritic patient who has become socially isolated except for a few friends. She is seeking ways of getting along better with others interpersonally. "I give a lot to my friends, but I expect a lot in return. Unfortunately, it seems like many of them don't recognize my caring and I react by getting angry with them."

   Therapist confrontation:

3. Robert, a cardiac patient, is recently divorced, has lost his job, and is broke. He keeps joking about it.

   Therapist confrontation:

From Cole, M. B. *Group dynamics in occupational therapy: The theoretical basis and practice application of group intervention* (3rd ed.). Thorofare, NJ: SLACK Incorporated. © 2005 SLACK Incorporated.

Generalizing

In client-centered theory, the meaning of occupation is a central concern. The generalizing stage of the group is devoted to deriving the meaning of a small slice of life, the group experience. The therapist should encourage the members to verbalize the meaning of the experience for them. Looking at similarities and differences in what is meaningful will help reinforce the values of each member. Using our "Circle of Feelings" example, some members might find meaning in becoming more aware of their own inner feelings, while others might value the opportunity to learn how others really see them. It may surprise some members to find themselves able to express feelings verbally, while others may be more guarded and unwilling to disclose their inner feelings to others. Some people seek the understanding of others through self-disclosure and these people find meaning in close relationships with others. For other people, the impression they leave with others might be more important, the "never let them see you sweat" approach. Therapists need to be careful not to judge any value as right or wrong. Accepting differences among members is an important norm to promote during this step.

Application

In this step, meaning is expanded and personalized. In client-centered groups, a connection needs to be made between the group activity and the goals of each individual member. The therapist asks each member in turn to discuss how he or she could apply this group experience to his or her own life. It will be important for the therapist to use concreteness and to get each member to give a specific example. This step provides an opportunity for therapist and clients to collaborate in identifying outcomes. These may take the form of greater self-awareness, new learning, skill development, greater self-understanding, new choices, or new solutions or strategies for stated problems. Enabling clients to verbalize the possible benefits or outcomes of group activities reinforces the value of occupational therapy group interventions. However, therapists should be careful to also accept negative or neutral comments and to use these as an opportunity to re-evaluate, problem solve, and collaborate with the group members to plan more relevant activities.

Summary

The summary, as with every step, should involve the group members whenever possible. They are presumed capable of analyzing the entire group experience and judging which parts are most significant. The therapist's role is to encourage them to do this, and not to do it for them. When the therapist asks for a summary of the group, about 5 minutes before it is time to end, members will quickly learn that this is what is expected and may eventually do it spontaneously.

Designing Client-Centered Group Interventions

Yalom in his *The Theory and Practice of Group Psychotherapy, Fourth Edition* (1995) describes a basically existential humanistic approach. Clients are treated in groups not only because it is practical, but because of the many unique advantages that only a group can offer in treatment. The goals for an individual have mostly to do with increasing self-understanding, self-worth, and self-actualization. In the group setting, members are expected to discuss their own lives, their problems, and their successes. Through their self-disclosure, members develop relationships with one another and learn to trust one another. The feedback and support they give one another is of far greater value than what they can get from any individual.

Furthermore, many of the therapeutic factors described by Yalom (instillation of hope, universality, altruism, group cohesiveness, and interpersonal learning) will help the members achieve their goals. The therapeutic factors are those aspects of groups that make them therapeutic. Instillation of hope conveys the positive expectation members have at the outset of groups that the group experience will help them. Clients in group intervention often feel great relief when they discover that their problems are not unique, that others share their misery (universality). Altruism implies that clients benefit not only by receiving from others, but also from giving. Learning to give to others in the group may in fact be the most important lesson of all. Group cohesiveness has been described as the final and most desirable stage of group development. It is an attraction for each other that is shared by all its members. Cohesiveness makes possible all the positive, productive work that can be accomplished by the mature group described in Chapter 2. Interpersonal learning incorporates a broad range of factors about the give and take of emotional and social relationships to one another. The reader is referred to Yalom (1995), Chapters 1 and 2, for further discussion of the therapeutic factors of groups.

Client-centered groups work best when members have a moderately high cognitive ability. It is the approach suggested for personal/professional growth of student groups or staff groups. A certain level of self-awareness is expected, and members should be able to communicate their self-perceptions to the group reasonably well. In short, members must be capable of insight. Insight means not only acknowledging one's own problematic behavior but having some understanding of the reasons behind it.

However, client-centered theorists warn that therapists should not underestimate the ability of cognitively disabled individuals to express their goals and preferences. Therefore, groups should be adapted to match the level of client understanding and insight, and therapists should enable whatever participation the members can contribute. For example, Ross (1997; Ross & Bachner, 2004) uses five-stage groups with a sensory integrative focus for clients with severe cognitive disabilities. Regarding groups with institutionalized clients, she writes:

> Relating to others without the use of words is very interesting. A connection made between two persons when no words have been spoken but only action takes place is a golden moment, perhaps the more poignant because it feels so stark. It was observed whenever group members showed more awareness and shared or passed items to one another for the first time. It was seen when a man in a group, the victim of Alzheimer's disease, suddenly intercepted a large, soft ball before his male neighbor could reach it, but then handed it to a withdrawn woman sitting next to him so she would have a turn. It is observed in the sudden smile, the unconsciously straightened posture, or the unsolicited hug that comes for the first time from someone who avoided contact or response. When a string of such golden moments happens, a marvelous feeling occurs and illuminates my understanding of how to proceed further. It is easy to become addicted to encouraging the feeling of flow. (2004, unpublished manuscript)

The skilled group leader can adapt the seven-step format using a client-centered approach with many different levels of client ability, disability, and circumstance.

Activity Examples

The Activity Examples at the end of this chapter are designed for use in the evaluation process of occupational therapy. They maybe used to help clients to identify and better define their occupational difficulties, to clarify and better communicate their goals and priorities, and to build trust and support within the safety of a therapeutic group. Some of the group activities help clients to explore contextual factors and/or to identify barriers to participation, and use group feedback in developing strategies for the removal of barriers and the creation of enabling environments.

Bibliography

American Occupational Therapy Association. (2004). *The reference manual of the official documents of the American Occupational Therapy Association* (10th ed). Bethesda, MD: Author.

Canadian Occupational Therapy Association. (1991). *Occupational therapy guidelines for client-centered practice.* Toronto, Ontario: Author.

Canadian Occupational Therapy Association. (1997). *Enabling occupation: An occupational therapy perspective,* Toronto, Ontario: Author.

Cole, M., & McLean, V. (2003). Therapeutic relationships redefined. *Occupational Therapy in Mental Health, 19*(2), 33-56.

Corey, G. (1986). *I never knew I had a choice* (3rd ed.). Monterey, CA: Brooks/Cole.

Corey, G. (1991). *The theory and practice of counseling and psychotherapy* (4th ed.). Monterey, CA: Brooks/Cole.

Corey, G. (1996). *The theory and practice of counseling and psychotherapy* (5th ed.). Monterey, CA: Brooks/Cole.

Crepeau, E., Cohn, E., & Schell, B. (Eds.). (2003). *Willard and Spackman's occupational therapy* (10th ed.). Philadelphia: Williams & Wilkins.

Dixon, S. (1987). *Working with people in crisis* (2nd ed.). St. Louis: Mosby.

Egan, G. (1994). *Exercises in helping skills.* Monterey, CA: Brooks/Cole.

Egan, G. (2001). *The skilled helper* (5th ed.). Monterey, CA: Brooks/Cole.

Fearing, V., Clark, J., & Stanton, S. (1998). The client-centered occupational therapy process. In M. Law (Ed.), *Client-centered occupational therapy.* Thorofare, NJ: SLACK Incorporated.

Hasselkus, B. (2002). *The meaning of everyday occupation.* Thorofare, NJ: SLACK Incorporated.

Law, M. (Ed.). (1998). *Client-centered occupational therapy.* Thorofare, NJ: SLACK Incorporated.

Maslow, A. H. (1968). *Toward a psychology of being* (Rev. ed.). New York: Van Nostrand Reinhold.

Matheson, L. N. (1998). Engaging the person in the process: Planning together for occupational therapy intervention. In M. Law (Ed.), *Client-centered occupational therapy.* Thorofare, NJ: SLACK Incorporated.

May, R. (1977). *The meaning of anxiety* (Rev. ed.). New York: Norton.

May, R., & Yalom, I. (1989). Existential psychotherapy. In R. J. Corsini & D. Wedding (Eds.), *Current psychotherapies* (4th ed., pp. 363-402). Itasca, IL: F.E. Peacock.

Rogers, C. (1961). *On becoming a person.* Boston: Houghton Mifflin.

Rogers, C. (1967). The conditions of change from a client-centered viewpoint. In B. Berenson & R. Carkhuff (Eds.), *Sources of gain in counseling and psychotherapy.* New York: Holt, Reinhart, and Winston.

Rogers, C. (1975). Empathic: An unappreciated way of being. *The Counseling Psychologist, 5*(2), 2-9.

Rosenfeld, M. (1997). *Motivational strategies in geriatric rehabilitation.* Bethesda, MD: American Occupational Therapy Association.

Ross, M. (1997). *Integrative group therapy: Mobilizing coping abilities with the Five Stage Group.* Bethesda, MD: American Occupational Therapy Association.

Ross, M., & Bachner, S. (Eds.). (2004). *Occupational therapy with the developmentally disabled.* Bethesda, MD: American Occupational Therapy Association.

Urbanowski, R., & Vargo, J. (1994). Spirituality, daily practice, and the occupational performance model. *Canadian Journal of Occupational Therapy, 61,* 88-94.

White, R. (1959). Motivation reconsidered: The concept of competence. *Psychoanalytic Review, 66,* 197.

Yalom, I. (1995). *The theory and practice of group psychotherapy* (4th ed.). New York: Basic Books.

Client-Centered
Activity Example 3-1
Self-Awareness

Directions: Fill out all the information listed on the worksheet. Then select what parts you would like to share with the group.

I am (name you prefer):

Some of my needs are:

Some of my hopes are:

I would describe myself as:

Some things that are important in my life now are:

Some things that may become important to me are:

Three things I am trying to achieve are:

I am good at:

Some things I would like to improve about myself are:

I run away from:

I feel confident when:

I am proud of:

My most striking quality is:

Client-Centered
Activity Example 3-2
Positive Attitudes

Materials: Magazines (at least two per client) with pictures on a variety of subjects.

Directions: Select from these magazines pictures of negative scenes, problems, or situations. There is no required number, so find as many as you like. You have 15 minutes for this task.

Procedure: Each member presents his or her pictures and describes the negative situation. Then the group is asked to point out all the positive aspects of the pictures. For example, appearance or personal hygiene of the people, weather conditions, communication and support available, etc. Then the group can choose a few situations to problem solve. Answer the question: "What can be done to give this situation a happy ending?"

From Cole, M. B. *Group dynamics in occupational therapy: The theoretical basis and practice application of group intervention* (3rd ed.). Thorofare, NJ: SLACK Incorporated. © 2005 SLACK Incorporated.

Client-Centered
Activity Example 3-3
Leisure Collage

Materials: Magazines on varied topics, scissors, glue, white paper, and markers.

Directions: Cut pictures of things you like to do from these magazines and then arrange and paste them on the paper. You have 20 minutes to do this task. After you have finished pasting, use a marker to label each picture with a word ending in "ing" (e.g., eating, talking, playing volleyball, singing).

Client-Centered
Activity Example 3-4
Saying Goodbye

Materials: Writing paper and pens.

Directions: At some point in our lives, we have all had to leave someone we love. Either we left, or we got left behind (i.e., a best friend moving away, a lover finding a new love, a relative's death, a child going away to school). Often we do not have the chance to say the things we want to say before the separation. So here is another chance. Take the next 15 minutes to write a letter to a loved one, telling him or her the things you would like the person to know. Begin with "Dear _____" and end with some form of goodbye.

From Cole, M. B. *Group dynamics in occupational therapy: The theoretical basis and practice application of group intervention* (3rd ed.). Thorofare, NJ: SLACK Incorporated. © 2005 SLACK Incorporated.

Client-Centered
Activity Example 3-5
My House

Materials: Worksheets, rulers, colored markers, and pencils with erasers.

Directions: Imagine you are going on a 1-month vacation and will live in a small house on the beach by yourself. The beach has a path that leads to town where you can buy food or other supplies. Visualize what the house would look like. You arrive in a taxi with your bags. You step onto the deck, unlock the front door, and walk in. What would you like to see? Now fill in the floor plan on the worksheet with whatever you would like in your house. Some suggestions are sofa, bed, dresser, rug, television set, bookshelf with books, refrigerator, stove, washer, dryer, bicycle, sailboat, etc. (Figure 3-2).

While doing this activity, think about what necessities you will need and also what items you would like to help you enjoy your vacation. You may assume there are other people to socialize with at the beach, but they will not be staying with you. You are the only one living in your house.

From Cole, M. B. *Group dynamics in occupational therapy: The theoretical basis and practice application of group intervention* (3rd ed.). Thorofare, NJ: SLACK Incorporated. © 2005 SLACK Incorporated.

Figure 3-2. "My House" design (for use with Activity Example 3-5).

Client-Centered
Activity Example 3-6
My Ideal Job

Materials: Worksheets and pencils.

Directions: Suppose you had the opportunity to be trained to do whatever job you want. What would be your ideal job? To help you define your ideal job, first circle your answers to the following questions. If you circle more than one, write "first choice" or "second choice" next to the answer.

1. What work setting do you prefer?
   Contemporary office
   Well-equipped workshop
   Home-like setting
   Outdoors
   Other

2. What other people would you prefer to work with?
   Work by yourself
   Be part of a working team
   Be the expert who gives help and advice to others
   Be your boss' right-hand man/woman

3. What skills do you prefer to use while working?
   Manual skills, work with hands or tools
   Artistic or creative skills
   Intellectual skills, knowledge, and ideas
   Political skills, strategies, or persuasion
   Technical problem-solving skills

4. What rewards would you seek from your job?
   Lots of money
   Satisfaction from helping others
   Having others recognize your skills
   Achieving your own potential

5. How much risk are you willing to take in your job?
   Prefer doing something familiar with regular pay
   Do not mind being paid on commission
   Willing to try new ideas, even if they are not a sure thing
   An element of danger might make work more exciting

From Cole, M. B. *Group dynamics in occupational therapy: The theoretical basis and practice application of group intervention* (3rd ed.). Thorofare, NJ: SLACK Incorporated. © 2005 SLACK Incorporated.

Client-Centered
Activity Example 3-6
My Ideal Job (continued)

Now consider your answers to those questions and circle the jobs that might fit your criteria from the list below.

Salesperson in a small clothing store

Licensed electrician

Mechanic

Nursery school teacher

Medical technician

Nurse in a large hospital

Medical receptionist in a doctor's office

Advertising artist

Newspaper reporter

High school coach

Hairdresser

Interior decorator

Telephone lineman

Insurance claims adjuster

Traveling salesperson for a large company

Chef in an expensive restaurant

Hostess in an expensive restaurant

Manager of a small delicatessen

Manager of an expensive antique shop

Home health nurse

Musician in a band

Public relations representative for a hotel

Counselor in a drug rehabilitation center

Landscape designer

From Cole, M. B. *Group dynamics in occupational therapy: The theoretical basis and practice application of group intervention* (3rd ed.). Thorofare, NJ: SLACK Incorporated. © 2005 SLACK Incorporated.

Client-Centered
Activity Example 3-7
Draw Your Wall

Anne Golensky, MS, OTR, is acknowledged for creating this activity for use with recovering alcoholics.

Materials: White drawing paper and sets of colored markers.

Directions: The purpose of this activity is to discover the barriers we face that prevent us from moving toward self-actualization. Members introduce themselves and each completes the sentence "Something I've always wanted to do is _____ ." Then, with paper and markers, members draw their "wall," which symbolizes the things that hold them back from achieving their dreams.

Client-Centered

Activity Example 3-8

Primary Concerns

Materials: Three 3- x 5-inch index cards for each member, pens, and area telephone directories.

Directions: This activity is for acute inpatient groups. Members introduce themselves giving names and stating one reason they are in the hospital. They may briefly discuss where they intend to go when they leave, if known.

Write on each of three index cards the following information:

Card 1—What are you most concerned about at this moment?

Card 2—What are you most worried about after you leave the hospital?

Card 3—Who can you count on to help you with your concerns after you leave this group? List names and phone numbers of your doctor, a pharmacy near your residence, your closest family members and friends, and any other resources available to you. (Phone numbers may need to be filled in afterwards.)

From Cole, M. B. *Group dynamics in occupational therapy: The theoretical basis and practice application of group intervention* (3rd ed.). Thorofare, NJ: SLACK Incorporated. © 2005 SLACK Incorporated.

Activities Wheel

Materials: Worksheet with two circles representing 24-hour days. A calculator on hand would be helpful.

Directions: For each hour, fill in the name of the activity you are typically doing at that time of day. Then, total the hours for each general category at the bottom of the circle. Finally, approximate the percentage of the total for each category.

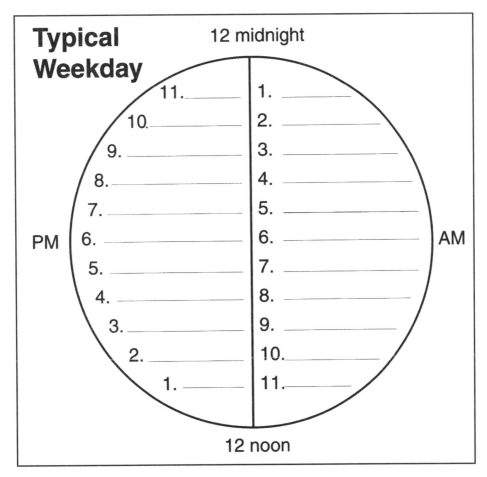

Work/Obligations: _____
Time: _____

Self-Care/Caregiving: _____
Total Time: _____

Leisure/Relaxation: _____
Total Time: _____

Other: _____
Total Time: _____

Sleep/Rest: _____
Total Time: _____

Activities Wheel (continued)

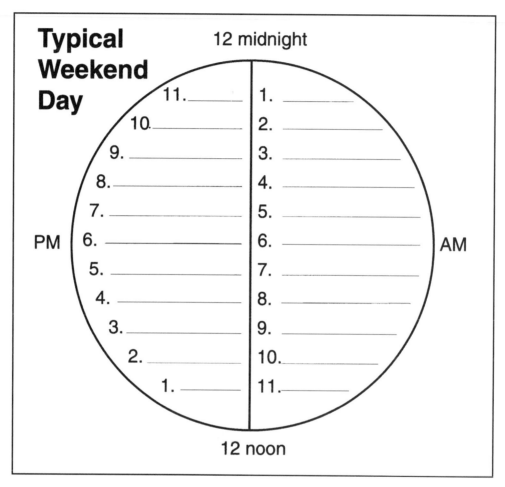

Typical Weekend Day

12 midnight

11._____ 1._____
10._____ 2._____
9._____ 3._____
8._____ 4._____
7._____ 5._____
PM 6._____ 6._____ AM
5._____ 7._____
4._____ 8._____
3._____ 9._____
2._____ 10._____
1._____ 11._____

12 noon

Work/Obligations: _____   Self-Care/Caregiving: _____
Time: _____   Total Time: _____

Leisure/Relaxation: _____   Other: _____
Total Time: _____   Total Time: _____

Sleep/Rest: _____
Total Time: _____

Client-Centered
Activity Example 3-10
Purpose in Life Chart

Things I love:

1.

2.

3.

4.

5.

Things I am proud of:

1.

2.

3.

4.

5.

Things I want to strive for:

1.

2.

3.

4.

5.

Things I can do today to feel better about myself:

1.

2.

3.

Things I hate:

1.

2.

3.

4.

5.

Things I am ashamed of:

1.

2.

3.

4.

5.

Things I never want to become:

1.

2.

3.

4.

5.

Chapter 4

Groups as Social Contexts

The American Occupational Therapy Association ([AOTA], 2002) framework, Domain and Process, defines the general overarching outcome of the occupational therapy process as "engagement in occupation" to support "participation... in desired roles or life situations in home, school, workplace, and community" (p. 611). Social participation is an area of occupational performance defined in the framework as "activities associated with organized patterns of behavior that are characteristic and expected of an individual or an individual interacting with others within a given social system" (p. 621). Occupational therapy group interventions are ideal for preparing clients for many levels of social participation. Some of the natural groups in which individuals participate are families, peer or friendship groups, classes, sports teams or recreational groups, work groups, church groups, and community organizations. This chapter explores the design of group interventions for some of these naturally occurring client groups, using various theoretical perspectives, including role theory, social supports theory, systems theory, family theory, Mosey's ontogenesis theory, and teams and teamwork. New research on Mosey's group adaptive skills (see Appendix C) includes a measure of social participation designed by Mary Donohue, which is based on Mosey's definition of group interaction skill (Donohue, 2003).

Identifying Groups of Frameworks

The *Occupational Therapy Practice Framework* defines clients as "a) individuals (including others involved in the individual's life who may also be served indirectly such as caregiver, teacher, parent, employer, spouse), b) groups, or c) populations (i.e., organizations, communities)" (AOTA, 2002, p. 630). This expanded definition of the client allows occupational therapists to design group interventions on a variety of levels.

- Groups of individuals: The occupational therapist identifies three to eight clients with common problems, disabilities, and/or goals to participate in a specific group or series of groups designed to meet one or more of the goals identified. In this type of group, individual goals will serve as the outcome measures, and the client members will actively participate in the task selection process. The seven-step format described in Chapter 1 was designed for groups of individuals with similar goals.

- Preselected groups: In these groups, the occupational therapist evaluates the group as a whole and recommends and plans group interventions that address targeted outcomes. Examples might be clients with mental retardation who share a group home or a group of clients with dementia who attend a day care program. In this type of group, the occupational therapist may collaborate with other professionals, caregivers, or family members in addressing desired outcomes. The seven-step format for group leadership may also be adapted for this type of group.

- Populations: The occupational therapist may be asked to evaluate an entire population and to design group interventions that address the population as a whole. An example of this might be designing wellness programs for elderly seniors living in a community. The community senior center might be the "client" with whom the occupational therapist collaborates in setting goals and selecting strategies. Community organizations whose purpose is to enhance the quality of life for underserved populations, such as the homeless, or other specialized groups may benefit from occupational therapy consultation. Occupational therapy consultants use group leadership skills in collaborating with organizations to identify problem areas, educate regarding evidence-based interventions, develop strategies for intervention, and enable and structure occupations related to targeted outcomes (e.g., fund raising, advocacy, mentoring, creating support groups).

- Client families: Another potential group intervention might be designed in collaboration with an individual identified client and the family members and significant others who participate in his or her care. This new area of practice uses knowledge of group dynamics theory and research on social contexts to collaborate with entire family groups to assist them in making adaptations and planning activities to enable the identified client to participate in family life.

- Teams and teamwork: Latella (2002) defines a team as "two or more individuals working together toward the achievement of specific goals" (p. 96). Interdisciplinary health care teams, work groups, and sports teams are examples. Often teams have social structures based on power and extrinsically defined roles. Teams may benefit from consultation to help them improve communication and may collaborate with one another through activities that build understanding and trust. For example, an occupational therapist consulting with work groups might use group problem-solving strategies to create social and physical contexts that enable occupation and prevent injury and stress.

Theories Contributing to Groups as Social Contexts

Context as Focus

A new focus of the document is the consideration of context in evaluating and implementing occupational performance. This approach uses a systems-oriented focus. Research tells us that people perform occupations differently in different situations. For example, persons with Alzheimer's perform self-care tasks more independently when these tasks are done in a familiar environment. Both existing and developing theory offer occupational therapists expertise in evaluating environments to eliminate barriers and safety hazards and optimize occupational performance. This knowledge has expanded our practice by applying it to many community settings, including home, school, work, religious, and recreational settings (both built and natural).

The place we choose for our group sessions should bear relevance for the clients and consider the factors that will impact their participation. When confidentiality is an issue, private areas free of distraction, which encourage careful listening and development of trust and empathy, are best. When adaptations are needed, groups can be more successfully run in real-life settings, where clients can readily observe and evaluate problems in adaptation within specific contexts (such as assessing social skills while dining in a restaurant).

In group work, the most relevant aspects of context for clients are social and cultural. The *Occupational Therapy Practice Framework* defines social context as "availability and expectations of significant individuals, such as spouse, friends, and caregivers (and) includes larger social groups that are influential in establishing norms, role expectations, and social routines" (AOTA, 2002, p. 623). There is some overlap with the definition of cultural context, which is defined as:

...customs, beliefs, activity patterns, behavior standards, and expectations accepted by the society of which the individual is a member. (Cultural context) includes political aspects, such as laws that affect access to resources and affirm personal rights. (It) also includes opportunities for education, employment, and economic support. (AOTA, 2002, p. 623)

Therefore, cultural and social contexts are difficult to separate. The reader is referred to Chapter 13 for some examples of groups dealing with cultural issues specifically.

Role Theory

The concept of roles comes from social psychology (Mead, 1934; Sullivan, 1953). The occupational therapy framework defines a role as "a set of behaviors that have some socially agreed upon function and for which there is an accepted code of norms" (Christiansen & Baum, 1997, p. 603). They "form the nucleus of social interaction" by defining the rules and procedures. "Smooth social interaction requires role reciprocity, or the effective role performance of each member of a group" (Christiansen & Baum, 1997, p. 56). Three types of group roles described in Chapter 2 are task roles, group maintenance roles, and individual roles. Task roles help the group get its work done, while maintenance roles address psychosocial issues. Individual roles are viewed by Benne and Sheats (1978) as meeting individual needs while interfering with overall group cohesiveness.

Roles may also be viewed as prescribed sets of behaviors and expectations that situate the person structurally (meaning position in the unit) or functionally (meaning performance demands associated with that structural role) within the social entity (Schaber, 2003, personal communication). Family roles can include spouse, sibling, mother, father, daughter, son, and grandparent as well as extended family members. Each role implies a set of expectations coming from society, one's culture, and one's self. Each has a set of occupations that accomplish an agreed-upon function. For example, caregiving, feeding the family, doing laundry, and keeping a clean house are occupations typical of a mother. The performance of these occupations and how they are carried out is influenced by both self-expectations and cultural expectations.

Occupational therapy group interventions can use social context to support role competence and reciprocity among client members. Group activities that encourage role reciprocity involve all members taking different roles in a shared task, such as giving a holiday party, preparing a meal, or taking a trip. The task-oriented groups described in Chapter 5 are examples of enabling engagement in occupations through role reciprocity. Using this approach, clients engage in planning and preparation, implementation of their various roles, and evaluation of the group task. This type of group helps members work on issues such as decision making, planning ahead, problem solving, communication, and cooperation with others.

Roles also serve as a basis of commonality in forming client groups. Clients who identify significant problems with work roles, for example, may be grouped together to deal with common areas of interest, such as accepting supervision, issues of authority, getting along with coworkers, or coping with job stress. Role identification occurs when a role is internalized. We call ourselves students, workers, or family members because we see ourselves occupying these social positions and performing the occupations associated with these roles (Kielhofner, 2002).

Role theory helps to explain a few problems with occupational performance, such as role conflict, role overload, and role confusion. Role conflict occurs when a person finds him- or herself having to choose between meeting one role expectation or another. The mother who is called home from work to care for a sick child is an example of a role conflict. She must either ignore the sick child, or leave her work undone. Role overload can occur when a person takes on more roles than he or she can handle. For example, a "workaholic" might work night and day, yet never seem to be able to meet all of the obligations demanded by his or her multiple social roles.

Roles can provide scripts that define our social interactions and behaviors. For example, our occupations, mode of dress, and style of interaction will be different when we are at work than when we are home with our families. Role confusion can occur when a husband and wife start a business together or when a boss invites an employee out for dinner.

Group interventions can help clients problem solve role confusion, conflict, and overload as well as other role behaviors that are creating difficulty. Groups can be organized around enabling clients in choosing roles that are meaningful for them, performing roles more effectively, or preparing for roles they perceive as helping them to achieve valued goals. For example, a client might choose the role of a student because he or she perceives that role as a stepping stone to acquiring a better job.

Table 4-1	Extrinsic Sources of Support and Relationships

- Immediate family
- Extended family
- Friends
- Acquaintances, peers, colleagues, neighbors
- People in positions of authority
- People in subordinate positions
- Personal care providers
- Strangers
- Domesticated animals
- Health professionals

Adapted from World Health Organization. (2001). *The international classification of functioning, disability, and health.* Geneva: Author.

Some roles help us organize and sequence the occupations we need to perform in order to achieve a higher social status.

Social Support Theory

People need social support on a variety of levels. Social support has been defined as "the experience of being cared for and loved, valued and esteemed, and able to count on others should the need arise" (McColl, 1997, p. 412). On a personal level, sources of this type of support may be perceived as coming from spouses, parents, or significant others. Some people need a great deal of support, and others have difficulty accepting or giving support. Social support is best thought of as a reciprocal process. Persons with mental illness often need excessive amounts of support, but cannot offer anything in return to those who give it. Group interventions can provide training and practice in giving and receiving social support. McColl (1997) reviews the evidence on the usefulness of social support for persons with disabilities. According to McColl, persons with disabilities tend to have smaller social networks, and often rely on only a few or one individual for most of their social needs.

Group interventions can deal with the above problems in two ways. The first uses the group format to assist clients in understanding the reciprocal nature of social support and providing opportunities to practice meeting each others' social and emotional needs. Another approach is to organize ongoing support groups for persons with disabilities in the community. The "clubhouse" concept for persons with mental illness and the 12-step groups

for alcohol and drug abuse survivors are examples of such support groups. However, there is a great need for organized support groups in addition to these. The "Healthy People 2010" initiative calls for the promotion of health for persons with all types of disabilities through social participation as well as surveillance and health promotion programs (U.S. Dept of Health & Human Services, 2000/2001). Occupational therapists have the knowledge and training in group facilitation needed to initiate community support groups for many different disability or at-risk populations.

Caregivers also need social support. Occupational therapists can organize groups that support caregivers, provide needed education, and enable them to make environmental changes to increase safety, security, and occupational performance for the disabled client. Occupational therapists should also be knowledgeable about sources of social support in the larger community or through public or national sources. When gaps in available services are found, advocacy and political or community action may be needed to overcome barriers or meet specific needs.

The *International Classification of Functioning, Disability, and Health* (World Health Organization [WHO], 2001) lists extrinsic sources of support and relationships (Table 4-1).

Group interventions can be organized to include some of these potential supports, or clients can develop strategies for building their social networks in order to better meet their needs. Social support involves Yalom's therapeutic group factors of universality and altruism (1995). Groups can provide social support to clients in crises, comforted by the knowledge that they are not alone and drawing upon their own innate need to belong, to be needed, and to help others. Occupational therapy groups can focus on developing skills in forming closer, more meaningful relationships with others so that social support will be available for each member, should the need arise.

Social support can take different forms. Three types have been identified by McColl (1997):

1. Practical
2. Informational
3. Emotional

Clients need different types of support at different times. Practical support includes tangible or instrumental tasks like fixing lunch and doing laundry. Clients report this type of support as the least helpful because it is caretaking rather than enabling occupation. Informational support is the type most often sought from formal or societal level sources, such as how to apply for Medicare. Emotional support was found to be most helpful in crisis situations.

Systems Theory

Systems are structures for understanding things that interact. Systems exist in many diverse areas of study, such as biology (musculoskeletal system) and sociology (political systems). Bertalanffy, a biologist, applied general systems theory to living things, which he called open systems. Bruce and Borg (1991) use the example of a baseball team to explain the concept of group as an open system. The team is composed of different individual players, each with a specified role. Yet when they play ball, the team can be understood as an interdependent whole. All systems are composed of four elements:

1. Input
2. Throughput
3. Output
4. Feedback

In an open system, throughput allows the system to change and adapt as a result of feedback. Bruce and Borg (1991) proposed general systems theory as a model for understanding the interactions of occupational therapy groups.

Kielhofner (2002) elaborates on the human open system by dividing "throughput" into three subsystems:

1. Volitional
2. Habituation
3. Performance

These subsystems help explain how the person adapts to changes in the environment by using feedback to learn new strategies and to alter one's responses (output). When applied to groups, occupational therapists facilitate shared experiences in ways that enable adaptations in occupational performance as a result of giving and receiving feedback from other members.

Similarly, we can use systems theory to understand the operation of social systems on many levels. The welfare system, for example, follows national policies in dispersing funds and benefits to those persons who meet specific criteria, whether poverty or disability. States have different guidelines for services offered to welfare recipients, and cities have still different policies and procedures. Local officers assist potential recipients when entering the system, and certain rules need to be followed by recipients in order to remain in the system. Large bureaucratic systems like this can present problems for individuals. For example, once a person with a disability enters the system, he or she cannot secure paid employment without losing benefits. This fact provides little motivation for clients to participate in the worker roles of their peers, even if they find themselves capable. The welfare system exemplifies a societal level social context.

The levels of social context have been defined as:

- Immediate
- Proximal
- Community
- Societal (Spencer, 1998)

Immediate scale social contexts focus on clients and their caregivers or other persons in their household. Not surprisingly, caregiver attitudes and values have the most powerful influence upon the occupational performance of persons with disabilities (Mattingly & Fleming, 1994). Occupational therapists could create groups that include clients and their caregivers to help resolve cultural and ethical differences regarding occupational issues, such as which occupations the client can do safely and which require caregiver assistance.

Proximal scale social contexts include social environments frequented by the client outside the home, such as a classroom, workplace, or clinic. Occupational therapists need to understand the social systems in each of these settings, including roles, expectations, occupational patterns, and rules for interaction. Many cultural factors overlap these social factors. Occupational therapists can consult with groups of workers, students, or day care attendees to facilitate communication; improve factors that enable occupational functioning of workers/clients; and minimize or recommend removal of barriers to social participation. Consultation with employers, teachers and administrators, or community day care staff might have similar goals but may present challenges with the client-centered approach. In consultation, a somewhat different approach has been suggested by Townsend and Landry (2005). Enabling guidelines in working with social groups should include the following:

- Participation: Invite recipients of service to be involved in the group process.
- Collaboration: Share the power of problem solving and decision making.
- Advocating for change: Involve group members in organizational change, such as changes in policy to prevent burnout or reduce stress.
- Empowerment and justice: Awareness of inequities and promotion of a more inclusive society.

Community scale social contexts include both social networks and multiple formal and informal services. Communities often provide services such as home-based medical services, transportation, delivery services, and senior services. Groups can explore community resources and share information. The occupational therapist should be prepared to recommend or facilitate access to community services that will enable social participation. For example, many churches offer assistance, visitation, and social activities for persons seeking engagement in occupation at the community level. Community organizations may be viewed as potential "clients" for occupational therapists. Potentially, a need exists for most organizations to recognize and eliminate barriers to participation for persons with disabilities.

Family Groups: Clients in Context

The disciplines of family therapy and family science have done substantial research on the family-centered approach, which views the family group as one entity rather than a group of individuals (Schaber, 2003, personal communication). Reviewing this extensive body of literature is beyond the scope of this chapter. The application of

small group theory, the Fundamental Interpersonal Relations Model (FIRO), has been applied to families and redefined as the Family FIRO model and serves to inform occupational therapists intervening with families with Alzheimer's disease by highlighting the unique needs of the family member (Schaber, 2002). The FIRO model is based on the theory of Schutz (1958), who proposed that each individual has three interpersonal needs: inclusion, control, and affection that can be met through group membership. Earlier (see Chapter 2) these needs formed the basis of the developmental stages of groups. Here, the theory applies to the family member in the family group. "Families as context" serve as the needs satisfier in evaluating and working with clients who are dependent on their families for daily care. Schaber (2003, personal communication) points out that this application does not replace the family-centered care model, but offers an understanding of the function of the family and can enhance the interviewing process. It is not intended to replace family therapy and is not a social work approach. Rather, it provides a way to examine the social context in which an identified client engages in occupations and explores their meaning within the context of family relationships.

Practically speaking, the occupational therapy family intervention most likely begins with an identified client. We will use the example of a grandmother with dementia, living with her daughter who serves as the primary caregiver. From a systems perspective, the progression of chronic disease in one family member affects all of the other members in some way. Therefore, instead of focusing only on Grandma, the occupational therapist defines her client as a family with dementia. Schaber (personal communication, 2003) suggests that the primary caregiver select the members who will participate in the occupational therapy group intervention. From Grandma's perspective, this group may include a son-in-law, several grandchildren, brothers or sisters who live nearby, nieces and nephews, or close friends and neighbors who are willing to participate. Schaber cautions that occupational issues do not always flow in a sequential manner and that issues of inclusion, control, and affection often need to be addressed simultaneously. Accordingly, the sequential structure described below may need to be altered to address changing family priorities.

The following is a proposed structure for six weekly occupational therapy sessions with a hypothetical family group, using the group protocol method described in Chapter 11. The sessions will include all seven steps of group facilitation, but the occupational therapist shifts their order, dealing with feelings, ideas, and practical applications repeatedly throughout the session. Working with families in the home environment, the activities (or occupational interventions) may not take place during the family session at all. In this example, the occupational interventions are collaboratively planned during the sessions, but occur at other times, and are processed after the fact the following week. Each session, therefore, begins with sharing how the "homework" activity went, and processing (i.e., how they felt about it), generalization (i.e., what they learned from it), and application (i.e., how they might alter strategies or plan additional changes) flow naturally through facilitated discussion. Each session ends with an outcome, which serves as an occupational intervention for the family to try out during the following week. In other words, the "activity" that was described in Chapter 1 as Step 2, actually occurs before each session begins.

Example of a Family Group Protocol

Session 1: Inclusion

The initial session serves as an evaluation of the entire family system in regards to the occupations of Grandma. What are the ways that Grandma is included or excluded from participation in family life? What are the barriers to inclusion from various members of the group? What are Grandma's feelings about inclusion or exclusion? Which member of the family best represents Grandma's wishes and preferences if she cannot voice them herself? Using the client-centered approach, the family collaborates with the occupational therapist to identify some specific occupations that address the need to belong. The group chooses an experimental activity for the following week and discusses ways the family members might enable Grandma's participation through occupations. For example, Grandma might help prepare a Sunday family dinner by using routines with which she is already familiar, such as setting the table or peeling apples for pie.

Session 2: Enabling Control

After reporting on the experimental activity and problem solving as needed, this session focuses on additional areas in which assistance is needed to enable autonomy in daily care. What occupations

can Grandma continue to perform on her own with some assistance from family members? Using specific activities selected by the client and family, therapist expertise may be shared with the family regarding what is possible for Grandma to do for herself safely and ways that caregivers could facilitate Grandma's continued independence in self-care or contribute to performance of instrumental activities of daily living. The session might include watching Grandma perform one task while the occupational therapist models the use of appropriate cues to enable autonomy and choice over activity involvement. The group will problem solve around what assistance is needed and which family member will provide it. The outcome of this session may be a schedule of supervision or assistance involving different family members.

Session 3: Balancing Control and Safety

In the case of dementia, safety concerns may arise regarding which occupations Grandma wants to do versus what she is able to do safely. Here again, therapist expertise may be shared regarding the effects of moderate stage dementia. She might use an Allen's Cognitive Levels Screen to evaluate Grandma's cognitive level and use this theory to predict potential safety issues. For example, if Grandma wants to cook, she needs to be able to understand the consequences of unsafe use of a stove and remember to take safety precautions. Family members may report problems like letting things burn or forgetting to use a potholder. Problem solving might include home adaptations to address specific safety issues involving Grandma. In recommending changes made to the environment, the occupational therapist considers the needs of the entire family. For example, disconnecting the stove will probably not be an option, since the rest of the family uses the same stove for cooking. Restricting access to the kitchen during periods when Grandma is unsupervised might be more workable. A house tour and a list of possible adaptations for safety and to maximize Grandma's opportunities for choice may be an outcome of this session.

Session 4: Control, Resolving Conflicts

Review the past week in which family members have rearranged environments and made home modifications as discussed during the previous week. What tasks can family members help Grandma do, and which are still causing problems? Some areas to explore are the following:

- Who provides care and when?
- What self-care routines can Grandma learn to do independently?
- What are some attitudes toward giving/receiving assistance?
- What expectations have been met/not met?
- How is care being received? Are caregivers feeling appreciated?
- What might be some financial issues regarding paid caregiving or supervision?
- What barriers to inclusion in family life still exist?
- Any other problem areas client and family members bring to the table.

Family members need to discuss strategies for resolving the most important conflicts as a family group. Collaborative decision making can be facilitated by the occupational therapist around the activities that are posing problems for family members. Some of the following strategies may be suggested:

- Deferring to Grandma when the risk is low
- Giving Grandma a realistic role to play in family activities
- Using environmental adaptation to manage risk
- Giving choices and/or making compromises
- Allowing Grandma to express self/emotions in nonverbal and verbal ways
- Getting Grandma her own pet
- Finding ways to communicate with Grandma during times she is left alone
- Allowing noninvolvement of members or relief of overburdened members

An outcome might be each member thinking of one way to show respect and affection for Grandma or to modify nonproductive responses while engaging in occupations with Grandma during the upcoming week.

Session 5: Expressing Affection Through Occupations

Problem solving issues of control paves the way for the family to resolve conflicts that interfere with the expression of affection between Grandma and members of her family. This session centers on occupations that help family members learn from Grandma. Family members can learn from Grandma, drawing on her life skills and accom-

plishments to raise the status and respect she enjoyed before the cognitive decline. Some examples might be writing down family recipes, retrieving photographs of ancestors and writing or tape recording stories about them, reframing old photos, or making scrapbooks. Recalling family history through reminiscence serves several purposes. It reaffirms Grandma's ties with family members, giving her a unique role as family historian, while providing a context of positive interactions with children and grandchildren. Whatever Grandma's special experiences and interests were, these can be shared through storytelling and sharing expertise (worker roles, living in another country, living in a specific period in history, doing needlework, cooking, gardening, or singing). In later stage dementia, family photographs can be labeled in clear letters to remind Grandma of each person's name, relationship, and approximated date. This is especially helpful for persons with large families and assists nonfamily caregivers in understanding the older client's stories or clearing up confusion about when in her life history different events occurred. An outcome of this session might be a schedule when each interested family member might share a chosen reminiscence activity with Grandma during the following week.

Session 6: Measuring Outcomes

This session will review all of the previous sessions. What were the desired outcomes with regard to inclusion, control, and affection? What has changed since the first session? What problems remain? A review of self-care routines and participation in family activities may be complied. A tour of the house to observe environmental adaptations might be useful in confirming what was changed and its effect on Grandma's occupational performance and avoidance of problems. The occupational therapist might share expertise about the progression of dementia, its current severity, and what the subsequent stages are likely to entail. Possible preventive strategies may be discussed, such as Grandma wearing a "safe return" bracelet with her name, address, and telephone number engraved on it if she becomes prone to wander. Possible supports in the community might be identified, both social activities for Grandma and respite for caregivers. Finally, a plan for follow-up or a way to identify need for future intervention can be discussed.

Mosey's Group Interaction Skills: A Measure of Social Participation

Mosey (1986) addressed group behaviors through her recapitulation of ontogenesis theory, which outlined five subskills of group interaction skill. Group interaction involves the ability to be a productive member of a variety of primary groups, including taking appropriate group membership roles, engaging in decision making, communicating effectively, recognizing and behaving according to group norms, contributing to goal attainment, assisting in resolving conflicts, and working toward group cohesiveness (Mosey, 1986, p. 435). The five subskills are organized into a sequence of developmental groups, which are described more fully in Chapter 5 (also see Appendix B and C). They are:

1. Parallel groups (18 months to 2 years)
2. Project groups (2 to 4 years)
3. Egocentric cooperative groups (5 to 7 years)
4. Cooperative groups (9 to 12 years)
5. Mature groups (15 to 18 years)

Donohue (1999) has reviewed and analyzed the theoretical foundations of Mosey's concepts of these five levels of group interaction skill and adds the following new assumptions:

1) most people function at two or more levels of developmental group interaction, 2) there is a relationship between the nature of the activity and the level of function, and 3) adults function at lower developmental levels of group interaction if the activity requires it. (p. 35)

Donohue also suggests extending the age range of the mature group to end in adulthood.

The Group Profile

The Group Profile (Donohue, 2003) is an assessment tool designed for evaluation of levels of activity group participation. Based on Parten's (1932) and Mosey's (1968) descriptions of levels of group interaction, the Profile incorporates five levels of group function among group members around the task involvement (Donohue, 1999). The Profile's five levels of group performance measure the five levels of group participation mentioned above.

Examples of activities associated with group interaction levels of behavior are given in Table 4-2.

Rating the Group Profile

The items of the Group Profile measure three categories of group participation:

1. Group membership
2. Group interaction
3. Group activity behavior

Items are ranked in a five-point Likert scale (never to almost always). The Group Profile typically measures group participation across one, two, or three levels of group function within a single session or across multiple activity sessions.

For example, a group of 10-year-olds playing an after school pickup game of baseball on their own, who once in a while express emotions about the rules could be described as at a Level 2-Sometimes, and at Level 3-Frequently and a Level 4-Rarely. The Profile gives an overview of their behaviors during a session or across multiple sessions. In another example, an independent activities of daily living group, psychiatric patients discuss budgeting for the month and expressing distress over their limited disability funding, might be rated at Level 3-Most of the Time and at Level 4-Sometimes to indicate a range of their behaviors.

Therapists using the Group Profile rate the behavior of members by placing check marks and comments on a grid form while observing a group session. The frequency of behaviors related to the three areas of member role, interaction, and activity are then rated using the five-point scale. A training worksheet defining each level is provided in the instruction manual.

Groups usually interact at multiple levels of participation in one session and across sessions, with the exception of a group of 2-year-olds on parallel play. To achieve a Profile measurement of the range of participation, all of the level ratings observed during the group session are mentioned. Various activities can influence the level or type of group participation, despite the group's highest potential or developmental level. A mature group may choose to perform exercises in a parallel mode while participating in an aerobics class. Groups can choose to interact at a range of levels of participation suitable for a given activity, depending on the goal. A developmentally mature group may watch a movie video together, express feelings or opinions about the video, and share a bowl of popcorn, thereby demonstrating behaviors of Levels 1, 2, and 4 during the viewing. Since the activity selected affects the members' group role and interactive behaviors, the group activity's potential for stimu-

Table 4-2	Donohue's Group Profile (2003): Examples of Activities and Behaviors

Group Profile Levels	*Examples of Activities and Behaviors*
1. Parallel Level Group	3 year olds playing separately next to each other in a sandbox Adults standing in rows next to each other doing movement to music in a movement group
2. Project/Associative Level Group	4 year olds playing telephone for 2 minutes 5 year olds building blocks together to make a fort—5-minute interaction Adults engaged in a "Pass the Ball" game identifying names of members—15-minute interactive exercise
3. Egocentric Cooperative Level Group	7 year olds role playing in costumes with mutually designed guidelines for role interaction Adults in an activities of daily living group washing, cutting, mixing, serving, and eating fruit in a salad
4. Cooperative Level Group	16 year olds discussing feelings about musical lyrics while making decorations for a parade float Seniors discussing feelings about peers' illnesses, memories of the past, and process of dying
5. Mature Level Group	20-year-old college students take turns coaching each other in a computer science course 40-year-old parents of children with learning disabilities coach each other on methods of intervention for their children in a parents' support group

lating behaviors at each of the five levels is also rated. Currently, the Group Profile is pending publication (Mary Donohue, PhD, OTR, August 2003, personal communication).

The Group Profile provides one of the first occupational therapy-based measures of social participation in groups. Students have used the Profile with fieldwork I sites, family groups, self-help groups, and community groups to evaluate multiple factors that are observed simultaneously: activity, interaction, and leadership. This assessment tool has the potential to provide the basis for linking the interaction and process skills of individual clients with the naturally occurring groups available to such clients in their communities.

Teams and Teamwork

Occupational therapists often work as members of interdisciplinary teams. From a medical perspective, the purpose of the team approach is to discuss client problems from several perspectives and to coordinate a treatment plan. Latella (2002) defines a team as "two or more people working together toward the achievement of specific goals" (p. 96). Latella applies Holpp's (1999) organization of teams, according five "Ps" to describe a health care team:

1. Purpose
2. Place
3. Power
4. Plan
5. People

The team's purpose is its vision of what is to be achieved, which usually reflects an organization's mission statement. In the case of health care teams, the vision is holistic, high quality assessments and interventions for clients. Place refers to the relationship of the team to the entire organizational structure. A health care team is one part of the structure of a hospital or home care agency, for example. Power refers to leadership style and degree of shared leadership among members. In a medical model, health care teams are usually led by a physician, psychiatrist, or medical director, with input from members structured around each case/client. Plan refers to the structure of the team and how members work together.

According to Latella, three approaches are used by health care teams:

1. Multidisciplinary
2. Interdisciplinary
3. Transdisciplinary

In the multidisciplinary approach, members of various disciplines work together but maintain separate and distinctive roles. Collaboration and coordination are not typically a part of this approach. An interdisciplinary approach allows more flexibility in member collaboration and shared assessments, reports, goals, and intervention plans. The transdisciplinary approach involves all team members "blurring" roles by crossing boundaries predetermined by their disciplines. This model maximizes the effectiveness of each member, and leadership rotates according to client needs and priorities (Latella, 2002, p. 97). People are the members of the team. Typical health care teams average five members and may include doctors, nurses, social workers, speech therapists, physical therapists, and occupational therapists. Team membership may be stable within an organization or may shift according to needs, goals, or other criteria. Occupational therapists can combine this model with their knowledge of group dynamics to better understand the interactions of teams in their own practice.

From a business perspective, Luthans (1995) offers a somewhat different view of teams as "highly cohesive groups that... given positive leadership, will have the highest possible productivity" (p. 251). According to this author, teams differ from traditional work groups in several ways. Work groups have a strong leader who delegates the work to members and holds each individual accountable for what he or she produces. Meetings of work groups are marked by efficiency, low cohe-

siveness, and a focus on overall organizational goals. In contrast, teams use shared leadership and work together to produce collective outcomes. Team meetings are highly interactive, use group problem solving, and are mutually accountable for decisions and outcomes. Good teamwork depends upon maintaining group cohesiveness, honest feedback, and open communication within all levels of management. Teams work best when self-managed (no appointed supervisor in charge) and given responsibility for the real work of the organization.

Many parallels may be drawn between this view of teams in business and groups in occupational therapy. Both rely on skilled and well-trained leaders who value and enable the unique contributions of each member. While goals may vary, the process of facilitating sessions or meetings includes similar principles. The group interacts openly to deal with the issues of the day, each member shares his or her perspective or expertise, problems are defined and clarified, and the group reflects upon possible solutions or outcomes.

Teams exist in many workplace, educational, and community settings. Gersick (2003) points out that most "organizations use teams to put novel combinations of people to work on novel problems and use committees to deal with especially critical decisions; indeed, organizations largely consist of permanent and temporary groups" (p. 59). Clients may have difficulties related to team membership. Deficits in communication and interaction skills, as well as poor self, social, or cultural awareness, may interfere with successful occupational performance related to team roles. Participation in occupational therapy groups may be structured so as to prepare clients to become better team members in whatever life contexts they choose.

Summary

The purpose of this chapter is to broaden the student's perspective on the kinds of groups that might now be included in occupational therapy's domain of concern. Groups form an integral part of our clients' participation in daily life. This chapter reviews both occupational therapy approaches to working with groups from the perspective of the Occupational Therapy Practice Framework, and theoretical perspectives regarding some of the naturally occurring groups in which our clients participate, including family groups, community organizations, and work teams. It is hoped that when students become entry-level graduates, they will help to define and expand some of the new roles suggested in this chapter for occupational therapists dealing with groups in community settings.

Bibliography

American Occupational Therapy Association. (2002). Occupational therapy practice framework: Domain and process. *American Journal of Occupational Therapy, 56*, 609-629.

Benne, K., & Sheats, P. (1978). Functional roles of group members. In L. Bradford (Ed.), *Group development* (2nd ed.). La Jolla, CA: University Associates.

Bruce, M. A., & Borg, B. (1991). *The group system: The therapeutic activity group in occupational therapy.* Thorofare, NJ: SLACK Incorporated.

Christiansen, C., & Baum, C. (1997). *Enabling function and well-being* (2nd ed.). Thorofare, NJ: SLACK Incorporated.

Donohue, M. (1999). Theoretical bases of Mosey's group interaction skills. *Occupational Therapy International, 6*(1), 35-51.

Donohue, M. (2003). Group Profile: Studies with children: Validity measures and item analysis. *Occupational Therapy in Mental Health, 19*, 1-23.

Donohue, M., & Greer, E. (2004). Designing group activities to meet individual and group needs. In J. Hinojosa & M. L. Blount (Eds.), *The texture of life: Purposeful activities in occupational therapy.* Bethesda, MD: American Occupational Therapy Association.

Gersick, C. (2003). Time and transition in work teams. In R. Hirokawa, R. Cathcart, L. Samovar, & L. Henman. (Eds.), *Small group communication: Theory and practice.* Los Angeles: Roxbury Publishing Co.

Holpp, L. (1999). *Managing teams.* New York: McGraw Hill Co., Inc.

Kielhofner, G. (2002). *The model of human occupation* (2nd ed.). Baltimore, MD: Williams & Wilkins.

Latella, D. (2002). Teams and teamwork. In K. Sladyk (Ed.), *The successful occupational therapy fieldwork student* (pp. 95-101) Thorofare, NJ: SLACK Incorporated.

Law, M., Cooper, B., Strong, S., Stewart, D., Rigby, P., & Letts, L. (1997). Theoretical contexts for the practice of occupational therapy. In C. Christiansen & C. Baum (Eds.), *Enabling function and well-being* (2nd ed., pp. 73-102). Thorofare, NJ: SLACK Incorporated.

Luthans, F. (1995). *Organizational behavior* (7th ed.). New York: McGraw Hill, Inc.

Mattingly, C., & Fleming, M. (1994). *Clinical reasoning: Forms of inquiry in a therapeutic practice.* Philadelphia: Davis.

McColl, M. (1997). Social support and occupational therapy. In C. Christiansen & C. Baum (Eds.), *Enabling function and well-being* (2nd ed., pp. 411-425). Thorofare, NJ: SLACK Incorporated.

Mead, G. (1934). *Mind, self, and society.* Chicago: University of Chicago Press.

Mosey, A. C. (1968). Recapitulation of ontogenesis: A theory for practice of occupational therapy. *American Journal of Occupational Therapy, 22*, 426-433.

Mosey, A. C. (1970). *Three frames of reference for mental health.* Thorofare, NJ: SLACK Incorporated.

Mosey, A. (1986). *Psychosocial components of occupational therapy.* New York: Raven Press.

Parten, M. B. (1932). Social participation among preschool children. *Journal of Abnormal and Social Psychology, 27*, 243-269.

Schaber, P. (2002). FIRO model: A framework for family-centered care. *Physical & Occupational Therapy in Geriatrics, 20*(4), 1-18.

Schutz, W. (1958). The interpersonal underworld. *Harvard Business Review, 36*(4), 123-135.

Spencer, J. (1998). Evaluation of performance contexts. In E. Crepeau, E. Cohn, & B. Boyt Schell (Eds.), *Willard & Spackman's occupational therapy* (pp. 427-448). Philadelphia: Lippincott, Williams & Wilkins.

Sullivan, H. S. (1953). *Conceptions of modern psychiatry.* New York: W.W. Norton.

Townsend, E., & Landry, J. (2005). Interventions in social context: Enabling participation. In C. H. Christiansen, C. M. Baum, and J. Bass-Haugen (Eds.), *Occupational therapy: Performance, participation, and well-being.* Thorofare, NJ: SLACK Incorporated.

U.S. Dept. of Health & Human Services. (2000/2001). Healthy people 2010. Retrieved November 3, 2003 from http://www.healthypeople.gov/Document/ table of contents.html

World Health Organization. (2001). *The international classification of functioning, disability, and health.* Geneva: Author.

Yalom, I. (1995). *The theory and practice of group psychotherapy* (4th ed.). New York: Basic Books.

Section Two

Group Guidelines From Six Frames of Reference

Introduction

Once the basics of group dynamics and client-centered practice have been mastered, the therapist can modify Cole's seven steps to fit different clinical situations. The *Occupational Therapy Practice Framework* suggests that the occupational therapist select "theories and frames of reference" to guide clinical reasoning during both evaluation and intervention planning (American Occupational Therapy Association [AOTA], 2002, pp. 616-617). Thus, when planning groups for the purpose of evaluation or intervention within selected occupational domains, the occupational therapist must apply the theory or frame of reference that best fits the needs of a group of clients. This section reviews six frames of reference that best guide our thinking about group approaches and illustrates how each might adapt the group structure using Cole's seven steps.

Frame of Reference vs. Model

Multiple levels of theory exist in the occupational therapy literature. In 1997, Christiansen and Baum wrote that "there is little agreement among writers about how to describe organized knowledge in the field... the terms theory, model, frame of reference, and paradigm have been variously used to describe subsets of the profession's knowledge" (p.41). In 2004, this trend continues as Blount, Blount, and Hinojosa suggest that our understanding of theoretical issues in occupational therapy depends upon "who is doing the defining" (p. 36). Reed and Sanderson (1999) use the term *models* to describe a link or bridge between theory and practice. Models are devices for explaining what we observe, and these authors define two types: conceptual models and practice models.

Conceptual models explain "why the profession works as it does" (Reed & Sanderson, p. 201). Some have called these grand theories, overarching theories, umbrella theories, or occupational performance models (Baum & Christiansen, 2005). Some examples are Ecology of Human Performance (Dunn, McClain, Brown, & Youngstrom, 2003), Occupational Adaptation (Schultz & Schkade, 2003), the Person-Environment-Occupation Model (Stewart et al., 2003), and the Person-Environment-Occupation-Performance Model (Baum & Christiansen, 2005). These models tend to be generic, explaining how the concepts of person, environment, and occupation interrelate as a system. Generic models, according to Reed and Sanderson (1999), do not provide much direction for actual practice. Therefore, I have not reviewed these "overarching" occupational performance models, but have included only one, the Model of Human Occupation (Kielhofner, 2002).

Practice models, according to Reed and Sanderson (1999), "are used to explain how the ideas of the theoretical model can be implemented into a plan of action to provide services to clients" (p. 201). Mosey (1981) preferred the term *frame of reference* to describe this concept, which may be defined as "a set of compatible concepts from theory which together guide the therapist toward a specific focus, view of function and dysfunction, explanation for how change occurs, and strategies for evaluation and intervention." Mosey writes that "many authors...recognize that no theory can be directly applied. A theory must first be transformed through a linking structure into usable information" (Mosey, 1989, p. 195). Mosey suggests that our research should focus on the development, refinement, and evaluation of the effectiveness of frames of reference. Occupational therapy uses a method called "extrapolation" (Mosey, 1989, p. 197) to make theory usable, involving several steps as follows:

- Identification of appropriate theories
- Selection of useful concepts from theory
- Combining concepts and postulates from various compatible theories
- Reformulating of the selected concepts and postulates to provide guidelines for treatment (intervention)

In addressing the problem of planning and leading occupational therapy groups, I have used a similar technique in applying theory.

Identification of Appropriate Theories

First, I have identified six appropriate practice theories (frames of reference):
1. Psychodynamic
2. Behavioral cognitive
3. Cognitive disabilities
4. Developmental
5. Sensorimotor
6. Model of Human Occupation

These are not the only theories that could potentially be used. The psychodynamic and developmental chapters draw widely upon psychological theory. The behavioral cognitive and sensorimotor chapters draw mainly from the fields of neurology (including dynamical systems and motor learning theories), anatomy, and physiology (and related medical fields). The Model of Human Occupation, while identified by its authors as original to occupational therapy, draws upon systems theory which is used widely in business and was originally derived from physics. Most of the theoretical concepts that make up occupational therapy frames of reference have also been researched and applied in other disciplines. What makes these frames of reference different from similar theories in psychology, basic science, and medicine is that the

concepts were reorganized in a way that can guide us in planning and leading occupational therapy groups.

Selecting and Combining Useful Concepts

In describing each frame of reference, compatible concepts that are applicable to occupational therapy group intervention are selected from various theories. First, each concept or basic assumption is described according to the source or author where it originated. Then the relationship of the concepts to occupational therapy groups is facilitated through examples and learning exercises.

Combining Compatible Concepts

Compatible concepts are combined from various theories to formulate a point of view on function, dysfunction, change, and motivation. A frame of reference should guide our understanding of illness and disability in our clients. Before jumping into group intervention, occupational therapists should have some understanding of the state of health of the group members, and this understanding is different in each frame of reference. The definition of dysfunction can range from neurological malfunctioning in the sensorimotor frame of reference, to the presence of unconscious conflicts in the psychodynamic frame, to the lack of adaptive skill development in the developmental frame. Principles or postulates regarding change (Mosey, 1981) are the assumptions derived from theory that help us formulate how intervention will work. These are the "principles by which prevention of dysfunction occurs, function is maintained, interfering behavior is managed, and an individual is assisted in moving from a state of dysfunction to a state of function" (Mosey, 1981, p. 141). The *Occupational Therapy Practice Framework* might call this "enabling occupation" for "participation" in life (AOTA, 2002).

Mosey (1981) further suggests that principles of intervention begin with the function to be developed (e.g., trunk balance, self-esteem) and end with the nature of the external environment that is likely to enact this therapeutic change. In other words, these principles help us predict how change will occur and guide our designing of occupational therapy activities that will facilitate the development of function or occupational performance. For example, in using a developmental frame of reference for a group of older adults with Parkinson's disease, the postulate regarding intervention may be as follows: "A sense of integrity and acceptance of one's life and death may be facilitated by participation in group activities where past accomplishments are the focus." In a behavioral cognitive frame of reference for the same clients, "Socially acceptable eating habits may be learned through the use of weighted utensils combined with peer examples." Each of these frames of reference suggests a different definition of function and dysfunction, different goals to be addressed, and a different kind of activity. Thus, the important parts of occupational therapy group evaluation or intervention are addressed in the different frames. Within each chapter on frame of reference, concepts are applied to group structure, limitations, role of the leader, appropriate goals, and suggested activities as examples.

To provide the student with a concrete idea of how groups should be run in each of the frames of reference, the seven-step format for group leadership described in Chapter 1 is modified for each frame of reference covered. Suggested modifications to the introduction, use of activity, sharing, generalizing, application, and summary are described at the end of each chapter in this section. A chart reflecting differences in the structure of groups based on these six frames of reference may be found in Appendix E. It is hoped that with this breakdown, the application of theory will be, at least partly, demystified.

Bibliography

American Occupational Therapy Association. (2002). Occupational therapy practice framework: Domain and process. *American Journal of Occupational Therapy, 56,* 609-639.

Baum, C., & Christiansen, C. (2005). Person-environment occupational performance: An occupation-based framework for practice. In C. Christiansen C. Baum, & J. Bass-Haugen (Eds.), *Occupational therapy: Performance, participation, and well-being* (3rd ed.). Thorofare, NJ: SLACK Incorporated.

Blount, M. L., Blount, W., & Hinojosa, J. (2004). Perspectives. In J. Hinojosa & M. L. Blount (Eds.), *The texture of life: Purposeful activities in occupational therapy.* Bethesda, MD: American Occupational Therapy Association.

Christiansen, C., & Baum, C. (1997). The occupational therapy context: Philosophy, principles, practice. In C. Christiansen & C. Baum (Eds.), *Occupational therapy: Enabling function and well-being* (2nd ed.). Thorofare, NJ: SLACK Incorporated.

Dunn, W., McClain, L., Brown, C., & Youngstrom, M. (2003). The ecology of human performance. In E. Crepeau, E. Cohn, & B. Boyt Schell (Eds.), *Willard & Spackman's occupational therapy* (10th ed.). Philadelphia: Lippincott, Williams & Wilkins.

Hinojosa, J., & Blount, M. (Eds.). (2004). *The texture of life: Purposeful activities in occupational therapy* (2nd ed.). Bethesda, MD: American Occupational Therapy Association.

Kielhofner, G. (2002). *A model of human occupation: Theory and application* (3rd ed.). Baltimore: Williams & Wilkins.

Mosey, A. (1981). *Occupational therapy: Configuration of a profession.* New York: Raven.

Mosey, A. (1989). The proper focus of scientific inquiry in occupational therapy: Frames of reference. *Occupational Therapy Journal of Research, 9,* 195-201.

Reed, K., & Sanderson, S. (1999). *Concepts of occupational therapy* (4th ed.). Philadelphia: Lippincott, Williams & Wilkins.

Schultz, S., & Schkade, J. (2003). Occupational adaptation. In E. Crepeau, E. Cohn, & B. Boyt Schell (Eds.), *Willard & Spackman's occupational therapy* (10th ed.). Philadelphia: Lippincott, Williams & Wilkins.

Stewart, D., Letts, L., Law, M., Cooper, B., Strong, S., & Rigby, P. (2003). The person-environment-occupation model. In E. Crepeau, E. Cohn, & B. Boyt Schell (Eds.), *Willard & Spackman's occupational therapy* (10th ed.). Philadelphia: Lippincott, Williams & Wilkins.

Yalom, I. (1995). *The theory and practice of group psychotherapy.* New York: Basic Books.

Chapter 5

Psychodynamic Approaches

In previous editions, this frame of reference has been called psychoanalytic. The term *psychodynamic* expands the conceptual base of this as an occupational therapy frame of reference to encompass concepts from ego psychology, humanism, and human spirituality (Bruce & Borg, 2002). Historically, occupational therapy theorists have been acknowledging the usefulness of various forms of psychoanalytic theory in guiding our interventions with clients with mental illness. Diasio (1968) explores the psychoanalytic view of motivation and the environment. The Fidlers (1963) point out the importance of the unconscious and view activities as part of a communication process with human and nonhuman objects to effectively gratify instinctual needs. Mosey (1986), in considering analytical frames of reference, emphasizes the "structure for linking psychoanalytic theories, the symbolic potential and reality aspects of activities, and the process of altering intrapsychic content in the direction of providing a more adaptive basis for interaction with the environment." Llorens & Johnson (1966) refer to "socially acceptable, ego-adaptive functioning" in describing the effects of client involvement in activity groups, thus focusing on occupational therapy techniques that help develop and strengthen the functions of the ego. Fidler and Velde (1999) refer to the "dynamic of congruence, or match, of an activity with the nature and characteristics of the person" (p. xi). In recent years, both Fidler and Velde (1999) and Hasselkus (2002) have looked beyond the "purposeful" nature of activities and focused on their symbolic and metaphorical meaning in the dimension of spirituality.

Framework Focus

Psychodynamic theory addresses a person's ability to love and to work. It includes both self-identity and interpersonal relationships, which impact all the performance in areas of occupation in the *Occupational Therapy Practice Framework* (American Occupational Therapy Association [AOTA], 2002). The context areas have a special importance as these environmental factors continue to shape the "self." It would be a mistake to limit the use of this approach to treating those with primarily mental illness. Psychodynamic approaches are especially useful in dealing with human emotions and motivational issues for all clients, as well as exploring the symbolic meaning of occupations. Groups that use creativity as a projection of the self to promote self-awareness and insight are best understood from a psychodynamic perspective.

Why Study Psychoanalytic Theory?

Psychoanalytic theory has been out of favor, even in the field of mental health from which it originated. This fact is generally attributed to the lack of efficacy research and the slowness and abstractness of the therapeutic process itself. As an occupational therapy approach, it is probably due for a comeback, perhaps in a redefined form. One sign of this comeback is the emergence of spirituality as a concern in occupational therapy. This spirituality is not defined as religion, but as belief in the human spirit. The spirit, or essence, or soul of the person, is really not so different from the "ego" or conscious self discussed in psychoanalytic theory. Furthermore, the complexity of the psychoanalytic theory provides an explanation for many of the irrational, even bizarre behaviors we observe in persons with a variety of illnesses (e.g., suicide attempts, risk-taking behaviors, paranoia, self-starvation, or obsessive compulsive behaviors) that are otherwise unexplainable.

Following the early theorists, two general goals of occupational therapy groups will be considered: alteration of personality and development of ego skills. This chapter will first review the basic assumptions of psychoanalytic theory, which are useful in planning occupational therapy groups. Ego functions and their relevance to occupational therapy will then be reviewed. Finally, contributions from the occupational therapy literature will be summarized, and group leadership guidelines will be derived from these psychodynamic theoretical concepts.

Psychoanalytic theory, based on the work of Sigmund Freud in the late 19th and early 20th centuries, has had a profound influence on all theories of group intervention. Corey (1991) describes Freud as an "intellectual giant" whose work represents "the most comprehensive theory of personality and psychotherapy ever developed." In the 1990s, there was a tendency to underestimate the influence of psychoanalytic theory because many subsequent theorists have either developed it further or reacted against it. The current emphasis on brain biochemistry as a determinant of human behavior has overshadowed the importance of personality dynamics in our understanding of mental illness. New technology has enabled researchers to observe the physiological and biochemical functioning of the brain in ways never before possible, and thus new genetic links have been discovered.

However, for occupational therapists, these new scientific discoveries do not alter the fact that there are many mental illnesses currently being diagnosed for which psychoanalytic theory offers the only plausible explanation. For example, there is a growing interest in borderline personality disorder, which is thought to originate from a failure to separate from parents and achieve an autonomous sense of self at around age 2. If the parent does not allow the child to explore his or her environment and do activities of his or her own choosing in a safe environment, then as an adult, he or she is unable to derive any satisfaction from activities. Knowing this, the occupational therapist can offer clients with borderline personality disorder an opportunity to explore activities according to their own interest. Recent research shows that for some borderline clients, it is possible to strengthen autonomous functioning through participation in task-oriented occupational therapy groups (Greene & Cole, 1991).

For occupational therapists, psychoanalytic theory is also useful in the physical disability areas of practice. The concept of self-worth and the many defenses of the ego can help us understand why some of our clients use denial of their illness or resist our suggestions for intervention. It is important for occupational therapists to determine the symbolic meaning of illness or trauma in the structure of personality and how symptoms are incorporated into the client's perception of him- or herself. For example, Julia, an 83-year-old woman with osteoporosis and chronic arthritis, was in and out of doctors' offices all her life, with many failed attempts to increase her independent functioning in occupational therapy. Only at age 79, after her husband died, did she learn to perform self-care independently. In her earlier years, Julia's many illnesses symbolized her helplessness. Her dependency on her husband for personal self-care fulfilled her need for attention and love. The client's sense of self is vital to her acceptance or rejection of occupational therapy intervention, whether the illness is mental or physical.

The original form of psychoanalytic theory, sometimes called "id psychology" (Fine, 1979, p. 319), has been widely criticized by psychologists, social scientists, and occupational therapists during the past 20 years for its vagueness and its unsuitability for research. The link with psychoanalysis and its questionable appropriateness for treating many types of mental illness has added fuel to the fires of discontent. Psychoanalysis is a therapeutic approach developed by Freud in which individual clients are assisted in uncovering their unconscious conflicts by conversing with a therapist, a process that could take many years. Critics feel that one cannot research the unconscious, since it is not observable or measurable. A more current emphasis on ego psychology focuses on the conscious rather than the unconscious aspects of the personality and is therefore, by definition, more observable and measurable. The ego is best understood as the "self." A client's sense of self, his or her self-concept, can determine his or her degree of involvement in occupational therapy intervention. If a client sees him- or herself as a capable and worthwhile individual, he or she will be motivated to overcome disability. If Dean defines himself as an accountant, he will make the effort to overcome his depression to return to that occupation. In this frame of reference, the ego is seen as a powerful motivating force that can either resist or facilitate therapeutic change.

Bellak, Huruich, and Gediman (1973) operationalized the functions of the ego, making them more amenable for research purposes. They define 12 ego functions:

1. Reality testing
2. Judgment
3. Sense of self and the world
4. Control of drive, affect, and impulse
5. Object relationships
6. Thought processes
7. Adaptive regression in service of the ego
8. Defensive functioning
9. Stimulus barrier
10. Autonomous functioning
11. Synthetic integrative functions
12. Mastery/competence

These functions most applicable to occupational therapy will be further defined later in this chapter.

Basic Assumptions

The following is intended as a brief review of the original concepts of Freudian psychoanalytic theory. A more thorough understanding may be obtained by referring to other basic psychology texts. Psychoanalytic theory is exceedingly complex, and there are many variations currently in use. It must be remembered that Freud's theory provides an intellectual understanding of the personality and its development. The parts described as id, ego, and superego do not parallel structures or functions of the brain, nor do they represent distinct developmental stages. The purpose for which psychoanalytic theory will be used in this text is to define those concepts that help us understand the dynamics of illness, both mental and physical, and to develop intervention techniques to address these dynamics. Because of the focus on group intervention, many important aspects of Freudian theory will be left out.

Personality Structure

Freud organized personality into three parts: the id, the ego, and the superego. This structure is still accepted by many psychotherapists regardless of their discipline or theoretical preferences. While a balance of these components is considered ideal, the functions of the ego in this text will be empha-

sized because of their direct relevance to occupational therapy groups.

The Id

The id is seen as largely unconscious. It is the part of the personality that houses primitive drives and instincts, needs, and conflicts that the ego is unable to integrate. The id is the biological component of the personality and is thought to operate through primary process thinking. Primary process thinking is the earliest to develop in the infant. It is illogical and undisciplined and operates on the pleasure principle, demanding immediate gratification of needs and drives.

The Ego

The ego is the psychological component and has contact with the external world. It functions logically and works to achieve a balance between internal drives and external expectations. The ego operates through a secondary process, one that is learned through experience in reaching compromises and applying logic and discipline in an attempt to adapt to the environment.

The Superego

The superego is the social component of the personality that serves as an individual's moral code, his or her sense of good and bad, right and wrong. The superego is often illogical and unrealistic in its quest for idealism and perfection. The superego is the last part to appear in the developmental process, and its beliefs are learned from parents and from society.

Psychosexual Stages

Freud believed that personality is largely determined by one's early childhood experiences. Psychosexual stages of development, spanning a range of 18 years from birth to maturity, are differentiated by changes in the objects that potentially provide need satisfaction. An object is someone or something that gratifies or frustrates a need; objects can be human or nonhuman. The classic example of an object in the oral stage is mother's breast. A nonhuman substitute for mother's breast is the bottle. When a child's needs are gratified, he or she thrives and is able to develop and move on to the next stage. However, when the child's needs are continually frustrated, he or she develops a fixation that can remain in the unconscious and cause many of the problems in adulthood that we know as symptoms of illness. Freud's

Table 5-1	Freud's Psychosexual Stages	
Age (years)	*Stage (source of gratification)*	*Fixation Characteristics (potential problem areas)*
Birth to 1 year	Oral stage early: sucking late: biting	Theme: trust, dependency Regression: psychosis
1 to 3 years	Anal stage early: excreting late: retaining	Theme: control, autonomy Regression: neurosis, character disorders
3 to 5 years	Phallic stage genital interest penis envy	Theme: Oedipal/Electra complex
5 to 12 years	Latency stage sublimation of sexual drive superego develops	Theme: skill development social role development emergence of guilt
12 to adulthood	Genital stage puberty capacity for intimacy	Theme: sexual identity adult responsibility for love and work

psychosexual stages of development are outlined in Table 5-1.

The psychosexual stages are critical to our understanding of mental illness. In spite of current discoveries of the genetic and biochemical origins of some illnesses, most psychopathology is still explained in terms of Freud's levels of personality organization. In general, the earlier the conflict occurs, the more severe the illness. While there are not rigid parallels between the stages and the development of certain illnesses, fixations in the early stages are likely to result in faulty or incomplete development in later ones. For example, failure to develop self-control in the anal stage may result in the overdevelopment or misuse of defense mechanisms as the ego's attempt to compensate for lack of self-control in later stages.

When we, as occupational therapists, observe clients in our therapeutic groups who are unable to work together and get along with one another, a knowledge of how the clients have progressed through the psychosexual stages may help us understand the reasons why. In addition, the stages may offer guidelines as to what type of therapeutic intervention is needed. For example, trust is an issue dealt with in the oral stage. Groups in which members seem to lack a basic trust of one another might benefit from activities that assist clients in feeling more comfortable with self-disclosure. This self-disclosure can form the basis of establishing trusting relationships with the therapist and with one another.

Psychic Energy, Libido, Aggression, and Anxiety

In Freud's view, the amount of psychic energy is limited and must be shared by all three parts of the personality. This explains why people cease to function when too much energy is being used up in trying to deal with unresolved conflicts from the past. A healthy individual is able to resolve conflicts as they arise and therefore keep psychic energy available for the ego to grow and develop and interact effectively with the environment. In mental illness, psychic energy may be trapped in the id and may produce nonadaptive behaviors, which we call symptoms.

Two specific forms of psychic energy are described by Freud: the libidinal and the aggressive drives. Libido is the sexual energy that represents the urge to perpetuate life, to be intimate, to love, and to reproduce. This is also called the life-force and is demonstrated by a person's tendency to form relationships with other people. The aggressive drive is equated with the death-force and is associated with hostility, hatred, and the urge to destroy. It is expressed in the tendency to be self-sufficient and to keep others at a distance. Both the libidinal and the aggressive drives are part of the id, and both seek expression through objects. It is a function of the ego to control these drives and to allow their expression in ways that are socially acceptable. It is a function of the super-ego to guide an individual's libidinal and aggressive drives toward constructive and morally acceptable expression.

Anxiety, in Freud's view, is defined in relation to both drives and the ego's control function. Anxiety is an alerting response that lets us know that something is wrong and needs to be changed and that some action needs to be taken to get us out of danger. However, unlike the existentialists who view anxiety as a normal condition of life, Freud views anxiety as pathological. Freudian anxiety develops out of the conflicts over control of the available psychic energy within the personality itself. This anxiety goes beyond fear of realistic danger from the external world. It is the fear that the id may take over, forcing the individual to act irrationally or in ways that are morally wrong, or that the superego may take over, causing a pervasive sense of guilt and self-punishment. As long as the ego maintains control, anxiety can be safely held in check and dealt with realistically. High levels of neurotic anxiety, however, may necessitate the unconscious use of ego defense mechanisms to help reduce the tension and protect the survival of the ego. These mechanisms will be reviewed later in this chapter.

Occupational therapists may facilitate the expression of psychic energy through activities. This helps the client in a variety of ways. Through activities, the aggressive drive can be directed toward productive work, constructive homemaking, or toward competition in sports. The libidinal drive can energize the client to the development of social skills, nurturing skills, and cooperation with others. Various ego functions might be encouraged in occupational therapy groups, such as appropriate expression of feelings, both loving and aggressive, or the sharing of perceptions to help members develop a realistic sense of self.

Symbols, Projections, and Communication With the Unconscious

Rarely, except in episodes of psychosis, does the content of the unconscious become known. Psychoanalytic therapy's main thrust is to help an individual become aware of his or her unconscious conflicts and fixations, so that the mature ego can deal with them effectively and resolve them. However, the nature of primary process makes awareness of unconscious material very complex. Primary process is not organized or logical and is not remembered in words or complete thoughts. Highly emotional material may take the form of symbols that represent experiences that originally produced them. For example, a child who experienced the violent death of a parent in an automobile accident may have repressed the original memory. If, as an adult, he or she draws a car as part of an occupational therapy activity, he or she may suddenly re-experience an overwhelming feeling of grief and loss without knowing why. It is the therapist's role to help the adult client to interpret the meaning of the symbols he or she produces, and with the help of a psychiatrist, remember and work through the original traumatic experience.

Object Relationships

Object relationships were previously mentioned as the organizing principles of the psychosexual stages. Freud viewed object relations as the foundation of an individual's capacity to love and to work. The Fidlers (1963) define occupational therapy in terms of the development of relationships with human (therapist) and nonhuman (environment) objects. In human relationships, the client develops the ability to satisfy some of his or her basic needs, such as recognition, self-esteem, and belonging, through a therapeutic relationship with the occupational therapist. In the safety of a therapeutic environment, the client uses realistic feedback from the therapist or other clients to correct his or her unrealistic concepts and expectations of self and others. Nonhuman objects are related to the client's ability to work. The client can learn, in occupational therapy, to use the symbolic as well as actual properties of objects to help satisfy instinctual drives and needs. For example, Bob can satisfy his need to express hostility by flattening a ball of clay or sawing a piece of wood. Mary can express her compulsive needs by maintaining a perfectly clean and organized kitchen. Using this principle, occupational therapy activities can be selected according to the instinctual needs of group members.

Assumptions of Ego Psychology

Alfred Adler is credited with making the first significant break with Freud over the nature and importance of the ego (Fine, 1979). He believed that the ego is responsible for shaping the personality, rather than the person being shaped by biological forces and early childhood experiences. Another theorist who recognized the importance of the ego was Heinz Hartmann. Hartmann (1939) looked at the process of psychoanalysis and suggested that it was not a reconstruction of what once existed buried in the unconscious (the Freudian view). He saw that psychotherapy requires that the mature ego establish correct causal relationships and judgments of the emerging memories. The significance of Hartmann's work is in establishing the autonomy of the ego as separate from the id in psychoanalytic theory. Ego psychology has been developing since 1923 and has had many spokesmen, including Adler, Sullivan, Hartmann, Erikson, Lewin, and Rapaport (Fine, 1979). The common element is an emphasis on the ego. For the sake of brevity, not all the functions of the ego can be reviewed. Those selected for emphasis are:

- Reality testing
- Sense of self
- Thought processes
- Judgment
- Self-control
- Defensive mechanisms
- Competence/mastery

Reality Testing

Reality testing is perhaps the most important function of the ego in therapy. It is the ego's ability to use perception and judgment to differentiate between internal needs and external demands. This process involves the use of interaction with the environment and with others in shaping and reshaping one's views of self and the world. It is precisely this process that is responsible for adaptation to the environment. The ego becomes aware of needs and drives from the id, but delays their gratification until they can be satisfied in ways that are socially acceptable.

Consensual Validation

Reality testing is an integral part of the therapeutic use of groups. As members share their perceptions of themselves and the world with others in the group, they have the advantage of hearing the responses of others. It is through this feedback that group members gather evidence to support their self-other perceptions. When perceptions of others are clearly different from one's own, then one needs to question whether his or her own perceptions are realistic. The process of integrating one's own perceptions, views, or beliefs with those of others is called consensual validation.

For example, Lisa shared with the group a painful experience involving her father's rejection of her. Lisa believed she had to live with this rejection and was powerless to change it. Several other members recounted similar feelings about their own fathers, based on similar experiences. This feedback helped validate Lisa's feelings of rejection; based on clear evidence, she had a right to feel rejected; in her situation, anyone would. However, another member of the group, Roberta, also told Lisa how she had begun speaking to her father after a 7-year period of silence. Roberta was able to significantly improve her father-daughter relationship through some more adult conversations and sharing of feelings. This feedback made Lisa reconsider her position; perhaps she was not as powerless as she believed herself to be. The group helped Lisa to see which parts of her self-perception were real (being rejected) and which were not real (being powerless).

Exploring Outer Reality

Occupational therapy groups involving the use of concrete tasks provide another kind of reality testing, one on a sensory level. Manipulation of objects and materials provides sensory input: taste, touch, smell, vision, hearing, and proprioception (position, pressure, balance, etc.), which can lead on to challenge internal perceptions. Robert felt he had no energy and therefore could not complete a woodworking project. When the group members persuaded him to try it, however, the sensory stimulation provided by sawing and hammering the wood (proprioceptive and auditory) helped release the needed energy. Robert learned through experience that by engaging in appropriate motor activities, he was able to direct his energy to produce a positive effect on the environment (a completed project). If the group then also provides positive feedback on his wood project, Robert is further inclined to change his view of himself from ineffectual, "I can't," to effective, "I can!" It is important here for the occupational therapist to be aware of Robert's abilities in choosing a task, ensuring that his experience is likely to be a successful one.

Sense of Self

Many aspects of sense of self appear in the literature, and their meaning can be somewhat confusing. Three discrete aspects will be defined here:

- Self-concept
- Body image
- Self-esteem

Self-Concept

Self-concept or self-identity, is sometimes used interchangeably with the word ego. Developmentally, the idea of self originates when the infant begins to differentiate self from mother and then from the environment in general. Psychotic individuals are understood by ego psychologists to have regressed beyond the point where they are able to differentiate self from others. These psychotic individuals are said to have "poor" or "loose" ego boundaries. This factor makes psychotic clients particularly sensitive to their environment. When someone in the group is angry, for example, it is often the psychotic client who is first to notice it, although he or she may not express his or her awareness realistically or appropriately.

Following Freud's original formulations, the attempt was made to correlate the various clinical entities with the points of fixation in psychosexual development. Primarily, the oral stage is associated with psychosis, the anal stage with neuroses, and the phallic stage with hysteria. Ego psychologists have elaborated and changed this original oversimplified concept of mental illness, but have retained the idea that the ego or self-concept is fundamentally different in these three levels of psychiatric diagnosis. Psychological testing such as word association (Jung, 1910), interpretation of inkblots (Rorschach, 1921), and association with photographs (Murray, 1951) are a few of the earliest attempts to measure ego functions with particular regard to self-concept.

The idea that concept of the self is a common problem area for mentally ill individuals has led occupational therapists to make self-concept and its related ideas—body image, self-esteem, and self-perception—the focus of occupational therapy intervention. Groups using movement, dance, or physical sports and exercise may be helpful to clients in developing a realistic body image. Drawing and word association activities, often taking their cue from the various psychological tests, have been useful in promoting knowledge of the self. Self-esteem is better approached in occupational therapy through successful experiences and feedback from others. Person drawings in particular are a useful therapeutic tool, for both evaluation and intervention in occupational therapy.

Body Image

Body image is the perception of one's physical self that forms the basis of self-awareness. According to theories of child development, the earliest learning involves the association and differentiation of somatosensory sensations. These provide a kind of geographical knowledge of the body and how it works that defines "me." Body sense, according to Allport (1958), allows a child to develop a sense of personhood. It is the sensorimotor exploration of early play that helps the child define the boundaries of his or her body and distinguish "me" from "not me." In adulthood, body sense continues to provide a basic reference point from which environmental interactions take place. The sensory systems, for example, help people know how they feel. Influences from the body guide day-to-day behavior. For example, you may stay home from work because you feel fatigued, or you may go for a walk because you feel restless. The child achieves a sense of control over his or her body by reaching out to the environment to satisfy body needs: a bottle satisfies hunger, a toy satisfies need for pleasure, mother satisfies the need for comfort. As adults, we continue to reach out to the environment and to others based on our perceptions of our bodies and what we need.

Illness tends to produce distortions in body image, and this may be the source of problem behaviors. As occupational therapists, one of our goals is to determine whether our client's body image is realistic. Using activities that encourage clients to become aware of their feelings and sensations can help to correct body image distortions. Movement activities and person drawings are two examples of this.

Self-Esteem

Self-esteem describes the subjective feelings of one's own ability. As with sensorimotor, perceptual, and cognitive processes, feelings are innate and develop as the child matures. However, feelings or affects are intricately tied to objects, and their expression determines how people relate to one another and to their world. The idea that affects our ego states comes from Freud's 1926 work *Inhibitions, Symptoms and Anxiety* (Bellak, Huruich, & Gediman, 1973). Rapaport (1953) attempted to articulate a theory of affect, suggesting that affect originates as psychic energy and is seen as a signal emitted by the ego to indicate an internal feeling state needing to be noticed. Spitz (1959) offered a theory of affect development in the infant as:

- Crying
- Smiling
- Stranger distress or fearfulness

Language development then allows the child to express a multiplicity of feeling states of increasing complexity.

The expression of affect or emotion is an important function of the ego. As suggested by Rapaport, it is one of the ways the ego has to control and direct energy from the id. Acting out has been described earlier as a more primitive, less socialized form of expression of affect through action. Those with special talents are able to express affect through artistic media, such as painting, music, or poetry and drama. While these ways are socially acceptable, the most commonly acceptable way to express affect is by describing it verbally with words.

As occupational therapists, we often observe in our clients (and sometimes in ourselves) a lack of ability to communicate emotions to others. In the ego adaptive frame of reference, a common goal of occupational therapy groups is the appropriate expression of emotions.

Thought Processes

Thought processes are the cognitive functions of the ego having to do with:

- Attention
- Memory
- Learning and logical thought
- Compromise
- Problem solving

Attention

Attention is the ability of the ego to focus on something for a period of time. It requires not only alertness of the mind, but a readiness to take in new information. Information coming in through the sensory systems is screened for relevance, and the brain focuses on aspects of the environment to which a response is appropriate. Sustained atten-

tion, or concentration, is needed for the individual to participate in occupational therapy groups.

Memory

Memory is central to psychoanalytic theory, as seen in Freud's persistent efforts to recapture early childhood events. Rapaport (1942) recognized the relationship between memory and emotional factors. The ego was thought to censor memory in accordance with the intensity of associated emotional factors. In other words, events that were extremely painful are repressed; the ego stores them below the level of consciousness and they cannot be remembered at all. Or, the ego can alter the perception of a traumatic event so that the senses are numbed and the brain will not receive more stimuli than it can handle. In this case, the memory of the event would be inaccurate or unrealistic. The current metaphor most closely associated with memory is that of the computer, with information storage and retrieval as the primary activities. It is believed that one's memory process reflects individual styles of secondary process functioning. In other words, what someone remembers is dependent upon how he or she perceives and understands an event in the first place.

When an occupational therapist hears a client report a remembered event in a group, it becomes the task of the therapist to listen not only for the facts, but also for the emotional bias the client expresses. This is particularly important if the client's emotional response is problematic. For example, Shelley reported at the beginning of the group that something about the last group had been bothering her all week. Last week, during a serious discussion among several group members, Shelley had gotten up from her chair and stepped into the center of the group to kill a spider that was crawling on the floor. She felt "terrible" that her action would be viewed as a violation or mocking of the members whose discussion she had disrupted. The group's response to this confession was surprising. Two or three members remembered the incident in passing, but said it was "no big deal." The three members who were involved in the discussion had no recall of the event at all. The facts of the spider killing event were the same for everyone, but Shelley remembered them in the context of a strong emotional bias that put herself in a negative light. It was only with the feedback of the other group members that she was able to shed the bias and put the event in a more realistic perspective.

With most significant events in our lives, we do not have the advantage of the feedback of the others to help us correct our emotional bias. Hence, when past events not witnessed by the group are reported to the group, it is difficult for members or the therapist to separate the facts from the emotions involved. It is only in the context of "here and now" events that groups can be helpful in this way. This is one reason that it is suggested that our occupational therapy groups have a "here and now" focus.

Learning and Logical Thought

Learning is a skill of the ego that has been given little attention by followers of psychoanalysis, yet it is central to the notion of making therapeutic change. It has been noted by ego psychologists that intellectual development (learning) occurs most favorably in a warm, secure environment. This observation is helpful to occupational therapy so we can recognize the importance of creating and maintaining this kind of safe environment in our groups. Physical safety should be a given; this means that the OT removes any dangerous objects or factors from the environment (e.g., sharp objects, loose wires, wet or slippery floors). Psychological safety is provided when the occupational therapist maintains control through the establishment of group norms, such as mutual respect and prevention of verbal attacks on one another.

Problem Solving

The kind of thinking attributed to the ego is secondary process thinking. This is also called reasoning or logical thought. It is the ability of the ego to consider facts in the light of reality and put them to use in guiding behavior. Problem solving is a cognitive skill that requires the use of logical thought. In fact, all of the functions of the ego contribute to problem solving: accurate perception and reality testing, memory, and control of impulses as well as appropriate use of defenses. The process of solving problems is quite complex, but the ability to do so is often a deciding factor in whether our clients are considered to be competent in activities of daily living. Occupational therapists are often asked to evaluate a client's problem-solving ability. Observation of the client in a group activity is one way to determine this skill. For example, Rich, a client in a cooking group, was unfamiliar with the process of peeling and slicing carrots for a salad. However, since he had arrived late, that was the only job available. Rich picked up the knife and proceeded to chop the carrot, leaving the skin on and cutting only part way through with each chop. When another client handed Rich a vegetable peeler, Rich turned on the would-be helper and waved the knife at him in a somewhat threatening way. After a few more attempts to cut the skin off the carrot with the knife, Rich put down the carrot and abandoned the task. After observing Rich's behavior, the occupational therapist discussed the situation with Rich and determined that Rich's ability to solve problems was poor.

How can occupational therapy groups be helpful to Rich in learning to solve problems? Clearly, teaching him to use a vegetable peeler will only help temporarily in the specific situation. In general, Rich's tendency to act alone and reject help are the real issues that need to be dealt with. Group discussion following the cooking task helped Rich to understand what his options were in solving the carrot problem. Asking for help and being able to accept it in a nonthreatening way were agreed upon as goals for Rich in future group tasks.

Judgment

Judgment is another function of the ego that is often the focus in occupational therapy groups. Good judgment requires the following cognitive processes:

- Accurate and realistic perception of the situation
- Identification of intended behaviors and likely consequences
- Prediction of the behaviors' effect on others
- Control of response until options are considered
- An appreciation of what it takes to accomplish something

On a well-known psychological test, the client is asked the question, "What is the thing to do if you find an envelope in the street that is sealed, addressed, and has a new stamp?" The most acceptable answer is "Mail it" (Wechsler, 1981, p. 126). How one arrives at this response requires a complex process of perception, reasoning, and anticipation of consequences. Judgment is a cognitive skill of the highest order, and one of the most difficult to learn or teach.

Self-Control

Control was the earliest of the ego functions to be recognized, when Freud conceptualized the ego's main function to control the instinctual drives from the id. Impulse control may be seen as a derivative of this earlier conceptualization.

In occupational therapy groups, we often encourage impulse control in a number of ways. We expect group members to arrive on time and to remain attentive for the length of the group, usually 50 to 60 minutes. We expect members to consider others in the group, listening to them, waiting their turn to speak, sharing tools and materials, passing the glue or the scissors. In a cooking group, we would ask members not to taste the food with their fingers and to wait to begin eating until the whole group is seated. On a shopping trip, we ask our clients not to taste items in the store, not to buy items impulsively, and to wait to light their cigarette until they have finished shopping. Following social norms and interacting effectively in groups requires good control of impulses.

Defense Mechanisms

Defenses are broadly understood as a way of warding off anxiety and ensuring the safety and preservation of an intact ego. The strengthening of healthy defenses is a common goal in occupational therapy groups. In addition, the concept of defenses helps us as occupational therapists to understand better our clients' responses to activities. Through our recognition of defenses in our clients, we as occupational therapists are better able to plan activities and make therapeutic interventions in our groups to help clients achieve a healthy balance in their lives. Defense mechanisms are an important part of the structure of the ego. Early psychologists focused on this aspect when developing the techniques of psychoanalysis. The goal of psychoanalysis was to break through a person's defenses so as to uncover the memory of critical childhood events.

Kaplan and Sadock (2003, pp. 208-209) have classified defense mechanisms into four categories:

1. Narcissistic defenses: Projection, denial, and distortion

2. Immature defenses: Acting out, blocking, hypochondriasis, introjection, passive-aggressive behavior, regression, schizoid fantasy, and somatization

3. Neurotic defenses: Controlling, displacement, dissociation, externalization, inhibition, intellectualization, isolation, rationalization, reaction formation, repression, and sexualization

4. Mature defenses: Altruism, anticipation, asceticism, humor, sublimation, and suppression

The contemporary ego psychologists view mature defenses as performing a healthy adaptive function, and these will be most relevant to our work in occupational therapy. Those defenses that are dealt with most often in occupational therapy are reviewed here. The reader is referred to Kaplan and Sadock (2003) for a more thorough description of the above defenses.

Sublimination

Sublimation was identified by Anna Freud in 1936 as a healthy and acceptable rechanneling of libidinal and aggressive drives into constructive activity. While sublimation is no longer a focus in psychological literature, the concept remains central to occupational therapy because of its implications regarding activity, creativity, and tasks or work. As occupational therapists using a psychoanalytic frame of reference, we continue to see clear evidence of this rechanneling of energy. The concept allows us to understand why work is such a central part of living, and why the loss of the work role produces both aggressiveness and anxiety and a sharp decline in one's self-worth. Neutralization (Hartmann's updated substitute for sublimation) refers to the de-energizing of the libidinal and aggressive drives. It is the "successful defense" by which the mature ego masters reality.

Projection

Projection is another defense, originating with Freud (1914), that continues to hold value in occupational therapy. The modern day variation was described by Melanie Klein (1948) as projective identification. In this mechanism, parts of the self are split off and projected onto an external object or person. Projection provides the ego with a means of getting rid of bad parts of the self. Sam is angry with his boss, but he believes the anger is bad, so he projects the anger onto his boss. Now Sam can like himself and feel justified in believing his boss is the bad guy who gets angry. Good parts of the self may be projected also, to avoid separation or keep them safe from the bad parts. Projection at higher levels leads to misinterpreting the motives, feelings, attitudes, or intentions of others.

Projection as a concept is used extensively in occupational therapy in the form of projective techniques. Projective techniques are generally creative modalities, such as drawing, sculpture, poetry, creative writing, or drama, that allow/encourage a person to express the hidden parts of the self. A client is said to project parts of him- or herself, particularly affects such as anger or love, in the form of symbols or shapes in art or characters and situations in writing or drama. When done in adulthood, these images or fantasies are then open to interpretation by the mature ego. As therapists, we encourage our clients to apply logic and mature judgment to the products of their projective creations when we ask them to explain them to their fellow group members. One Vietnam veteran participating in an occupational therapy projective arts group was asked to explain his elaborate drawing of the atrocities of war. The guns, the dead body parts, and the destructive remains of buildings symbolized for him the bad parts of himself which he found so hard to accept.

Regression

Regression was also an emphasis of Freud's early work as it helped to explain "fixations" as a cause of mental illness. Regression is going backward from a later to an earlier stage of development. In 1964, Arlow and Brenner defined regression as "the re-emergence of modes of mental functioning characteristic of earlier phases of psychic development." They further state that regressions are usually transient and reversible.

Pathology is not determined by the depth of the regression (oral, anal, etc.) but by its irreversible nature, by the conflicts that it engenders, and by its interference with the process of adaptation. The importance of regression has recently been enhanced by its relation to borderline and psychotic conditions. Psychotic individuals are said to be regressed to the oral stage (birth to 1 year), the earliest stage in Freud's psychosexual stages of development. Borderline (character disorder) individuals are thought to be regressed to the anal stage (1 to 3 years) and fixated there. This view of regression may help to explain the behavior of our clients with these diagnoses in terms of the functioning of the ego. To do so, however, would require a thorough understanding of Freud's psychosexual stages of development.

Regression has another implication that is important for the occupational therapist in planning intervention. This is the concept of "regression in the service of the ego." Ernst Kris (1936) first used this term to imply a purposeful regression to earlier modes of functioning without the loss of overriding ego control. The artist who smears paint on a canvas to express extreme affect but retains the control to return to the normal world (while the psychotic client cannot) is a good example. The technique of "free association" or the uncensored, often illogical associations of words and images has been cited as another example.

The therapeutic usefulness of regression to the ego lies in its contribution to a clearer self-understanding. When we ask our clients to wedge clay or use finger paints, these processes reflect the typical (sometimes forbidden) fascination of the anal stage (smearing feces). Our therapeutic purpose for doing this is not to encourage regression, but to free the individual to express affect in an uninhibited way, with the hope of recapturing the innate urge toward mastery that may be trapped there. The client, after engaging in such a creative process, returns to a more mature level of functioning, but he or she retains an awareness of the affect discovered during the regression. This affect is essential if the client is to change the way he or she understands and uses activity as a part of his or her return to healthy functioning.

Acting Out

Acting out can best be defined as an action, usually repetitive and compulsive in nature, and often self-destructive, that serves the unconscious purpose of resolving a repressed internal conflict by external means. This is a popular way to explain self-destructive behavior in analytical terms. It reflects a primitive lack of control over actions that are typical of the infant and regressively present in psychosis and character disorder.

In groups, we often see emotions being "acted out" instead of talked about. For example, anger at someone in the group is expressed by walking out of the room and slamming the door. An action is substituted for a mature verbal description of a feeling state. Occupational therapist group leaders should discourage acting out responses. These are inappropriate and unproductive for both the client and other group members. The more mature ego skill of verbal expression of affect should be encouraged.

Identification

Identification, as a defense described by Freud, was meant quite literally as the taking onto one's self the characteristics of another. The concept originated as a logical outcome of the Oedipal conflict, in which sexual desire for the opposite sex parent is replaced by identification with the parent of like sex. Anna Freud (1936) described this phenomenon as "identification with the aggressor." The child's identification with the feared "aggressor" is used, in part, to explain the repetition of behavior patterns in families. Child abuse is an example when the abused child grows up to abuse his own children. Erikson (1950) contributed greatly to the popularity of this concept in his extensive discussion of the identity crisis occurring in late adolescence.

Competence/Mastery

Bellak et al. (1973) defines this function of the ego as adaptive performance in work and relationships and the subjective feelings of competence. R. H. White defines competence as "an organism's capacity to interact effectively with its environment..." (Bellak et al., 1973, p. 260). "Fitness to interact with the environment" in White's view, includes language and motor skills, cognition, and higher thought processes. The affect or feeling of efficacy is what White called "effectance motivation" (Bellak et al., 1973, p. 260), referring to the individual's tendency to put more effort and energy into producing responses that will have a desirable effect on the environment. The feelings of competence are the result of a well-developed ego and include a history of successful experiences in coping with the environment.

The ego's ability to cope is what rescues a person in times of illness or crisis. In an emotional crisis, many of the ego defenses described earlier may be viewed as coping mechanisms, protecting the ego from destruction by diverting psychic energy. In the case of physical trauma, the ego uses body sense and reality testing to determine what functions of the body remain intact. The ego's sense of self will often provide the motivation to find ways to compensate for lost functions. For example, a client with right-sided hemiplegia will learn to write with his or her left hand. Compensation is a coping strategy.

Another example of a coping strategy is energy conservation. When physical and mental deterioration occur, energy for use in everyday activities is severely limited. Careful planning before embarking on a task can prevent the client from wasting energy in needless movements. For example, after I had an operation, I was only able to stand up or walk for 15 minutes before stopping to take a rest. When preparing a meal, I had to learn to use the 15 minutes to gather absolutely everything I needed to make meatballs, then assemble them while sitting at the kitchen table. The cooking had to be done in an electric frying pan on the table, rather than at the stove. I had to learn to be satisfied with accumulating a mess around me, rather than cleaning as I went along, and to use a wet sponge to wipe my hands, rather than washing at the sink every few minutes. For clients with chronic disability, conserving energy is a coping skill that is absolutely essential for continued functioning at a level that is consistent with the client's self-identity.

Function and Dysfunction

A functioning adult is free of conflicts and fixations and is able to satisfy his or her needs and direct his or her drives in ways that fit in with the social environment and culture. A balance exists in the functioning individual that allows the psychic energy to flow freely between the id, ego, and superego. The ego is in control and defense mechanisms are not exaggerated, so that the individual with a healthy ego can use most of his or her energy to grow and develop and interact effectively with others. In Fidler's model, the healthy person is able to work productively with others to accomplish a task. As an adult, he or she has acquired all six of Mosey's adaptive skills (Mosey, 1981; see Appendix A). The defenses the individual uses are mature ones, like sublimation of aggression in work, identification with idealized others, and the suppression of immediate gratification. A healthy ego is synonymous with a strong sense of self; body image, self-identity, and self-esteem are realistic and can serve as the basis of adaptive function.

Dysfunction in the psychoanalytic frame of reference is defined in terms of inadequate psychosexual development, the presence of conflicts and fixations, and the imbalance of psychic energy among the three parts of the personality. These abnormal states can produce symptoms of neurosis, psychosis, or character disorder, which imply a disturbance in the ability to carry out activities of daily living.

Dysfunction can be seen as a lack of ego skills. This can take the form of poor reality testing, poor or unrealistic body image, poor self-identity, poor self-esteem, impulsiveness or passivity, unbalanced use of defenses, and an inability to cope. Assessment of the ego functions will guide our setting of goals in occupational therapy. Clients with similar goals may be treated together in groups.

Change and Motivation

Change occurs through the learning and performance of adequate ego adaptive skills. These skills can be learned within the social context of therapeutic groups, where the consequences of problem behaviors can be readily seen and discussed. Foundation skills can be worked on through simple, well-structured, reality-oriented tasks that focus on the development to sensorimotor, perceptual, and cognitive skills. Motivation can be enhanced through success experiences in occupational therapy.

Motivation comes from the directing of psychic energy toward the mastery of ego skills. When energy is bound up in dealing with conflict, persons may not be motivated to develop ego skills. As the ego is available to help reduce tensions and to satisfy needs through mature relationships and meaningful work activities, persons will be motivated to increase ego skill development. The occupational therapist can set up therapeutic groups that allow clients to practice adequate ego skills and experience successful and satisfying consequences for clients. A strong self-concept and high self-esteem are also motivating; these foster a sense of control and lead people to direct their energy toward even greater skill development.

Review of the Occupational Therapy Perspective

The next portion of this chapter will review three authors from occupational therapy whose work has reflected the principles of the psychoanalytic frame of reference: Gail Fidler, Lela Llorens, and Anne Mosey. Occupational therapy groups using this frame of reference became popular during the 1960s and 1970s, and consequently many of the published works of these authors began about then.

An important influence in occupational therapy at the time of the early writings of Fidler, Llorens, and Mosey was an intervention approach begun in England by Maxwell Jones (1953) known as the therapeutic community. The therapeutic community represented in the 1960s and 1970s a fundamental change in approach to interventions with mental illness. Both psychodynamic theories of personality and theories of sociology contributed to this unique approach, which called for the client role to change from a "sick role" to that of a responsible community member. Hospitals and institutions all over Europe and America began therapeutic communities on their psychiatric units, and occupational therapists were an integral part of this new approach.

Prior to the 1960s, occupational therapy, although administered in groups, had a task skill focus with an emphasis on the use of crafts and productive work skills. The rise of therapeutic communities called for occupational therapists to incorporate milieu principles into their intervention approach. Examples of these principles are:

- Those most affected by a decision should be involved in making it (Jones, 1953).
- "In the context of responsibility for self and others, clients will alter their self-perception from that of subordinate to that of peer group member" (Fairweather, 1964).
- Clients learn best when they are allowed to experience the consequences of their own actions.

Fidler's The Task-Oriented Group

In keeping with the times, Gail Fidler published her classic article "The Task-Oriented Group as a Context for Treatment" in 1969 (see Appendix A). She mentions several spokesmen for ego psychology in her rationale, such as Sullivan and Lewin, and points to the "emerging focus on ego functions and adaptive skills" (Fidler, 1969, p. 43). Fidler also alludes to a focus on the use of groups in therapy as "a dynamic force in facilitating learning and behavior change" (Lewin, 1945).

Fidler, in incorporating occupational therapy principles with those of the therapeutic milieu, pointed out the value of observing clients doing tasks. She noted that "as clients engaged in activities or created objects, they expressed characterological difficulties, and that attention to these problems as they emerged and were operant in the here and now, seemed to be of benefit to the client" (Fidler, 1969, p. 45). There appeared to her to be a relationship between problems encountered by a client in his or her activity experiences and those difficulties he or she encountered in the outside world. The assumption here is not unlike one made by the ego psychologists. If the client's difficulties either interpersonally or in task performance are made conscious, whether by experience itself, group feedback, or feedback from the therapist, the client can utilize ego skills to cope with the difficulties. The strengthening of ego skills, then, becomes the goal of the task-oriented group.

Although the task is defined as either an end-product or a service that is done by the group as a whole, Fidler points out that task accomplishment is not really the purpose. Rather, the task is intended to "provide a shared working experience wherein the relationship between feeling, thinking and behavior, their impact on others and on task accomplishment and productivity can be viewed and explored" (Fidler, 1969, p. 45). Through the task group experience, ego skills and deficits can be observed in the client. Clients demonstrate, in the process of participating in the group, their problems in interaction and in doing, and these problems can then be the focus of group problem solving. Through both therapist and group feedback, "alternate patterns of functioning can be considered and tested within the context of the here and now, to the end that such learning may induce ego growth and improve function" (Fidler, 1969, p. 45).

In other words, clients are expected to reflect on their behavior in the group and to come to some understanding of its consequence on other members and on task accomplishment. Behavior that is disturbing to others or counterproductive is identified as such, and presumably more adaptive modes of behavior are suggested and tried. The occupational therapist facilitates this process during the group; he or she intervenes as problems arise, points them out to the group, and helps the group problem solve. (See Appendix A for Fidler's article.)

Llorens' Occupational Therapy in an Ego Adaptive Milieu

Lela Llorens also wrote about occupational therapy programming using the psychoanalytic frame of reference. Her article *Occupational Therapy in an Ego-Oriented Milieu* with Johnson (1966) and her book *Developing Ego Functions in Disturbed Children* with Rubin (1967) present useful occupational therapy assessment and intervention ideas using this practice model. Llorens writes that "a program of occupational therapy designed to enhance and support adaptive functioning must provide for the development of ego skills, opportunities for practice, and support for mastery" (1966, p. 179). She describes occupational therapy groups in three phases of treatment:

1. Evaluation
2. Convalescence
3. Rehabilitation

In the evaluation phase, observation is emphasized. The group meets 3 consecutive days for 1 hour each day, and activities include orientation to occupational therapy, written completion of a background information sheet, and completion of a small mosaic tile tray. This small sample of behavior allows the occupational therapist to observe the client's mood, relationships, motivation, performance, and skills. Results of the evaluation show how well the client's ego is functioning in helping him or her adapt to the environment. Those whose egos are functioning less than normal are assigned to the convalescent phase of treatment.

The goals of the convalescent phase are to promote increased feelings of adequacy and to encourage independence in functioning. Modalities suggested to achieve these goals are sewing, needlework, art, leather work, metal work, and woodwork. Convalescent groups consist of five to 15 clients with two therapists. Some ego skills worked on in this phase are:

- Expression or sublimation of needs in an acceptable manner
- Attention span and work tolerance
- Reality testing and orientation
- Verbal and nonverbal communication of feelings

The therapist takes responsibility for planning in these groups according to the client's ability.

Clients whose egos are more highly functional are placed in the rehabilitation phase of occupational therapy treatment. Modalities for groups in this phase include more interaction: male and female interest groups, activities of daily living discussion group, graceful living, typing, and cooking. A less authoritative leadership style is used in these groups. Mastery is both the motivation and the goal.

Mosey's Adaptive Skills and Developmental Groups

Anne Cronin Mosey's concept of adaptive skills is also useful in the psychoanalytic frame of reference. While she frames the adaptive skills in a developmental context (recapitulation of ontogenesis), the skills themselves closely resemble many of the functions of the ego described earlier. According to Mosey (1970b):

...the term adaptive is used to indicate that these skills are acquired and utilized by the individual so that he may satisfy his inherent needs and the needs of others, interact with the environment in order to attain personal goals, and knowledgeably select those environmental demands he wishes to meet. (p. 134)

Mosey acknowledges the influence of psychoanalytic theory on the adaptive skills by accepting the concepts of conscious, preconscious, unconscious, complex formation, and regression, but adds the need for mastery as an important component. She proposes that fixation may be the result of deficient adaptive skill learning. She identifies six adaptive skills, which are learned in sequence, with some overlap and interdependence as the child matures:

1. Perceptual-motor skill
2. Cognitive skill
3. Dyadic interaction skill
4. Group interaction skill
5. Self-identity skill
6. Sexual identity skill

The idea that group interaction skill precedes and therefore needs to be mastered before self-identity or gender identity are possible is significant. For an elaboration on these, the reader is referred to Mosey's *Psychosocial Components of Occupational Therapy* (1986). (See Appendix C for a complete list of Mosey's adaptive skills and subskills.)

Summary of Mosey's Developmental Groups

Of particular interest to occupational therapists working with groups are the components of group interaction skill described by Mosey. She suggests five types of nonfamilial groups that simulate those which may be encountered in normal development. The intention of these groups is to provide opportunities to develop group interaction skills in the correct developmental sequence. Group interaction skill is "the ability to participate in a variety of groups in a manner that is satisfying for oneself and for one's fellow group members" (Mosey, 1970b, p. 273). The five types of groups are:

1. Parallel
2. Project
3. Egocentric-cooperative
4. Cooperative
5. Mature (Mosey, 1986)

(See Appendix B for Mosey's article describing these groups.)

Parallel Groups

Parallel groups are the lowest level, made up of clients doing individual tasks side by side. Preschool children may be observed in a similar process on a playground, one swinging, another climbing, another digging in the sandbox. Little interaction is required, and the therapist defines the task and provides clients with the necessary assistance and emotional support.

Project Groups

Project groups emphasize task accomplishment. Some interaction may be built in, such as shared materials and tools and sharing the work. Social interaction outside of the task is not expected. The therapist structures the group with tasks that require interaction of two or more persons to complete.

Egocentric-Cooperative Groups

Egocentric-cooperative groups require the members to select and implement the task. Tasks are longer term and social interaction is expected. Although the task serves to organize this group, members are expected to respond to one another's social and emotional needs. The therapist facilitates this process.

Cooperative Groups

Cooperative groups require the therapist only as an advisor. Members are "encouraged to identify and gratify each other's social and emotional needs in conjunction with task accomplishment" (Mosey, 1970b, p. 273). The task in the cooperative group may be secondary to social aspects.

Mature Groups

In mature groups, the therapist is a coequal member. The group members take on all the necessary leadership roles in order to balance task accomplishment with need satisfaction of the members.

Group Interventions

Occupational therapy writers have implied that ego functions can be both evaluated and developed (learned) in the context of task-focused groups. The task, in groups using a psychoanalytic frame, takes on greater importance than in humanistic groups. Even when the task is not the focus, it is the context in which discussion, problem solving, and therapeutic change take place. Therefore, the structure of the occupational therapy group in this frame is fundamentally different.

Structure and Limitations

After the introduction, the task predominates the group session, providing both the structure and the time frame for the group. Tasks can last for part of one session or go on for several sessions. A task might take 3 hours at one time. Discussion depends on problems that arise and how the therapist chooses to intervene. Evaluative discussion is left for the last 15 minutes of each session, with a longer evaluation reserved following the end of the task. This alternative structure is primarily based on Fidler's task-oriented group but has been expanded and further defined. Mosey's concept of developmental groups is reflected in the changing role of the leader. The leader gives more help and structure to groups that are less capable and less help to groups that have a higher level of ego functioning. The task group is not limited to high functioning clients. It can be adapted to fairly low levels of group interaction skill, with some changes in structure and the amount of help given by the leader.

Role of the Leader

Fidler defines the role of the occupational therapist as one of a facilitator. The leader's major goal is to make learning possible, and not to take over the group. Facilitation, then, requires that the therapist maintain and communicate a basic belief in the group's capacity to be "constructively self-determining" (Fidler, 1969, p. 46). This means he or she does not make decisions for the group or rescue the group from its difficulties. Rather, he or she intervenes in the group's process in ways that encourage the group to make its own decisions and solve its own problems. The therapist decides how much freedom he or she will allow the group to be self-determining, based on his or her assessment of the level of ego functioning of group members. There is a delicate balance between success and failure, and he or she should not permit the group to become immobilized with frustration when it is truly incapable of doing a task or solving a problem without his or her help. This kind of leadership requires a thorough understanding of group dynamics.

Goals

The goals of groups in the psychoanalytic frame are for clients to develop and practice ego skills. These skills, reviewed from the beginning of the chapter, are reality testing, body image, self-identity, self-esteem, sense of control, and the use of healthy defenses and coping strategies. Providing the foundation for these skills are cognitive, perceptual, and sensorimotor skills. Clients can be encouraged to develop and practice these skills within the group context through the shared working experience of tasks.

Examples of Activities

The group itself should decide on the task, using the resources of its members. Some of the successful task groups are reviewed here. Most tasks offer many opportunities to develop and reinforce ego skills. A few of these are highlighted for each group, but it is likely that many others are also possible.

A Group Newspaper

The group consisted of six Vietnam veterans who exhibited symptoms of substance abuse and post-traumatic stress syndrome. This was significant in their choice of a task. They decided that what was most meaningful to them was to "tell the world the truth" about Vietnam veterans. The group took a trip to the library, where books and articles on the Vietnam war and on post-traumatic stress syndrome were read and notes taken. From the notes, articles were written. Group members added their own stories, poems, and drawings, as well as old newspaper articles they had saved. The result was a 20-page booklet that was typed, copied, collated, and widely distributed to VA Hospital clients and staff by the group members.

In this group, members' common self-identity as "the unsung heroes" was reinforced. The task facilitated a sense of control by giving members a vehicle for expression of feelings and opinions that was acceptable in the social environment. Self-esteem was increased by the recognition of their work by others.

Easter Chocolates

The chocolates were really a combination of a product and service project. The group knew of a local residential school for handicapped children and wanted to do something for them. Since Easter was the next holiday, they decided to give them Easter candy. But they were on a limited budget, so they came up with the idea of making candy instead of buying it. Candy molds, baker's chocolate, sugar, and tin foil were the only purchases. Members were able to collect enough old Easter baskets to hold the wrapped candy. The candy was made in the shapes of eggs, chicks, and small bunnies. Members wrapped each piece in foil and placed them in the baskets. Two of the group members delivered the baskets to the staff of the residential school the week before Easter. A week later they were very proud to receive a big thank you letter from the children.

Self-identity and esteem were reinforced in this group through doing for others. Members learned that they were capable of producing a product that brought pleasure to others and were recognized for their altruism. Identification as a healthy defense was encouraged through nurturing the children (by giving candy) as perhaps they might have wished to be nurtured themselves.

A Walk to the Pet Store

The most important factor to this group was to get away from the hospital. They were psychiatric clients and not even allowed to walk around the grounds unescorted. In the task group, walking to the pet store gave them a way to go out as a group during scheduled group time, escorted by the occupational therapy staff. They decided on the destination because it was only a 15-minute walk, it was always interesting to see, and it would not cost any money. This task group gave them the opportunity to plan something together to meet their needs, restoring in them some sense of control. The sensory stimulation of walking and being in the outdoor environment also increased sensorimotor skills.

Cooking a Spaghetti Dinner

Almost every group seems to enjoy a cooking task. Its relatively short-term, provides enough work for all the members to participate, and satisfies a basic need for everyone—the need to eat. If possible, the group can do the menu planning and shopping, as well as the actual meal preparation. Since spaghetti and salad can feed the whole group for relatively little money, the group was able to afford soft drinks and dessert as well. This group made brownies from a mix before beginning the main course. Members were divided into salad makers, spaghetti makers, dessert makers, and table setters. The meal was enjoyed by the whole group and everyone was expected to help clean up.

This group requires many adaptive ego functions. Members identify with different roles to work on a realistic goal. They use their skills to cope with their part of the task and receive feedback from others about their performance (reality testing). All of the senses are stimulated through the cooking task, and impulse control is necessary when using the tools and equipment (knives, stove).

Group Car Wash

This task required the cooperation of the hospital or sponsoring institution to provide permission, a space to work, and a source of water. At the VA Hospital, the group took on the responsibility of writing letters to the various hospital administrators asking for permission. The letters were followed up with phone calls from the occupational therapist and other staff. Supplies included buckets, soap, rags, sponges, and a nozzle for the hose, most of which were borrowed from relatives and friends. Members prepared for the car wash 1 week ahead by making signs to post all over the hospital. On the day of the car wash, a few group members, accompanied by staff, went outside to post signs and arrows on the street and in the parking lot directing customers to the car wash location. Clients and staff took shifts of 2 hours each for 6 hours. At $3 a car, the group made almost $200, which they spent on a videotape player so the whole ward could watch movies on weekends.

Patience and perseverance were required in the planning of this extended task. There were many opportunities to reality test, reinforce body image (gross motor actions), self-identity (through working roles), and self-esteem (through the concrete result of their effort).

Group Leadership

In this frame of reference, as suggested earlier, the structure of the group is modified to include most of the discussion areas in the context of the activity or task. The activity, sharing, processing, generalizing, and application are not done as separate phases of the group, but are incorporated into the process of doing the task. Since the goal is to develop ego skills, the leader may stop the group whenever an opportunity for members to learn becomes evident. The evaluation portion should include all of the discussion phases of the group and should end with a summary.

Introduction

This part of the group can dispense with the warm-up and replace it with choosing a task. In beginning a task-oriented group, it is helpful for the leader to set forth some ground rules. Some of these will be specific, such as when and where the group will meet, for how long, and the practical limitations to their choice of task, such as availability of supplies. The leader also needs to set forth the expectation that the group will choose a task that they can all work on together, and that once decided, every member of the group is expected to contribute to task accomplishment. Three phases of a task group are introduced:

1. Planning
2. Doing
3. Evaluating

The time frame may vary according to the task, and a thorough discussion will be delayed until the task itself is finished.

Phase 1—Planning (Step 2: Activity, Part 1)

After a brief introduction by the facilitator, the planning phase begins with brainstorming.

Brainstorming

Brainstorming involves the suggestion of possible tasks for the group by all members. Cooking a meal, planning a group walk, learning to do needlepoint, and making Easter baskets for the pediatrics ward are some examples of group tasks. It is often useful for a member of the group to record the ideas. The therapist should caution the group not to make judgments of the ideas suggested during brainstorming, but just to collect a list of ideas.

Persuasion

The next step in planning is persuasion. Members consider the pros and cons of each suggestion and attempt to persuade the group to do one of them. Here the therapist may need to introduce the idea of meaningfulness. A task that is likely to succeed is one that has meaning for its members. It is very tempting for some groups to plan something easy to accomplish, but often the easy tasks hold little value for the members. This results in member residence in the doing phase. While the therapist should not under any circumstance influence the decision of the group, he or she should perhaps point out that a better decision will be made when the opinions of every member have been voiced and considered.

Interventions of the leader should be carefully thought out so as not to exert more authority than is necessary. Groups with poor ego skills will need more help than those with stronger ego skills. When in doubt, it is best to allow the group to experience the consequences of its actions and then to find something to be learned from whatever happens. Occupational therapists often have difficulty with allowing groups to "fail" or to turn out

badly. In the task-oriented group, however, it is often from the "failures" that clients can learn the most. Successful groups are of benefit in many ways also, but it is often the failures that promote real therapeutic change.

For example, I have sometimes observed in task-oriented groups with members of varied diagnoses, ages, and functioning levels an inability to make a group decision, even after 45 or 50 minutes of group discussion. Nothing is more frustrating to a group than sitting and doing nothing for an hour because nothing was planned. It is a mistake groups usually do not make twice. The planning session following such a group usually turns out to be quite productive.

Decision

After more or less persuasion, the group is expected to reach some kind of decision. Group decisions are made in several ways. Someone in the group can take a vote, with the majority ruling. Perhaps a consensus will be reached on the last suggestion discussed; if no one voices an objection, it may be assumed that everyone agrees. A client leader might emerge in the group whose preference might be deferred to by the other members, or a decision can be made by a process of elimination. However the decision is made, it must be considered at some point during planning to be final. Often the group needs for the decision to be acknowledged and approved by the leader in order to proceed.

Specific Planning and Division of Labor

Once a decision is made, how the task will be accomplished should become the topic of discussion. Questions about what equipment and supplies are needed, how these will be obtained, where the group should be held, and how necessary procedures will be learned are addressed. The facilitator, in this phase, often needs to be a resource to the group, offering his or her knowledge of supply sources, procedures, and space availability. In lower functioning groups, this information should be offered more readily; in higher functioning groups, the therapist may offer information only if asked. The discussion of procedures naturally leads to the division of labor (who will do what). It is best when all the planning and preparation can be done by group members. Often each client is charged with the responsibility of obtaining some item and bringing it to the group. Each member bringing one ingredient for a fruit salad or a pizza is an example of this. In this way, it is easily seen that the success of the group task is dependent on each member of the group remembering and carrying out his or her responsibility.

Phase 2—Doing (Step 2: Activity, Part 2)

It is usually most practical for the doing phase to be done at least a day or two later than the planning. This gives members a chance to prepare adequately. On the day of the activity, gathering and organizing is best left up to group members, although they may need some help. If moving right into activity is something that works for the group, then the leader should allow this. Generally, if careful planning has been done, then not a great deal of time is needed to organize the doing. As members proceed with doing the activity, the facilitator's role may expand to include consulting, advising, and providing information. The leader should be careful to offer these services only when asked or when group disorganization is imminent. It is the role of the facilitator, however, to look for problems and to bring these to the attention of the group along the way. As problems arise, the leader may apprise the group: "Mary seems to be feeling left out" or "Sam seems to be doing all the work." Care should be taken not to suggest solutions until it is evident that the group cannot cope with the problem on its own.

Phase 3—Evaluating (Steps 4 Through 7: Processing, Generalizing, Application, Summary)

Doing is not complete until the task is finished. However, evaluation of the group should be done before the end of every session. Sessions should be sufficiently long to allow for this process to occur. It is usually necessary for the leader to let the group know when it is time to stop doing and start talking. Discussion should focus on the process of the group and the role each member has chosen to play. The discussion phases of processing, generalizing, and application are incorporated into this evaluation phase of task groups.

Reflection of Behavior and Its Consequences

This should be verbalized if members are to learn from their experiences. Why was Mary feeling left out? Did she withdraw because she is shy? Was she seeking attention through nonparticipation? Was she uncertain about how to do her part of the task? Was she threatened by the perceived dominance of another member? How well did the group cope with Mary's problem? How did Mary feel? How did others feel about her? What other choices did the group have regarding Mary? These are the types of issues that should arise in evaluation of the group.

Feelings of Members About the Group

This "processing" aspect is an important part of evaluation. If Sam feels really good about the group, but Mary feels terrible, what are the reasons for this? Could Sam be feeling good because he is doing the whole thing himself and not allowing Mary an opportunity to contribute? How do other members see this? Suppose most of the members are bored with the task? What do they think makes it boring? How are they responsible for the boredom? What can they do about it? A leader should be very reluctant to allow a group to abandon a task part way through. Opportunities to learn should determine what is to be gained or lost from the abandonment. Most of the time the group can learn more from following through on a task, even if to do so is frustrating and problematic. However, if the group is overwhelmed by frustration, the members' anxiety may interfere with their ability to learn. This is another judgment call that may be difficult for the leader to make.

Evaluation of Task Accomplishment

Finally, an overall evaluation of task accomplishment is in order. How does the group feel about the result? How does it compare with what they hoped for/expected? What did each member contribute to its accomplishment? To what extent did planning affect outcome? It is in this phase that the relationship between thinking, feeling, and behavior is most evident, and the therapist should never miss an opportunity to emphasize it. Good planning (thinking) generally produces successful action (behavior) and results in good feelings about one's self and the group. Concurrently, bad planning often produces an unsuccessful outcome and promotes bad feelings about self and the group. Individual examples of this process might also be pointed out. In all cases, learning from mistakes should be emphasized, so that members develop the strength and skill for making things turn out better next time.

Occupational Therapy Group Interventions Using Symbolic and Transitional Objects

Task-oriented groups are an excellent example of occupational therapy intervention using the psychodynamic frame of reference. It is a context in which all of the ego skills discussed can be evaluated and worked on. However, it should be noted that it is not the only approach that works in this frame. Groups that use the symbolic meaning of activities or encourage self-expression through art, poetry, drama, dance/movement, or creative writing are alternative group goals. Occupational therapy groups that encourage exploring the unconscious and uncovering painful or conflictual memories to be resolved remain less popular, but an equally legitimate, application of psychodynamic theory.

Pet Therapy

One up and coming group intervention based on object relations theory is pet therapy. People create relationships with animals in order to satisfy needs, use skills, socially engage, and find meaning in life. Animals provide a means by which individuals can love and be loved unconditionally. The interactive nature of caring for animals is deeply satisfying to many individuals. Pets provide affirmation of the self and an unconditional source of need gratification. Animals can provide a sense of security through their protective nature. Furthermore, service animals have been shown to improve self-esteem, internal locus of control, and psychological well-being in individuals with severe ambulatory diseases (Latella, 2003).

Bibliography

Allport, G. (1958). *Becoming: Basic considerations for a psychology of personality.* New Haven, CT: Yale University Press.

American Occupational Therapy Association. (2002). Occupational therapy practice framework: Domain and process. *American Journal of Occupational Therapy, 56,* 609-629.

Arlow, J., & Brenner, C. (1964). *Psychoanalytic concepts and the structural theory.* New York: International University Press.

Bellak, L., Huruich, M., & Gediman, H. (1973). *Ego functions in schizophrenics, neurotics and normals.* New York: Wiley & Sons.

Bruce, M., & Borg, B. (2002). *Frames of reference in psychosocial occupational therapy* (3rd ed.). Thorofare, NJ: SLACK Incorporated.

Corey, G. (1991). *Theory and practice of counseling and psychotherapy* (4th ed.). Monterey, CA: Brooks/Cole.

Diasio, K. (1968). Psychiatric occupational therapy: Search for a conceptual framework in light of psychoanalytic ego psychology and learning theory. *American Journal of Occupational Therapy, XXII*(5), 50-57.

Erikson, E. (1950). *Childhood and society.* New York: Norton.

Fairweather, G. W. (1964) *Social psychology in treating mental illness.* New York: Wiley & Sons.

Fidler, G. (1969). The task-oriented group as a context for treatment. *American Journal of Occupational Therapy, XXIII*(1), 43-48.

Fidler, G. (1984). *Design of rehabilitation services in psychiatric hospital settings.* Laurel, MD: Ramsco.

Fidler, G., & Fidler, J. (1963). *Occupational therapy: A communication process in psychiatry.* New York: Macmillan Co.

Fidler, G., & Velde, B. (1999). *Activities: Reality and symbol.* Thorofare, NJ: SLACK Incorporated.

Fine, R. (1979). *A history of psychoanalysis.* New York: Columbia University Press.

Freud, A. (1936). *The ego and the mechanisms of defense.* New York: International University Press.

Freud, S. (1914). History of the psychoanalytic movement. In J. Strachey (Ed.), *The standard edition of the complete psychological works of Sigmund Freud.* London: Hogarth.

Greene, L., & Cole, M. (1991). Level and form of psychopathology and the structure of group therapy. *International Journal of Group Psychotherapy, 41*(4), 499-521.

Hartmann, H. (1939). *Ego psychology and the problem of adaptation.* New York: International University Press.

Hasselkus, B. (2002). *The meaning of everyday occupation.* Thorofare, NJ: SLACK Incorporated.

Jones, M. (1953). *The therapeutic community: A new treatment method in psychiatry.* New York: Basic Books.

Jung, C. (1910). The association method. *American Journal of Psychology, 21,* 216-269.

Kaplan, H., & Sadock, B. (2003). *Synopsis of psychiatry* (9th ed.). Baltimore: Williams & Wilkins.

Kernberg, O. (1983). Psychoanalytic studies of group processes: Theory and applications. In L. Grinspoon (Ed.), *Psychiatry update* (Vol. II, pp. 21-35). Washington, DC: American Psychiatric Press.

Klein, M. (1948). *Contributions to psychoanalysis 1921-1945.* London: Hogarth Press.

Kris, E. (1936). The psychology of characterature. *IJP, 17,* 285-303.

Latella, D. (2003). *Animals as a therapeutic modality: A curriculum model for occupational therapy.* Bridgeport, CT: University of Bridgeport Press.

Lewin, K. (1945). *Dynamic theory of personality.* New York: McGraw Hill.

Llorens, L., & Johnson, P. (1966). Occupational therapy in an ego-oriented milieu. *American Journal of Occupational Therapy, XX*(4), 178-181.

Llorens, L. (1976). *Application of a developmental theory for health and rehabilitation.* Rockville, MD: American Occupational Therapy Association.

Llorens, L., & Rubin, E. (1967). *Developing ego functions in disturbed children.* Detroit: Wayne State University Press.

Mosey, A. (1970a). *Three frames of reference for mental health.* Thorofare, NJ: SLACK Incorporated.

Mosey, A. (1970b). The concept and use of developmental groups. *American Journal of Occupational Therapy, XXIV*(4), 272-275.

Mosey, A. (1981). *Occupational therapy: Configuration of a profession.* New York: Raven Press.

Mosey, A. (1986). *Psychosocial components of occupational therapy.* New York: Raven Press.

Murray, H. A. (1951). Uses of the thematic apperception test. *American Journal of Psychiatry, 107*, 577-581.

Rapaport, D. (1942). *Emotions and memory.* New York: Harper.

Rapaport, D. (1953). On the psychoanalytic theory of affects. *IJP, 34*, 177-198.

Rorschach, H. (1921). *Psychodiagnostics: A diagnostic rest based on perception.* New York: Grune & Stratton.

Spitz, R. (1959). *A genetic field theory ego formation: Its implications for pathology.* New York: International University Press.

Wechsler, D. (1981). *Wechsler Adult Intelligence Scale* (Rev. ed.). New York: The Psychological Corporation.

White, R. (1967). Competence and the growth of personality. In *Science and psychoanalysis: Vol. XI: The ego.* New York: Grune & Stratton.

Psychodynamic

Activity Example 5-1

Out on the Town

Materials: Colored crayons or pastels and 9- x 12-inch white drawing paper for each member.

Directions: Imagine that it is Saturday night and you have big plans. Choose anyone you like to be your companion--a significant other, a relative, a friend, even someone you have not yet met. Write the name of this person at the top of the paper.

Next think about where you would like to be going—a romantic dinner, a concert, a play or movie, a sports event, a social event—really anything you can imagine.

Now draw yourself, as you imagine, ready to go out for the evening. Pay attention to how you would look, what you would be wearing, and what would be your emotional state. Choose colors that represent your emotions as well as your outward appearance. You have 20 minutes to complete this drawing, so do not worry about artistic perfection.

Psychodynamic
Activity Example 5-2
My Room

Materials: 8 1/2- x 11-inch white paper, pencils with erasers, and rulers for each member. Colored pencils may also be used.

Directions: Introduce yourself by saying your name, and recalling a name your parents called you before you were 5 years old, or recalling a toy you remember playing with as a child.

Use the paper, pencil, and ruler to draw the floor plan of the room you slept in as a child. Try to remember as much about the room as you can.

- What was its size and shape?
- Whom did you share it with, if anyone?
- What color was it (paint, wallpaper)?
- Where was the bed? The window? Other furniture?
- Where did you keep your clothes and belongings?
- How old were you when you began sleeping there?
- What do you remember doing in this room besides sleeping?
- What else was in the room (carpets, curtains)?
- How did the bed look (bedspread, pillows, stuffed toys)?
- How did it feel to be in the room (sunny, dark)?
- What did it smell like?
- What was on the floor?

When you feel that you have a sense of this memory, begin drawing. You have 25 minutes to complete this floor plan.

From Cole, M. B. *Group dynamics in occupational therapy: The theoretical basis and practice application of group intervention* (3rd ed.). Thorofare, NJ: SLACK Incorporated. © 2005 SLACK Incorporated.

Psychodynamic
Activity Example 5-3
Pass the Hat

Materials: A collection of various hats (e.g., sun visor, cowboy, baseball, ski hat, beret, etc.).

Directions: Choose a hat from the center of the circle and try it on. Think about who might wear this hat. As you introduce yourself, describe for what occasion you might wear a hat like this, if ever.

Put the hats back in the center of the circle. Now ask someone to volunteer to begin a story about a character wearing one of these hats. If no one volunteers, the leader may begin the story. After 1 minute, the first person stops and passes the hat to the next person in the circle. That person continues the story for 1 minute, and on around the circle. At any time during the storytelling, a member may choose to change the main character or add a new character by choosing a different hat. Ask members to describe interaction between the characters.

Discussion centers around the fantasized characters.

- Who did you like or dislike?
- Who do you know that any imagined characters reminded you of?
- Who are you vs. who might you rather be?
- How would you change if you could?
- Which hat fits most comfortably?
- What does your imagination say about yourself?

Psychodynamic
Activity Example 5-4
A Poem for Myself

Materials: Pens and paper for each member and an assortment of used greeting cards (e.g., birthday, anniversary, wedding, sympathy, get well, friendship) that contain some form of a short poem.

Directions: Ask members to choose a greeting card and read the poem to the group. Collect the cards and put them away. Give out pens and paper. Ask members to think about how they are feeling right now, and what kind of card they might like to receive from someone. Ideas for this may be shared and discussed.

You have 15 minutes to write the first draft of a poem to yourself. This may be written as if it were from someone specific, or may be anonymous. The poem does not have to rhyme. It does not have to be in complete sentences. However, it should contain some words of inspiration relating to your current emotional state. Possible themes include:

- Needing a friend
- Sharing a joy
- Feeling alone
- Praying for guidance
- Missing someone
- Wishing to be healed
- Finding something (or someone) that was lost
- Discovering the truth about yourself

From Cole, M. B. *Group dynamics in occupational therapy: The theoretical basis and practice application of group intervention* (3rd ed.). Thorofare, NJ: SLACK Incorporated. © 2005 SLACK Incorporated.

Psychodynamic
Activity Example 5-5
Introducing the Empty Chair

Materials: 3- x 5-inch index cards and pens. Members sit in a circle with one extra chair in the center.

Directions: Everyone has troubled relationships in their lives. Is there someone you wish you could become emotionally closer to or have more supportive of you? As you introduce yourself, say a few words about someone in your life with whom you might like to have a better relationship.

Now, on the index card, write the name of one such individual. Then write the answers to the following questions:

- How is this person related to you (relative, spouse, friend, parent, neighbor)? Write a few sentences about the quality of this relationship.
- Where and when did the relationship begin?
- How many years have you known this person?
- What activities did you share with this person? Describe one such activity.
- When and where was your last meeting?
- Describe the nature of your most recent interaction.
- What about your relationship with this person do you wish to change?
- What would make the relationship better?

Sharing: When members have finished writing, ask them to focus on the empty chair in the center of the circle and imagine the person each member has chosen seated in it. Members then take turns standing behind the chair and introducing their significant person to the rest of the group, giving details from their writing.

Discussion: Focus on mutual support and give-and-take of relationships. Encourage feedback and suggestions.

From Cole, M. B. *Group dynamics in occupational therapy: The theoretical basis and practice application of group intervention* (3rd ed.). Thorofare, NJ: SLACK Incorporated. © 2005 SLACK Incorporated.

Psychodynamic

Activity Example 5-6

Paint Your Day

Materials: Roll of bond paper large enough to cover the center of a 72-inch oblong table, 12 poster paints in a variety of colors, a paintbrush for each color, large jars of water, and sponges for cleaning up. No chairs are allowed.

Directions: Group members (no more than eight) introduce themselves and describe how they are feeling today. They are then instructed to do a group mural. The group members take a few minutes to organize how they will do the painting, such as if there will be a "top" and a "bottom" and how space will be divided. Members are encouraged to move around the table as they paint and to exchange colors as they wish. The subjects should relate to the feelings presented and should not be reality-oriented (e.g., garden scene, ocean scene). Abstract shapes and symbols are best. About 20 minutes usually suffices to cover most of the surface of the paper.

Discussion: This centers around how members interacted with each other, as shown in the group mural. Sharing will reveal each member's painted creations, as well as what they might mean to that individual. Overassertive or bold painting, color choices, and shapes and lines all reveal emotional states as well as personality traits. Group roles may also be identified this way (e.g., imitator, follower, orienter, elaborator, etc.). Refer to Chapter 2 for a review of potential group roles.

From Cole, M. B. *Group dynamics in occupational therapy: The theoretical basis and practice application of group intervention* (3rd ed.). Thorofare, NJ: SLACK Incorporated. © 2005 SLACK Incorporated.

Chapter 6

The Behavioral Cognitive Continuum

From a historical perspective, most of the cognitive frames of reference in occupational therapy are derived from "learning theory," which grew from the roots of behaviorism in the 1930s and 1940s. The works of Skinner, Pavlov, and others revolutionized the field of psychology by applying the scientific method to human behavior. This idea was directly opposed to the concept of the unconscious in psychoanalytic theories because behaviorists believed that only what was "observable and measurable" could legitimately be the subject of scientific study. Modern day thinking has mellowed the radical thinking of early behaviorism. Most current theories include cognition in the definition of observable behavior and acknowledge the internal control of the individual. However, some concepts from behaviorism remain useful and may be recognized in the occupational therapy practice of today. Therefore, this chapter begins with an overview of those behavioral concepts that still apply to group leadership in occupational therapy: behavioral objectives, conditioning and habits, shaping and chaining, rehearsal and practice, modeling, and reinforcement.

Next, the biomechanical approach is briefly reviewed. While this frame is not usually included in a behavioral or cognitive context, therapy in the biomechanical frame of reference relies on behavioral concepts such as practice and repetition, behavioral objectives, and the formation of good habits of posture and body mechanics and often requires external reinforcement. The biomechanical frame of reference also provides the background for certain cognitive behavioral techniques, such as biofeedback, progressive relaxation, and systematic desensitization, which are useful in groups when addressing issues like stress management, the management of pain, or the modulation of emotions. Frames previously described as "rehabilitative" or "acquisitional," including those of Denton, Mosey, and Trombly, are briefly included as their concepts contribute to group intervention.

Two different cognitive approaches are then described in this chapter. The first is "cognitive rehabilitation," developed by Abreu and Toglia (1987) and updated by Toglia as the "multicontextual approach" (1991) and the "dynamic interactional approach" (1997) to cognitive rehabilitation. Toglia's theory has recently moved away from its original focus on separate and distinct cognitive subskills toward a more integrated systems approach. This model uses the works of Luria, a noted Russian brain physiologist, and other current brain research to develop a more holistic approach to cognitive rehabilitation. This theory, as updated, is particularly well-suited to group intervention, especially as it impacts "metacognition," or the ability to monitor, regulate, and predict one's own functional performance.

The second set of concepts discussed in this chapter is cognitive behavioral therapy, recently dubbed "CPT" by Duncombe (1997). Duncombe has presented this approach as a legitimate occupational therapy frame of reference, which uses principles similar to those used in its psychological counterpart. Cognitive behaviorism is one of the most frequently used in mental or behavioral health settings for several reasons. It sounds simple and logical, it easily lends itself to advances in technology, such as computer programming and biofeedback, and it is appropriate and useful in

Table 6-1	Summary of Behavioral Cognitive Continuum			
	Behavioral	*Biomechanical, Rehabilitative*	*Cognitive-Perceptual Rehabilitation*	*Behavioral Cognitive, Dialectical Behavioral*
Theorists	Skinner, Pavlov, Lazarus	Trombly, Denton, Mosey, Fidler	Toglia and Abreu	Bandura, Beck, Ellis, Linehan
Client Applications	All populations	Physically disabled	Brain injury, stroke, mental illness	Mental illness, emotional aspects, character disorder
Concepts and Techniques	Goals and objectives, conditioning and habits, shaping and chaining, reinforcement, rehearsal and practice, role playing and role reversal, systematic desensitization, biofeedback	Strength, ROM, endurance, positioning prevention, restoration, compensation, adaptation, skill acquisition, lifestyle performance, biofeedback	Orientation, attention, visual processing, motor planning cognition, ADL, multicontextual treatment, metacognition, generalization, criteria for transfer of learning	Social learning, modeling, self-regulation, cognitive distortions, automatic thoughts, disputing irrational beliefs, cognitive restructuring, dialectical strategies
Occupational Therapy Group Themes	Graded tasks, social skills training, assertiveness, relaxation, stress, time or emotion management, coping skills training, conflict management	Group exercise, group games involving movement, graded strength and endurance, prevention education, work readiness, work hardening	Strategy themes (any of the six cognitive areas) in multiple contexts, group discussion of strategy generalizations, self-skill assessment in group	Psychoeducational modules/groups, reading/films and discussion, role playing groups, worksheets and discussion in interpersonal effectiveness, emotion regulation, distress tolerance and mindfulness

short-term intervention. Occupational therapists use the psychoeducational approach from cognitive behaviorism in treating clients on a verbal and symbolic level. To benefit from this approach, it is suggested that clients be capable of learning through logic and reasoning. The principal spokesmen for the cognitive behavioral therapies in psychology are Aaron Beck, Albert Ellis, and Albert Bandura. A more recent outgrowth of cognitive behaviorism used by occupational therapists, called "Dialectical Behavior Therapy," developed by Linehan (1993a) is described. This approach is widely used and is a basis of group intervention with psychiatric populations. Both Toglia and Linehan share the guiding principle that therapy should focus on the cognitive process and that changes in thinking will produce adaptive changes in client behavior.

Framework Focus

This group of approaches, some more behavioral, others more cognitive, were all developed through application of the scientific method to human behavior. They can be expressed in a continuum as shown in Table 6-1.

Behavioral approaches are most ideal when addressing the need for learning or changing client "performance patterns" in the *Occupational Therapy Practice Framework* (AOTA, 2002). "Contexts" will be examined in identifying "cues," which can either facilitate function or trigger maladaptive behaviors in any of the "performance areas of occupation." Cognitive behavioral approaches are the top choice when self-control and self-management are primary concerns. This approach includes theories of learning, which are especially useful in promoting client "performance skills," whether motor, process, or communication/interaction skills.

Basic Assumptions

Behavioral Concepts

This section selects for review those behavioral concepts that still appear as an integral part of occupational therapy: behavioral goals and objectives, conditioning and habits, shaping and chaining, reinforcement, and rehearsal and practice.

Behavioral Goals and Objectives

One of the most fundamental contributions of behaviorism is the concept of behavioral goals. Only observable behavior was thought to be an appropriate focus for intervention. Therefore, behavioral goals and objectives should always be observable and measurable. The early behaviorists taught us to identify problems narrowly and specifically, so that focused intervention could be designed and its effects measured. The goals for our occupational therapy groups should be written in specific, measurable terms, so that necessary documentation of progress is possible. Often these goals are set by the clients and therapist together, and progress toward the goals is openly discussed with the group. In cognitive behavioral groups, an evaluation of the group should be set up to see if goals are met. Worksheets 6-1 through 6-3 are designed to help students learn how to write behavioral goals.

Long-term goals are not always measurable. Sometimes when we set lifetime goals, such as "Be successful at my job," it is not clear what it is that success really means. Even when these goals are measurable, such as "become a millionaire by age 40," how these goals will be accomplished remains unplanned. Until these goals are broken down into smaller, doable steps, they will remain only

dreams. Short-term, measurable goals are the actions and behaviors that help us and our clients make dreams a reality. A measurable goal is one that describes behavior that can be observed. For example, your goal might be to improve self-esteem. How can you tell when self-esteem has improved? What behaviors would you look for? What actions could you take? Some possibilities might be standing taller, taking more care in dressing and hygiene to look your best, and verbalizing several positive aspects of yourself.

The measurable goals in Worksheet 6-2 are 2, 4, 9, 10, 12, 14, 15, 17, and 18. One key to writing a measurable goal is the language used. Words like "learn," "understand," "encourage," "improve," "handle," and "manage" are vague because they do not specify how these things can be accomplished. Measurable goals are usually specific, and they incorporate behaviors that can be observed. Words like "define," "list," "discuss," and "complete" refer to either words or actions that can be readily observed, heard, or read. In the cognitive behavioral frame of reference, thoughts are also considered to be behavior. However, thoughts must be verbalized in order to be measurable.

Conditioning and Habits

Pavlov has been credited with identifying classical conditioning as a process through which much of human behavior is learned. When a piece of chocolate candy is placed in the mouth, the mouth waters and the person experiences a pleasant taste sensation. The autonomic response is soon associated with the visual stimuli, so that it only takes a glance at the candy bar in the store window to make the mouth water. Likewise, many associations in the brain are formed that attach meaning to incoming stimuli. Pavlov was able to recreate this phenomenon in the laboratory, and he called it "classical conditioning." Much of today's advertising uses this principle (Corey, 1996).

Skinner (1953) identified a more complex, but less controlled form of learning, which he called "operant conditioning." According to this principle, behavior that is reinforced by the environment tends to be repeated, while behavior that is discouraged or ignored tends to become extinct or disappear. Humans are continually subjected to random or chance reinforcement as they go through life, causing maladaptive as well as constructive learning. Therapy, therefore, must involve the identification and control of environmental factors that reinforce a behavior, so that the stage can be set for positive behavior change.

Worksheet 6-1
Writing Long-Term Goals

Directions: Begin by writing your lifetime goals for yourself. Write at least one goal for each of the following categories.

1. Professional

2. Educational

3. Monetary

4. Family

5. Health

6. Social

7. Spiritual

8. Emotional

9. Recreational

10. Creative

Worksheet 6-2
Recognizing Measurable Goals

Directions: From the list below, circle the goals that you think are measurable.

1. Encourage decision making.

2. List one strength and one weakness.

3. Develop a better self-concept.

4. Discuss feelings about parents.

5. Relate better to authority figures.

6. Manage time better.

7. Conserve energy in cooking a meal.

8. Handle frustration.

9. Demonstrate pride in personal accomplishment.

10. Plan a weekend activity and carry it out.

11. Define assertive behavior.

12. Complete a task within time limit.

13. Relieve stress.

14. Eat a well-balanced diet.

15. Plan time to study for a test.

16. Take responsibility for behavior.

17. Attend school regularly.

18. Stay on a diet 80% of the time.

19. Understand yourself better.

20. Strengthen feminine/masculine identity.

From Cole, M. B. *Group dynamics in occupational therapy: The theoretical basis and practice application of group intervention* (3rd ed.). Thorofare, NJ: SLACK Incorporated. © 2005 SLACK Incorporated.

Worksheet 6-3
Making Our Lifetime Goals Measurable

Directions: In Worksheet 6-1, we wrote down some lifetime goals. First, go back to that list and check off which of those goals are measurable. Next, choose three goals from your list that are not measurable and write them down below. For each one, list several measurable short-term goals or steps to be completed.

Lifetime Goal 1

  1.

  2.

  3.

  4.

  5.

Lifetime Goal 2

  1.

  2.

  3.

  4.

  5.

Lifetime Goal 3

  1.

  2.

  3.

  4.

  5.

The development of habits is explained by the principle of operant conditioning. Persons repeat behaviors that are reinforced repeatedly until they become habitual, but once a habit is formed, reinforcement is no longer necessary. Habits are routine or customary ways of doing things. James (1985) explains that an "acquired habit, from a physiological point of view, is nothing but a new pathway of discharge formed in the brain, by which certain incoming currents ever after tend to escape" (p. 55). This statement implies that certain stimuli, when encountered in the environment, evoke predictable responses that have been "conditioned" or learned. Waking up in a familiar environment, most people can wash, dress, eat breakfast, and otherwise get ready for the day, without much conscious thought. James writes that "habit diminishes the conscious attention with which our acts are performed" (1985, p. 59). In the above example, the familiar objects in the environment serve as stimuli for the habitual performance of these necessary tasks, so that brain energy is reserved for the more challenging tasks at work or school. Using this principle, cognitive rehabilitation seeks to re-establish habitual ways of performing functional tasks after brain trauma. When familiar ways of accomplishing a task are no longer possible, new pathways must be formed through the rehearsal and practice of the most efficient alternative strategies.

Shaping and Chaining

Skinner once demonstrated, before a large audience, teaching a live pigeon to turn around using the technique of shaping. The pigeon's cage was set on the stage, where it could be readily seen. Using the principle of operant conditioning, he waited until the pigeon turned slightly in the desired direction and reinforced this behavior with a pellet of food. Each time the pigeon turned a little farther in the desired direction, it was reinforced again with a pellet of food. Within 2 or 3 minutes, the pigeon had learned to turn a full 360 degrees before being reinforced. The technique of shaping requires that each step in a sequence be reinforced until the entire task is learned. When occupational therapists analyze activities, we break them down into component parts, or steps. Instructing a client in using a reacher, for example, we may begin with the correct grip, then practice the movements of the handle, and finally, practice picking up first lighter, then heavier objects. We may use approval or praise after each step is done

correctly, without even realizing that we are using reinforcement to shape the client's behavior.

Chaining refers to the learning of steps in a specific sequence, so that each action serves as the stimulus to provoke the next action (James, 1985). When a sequence follows along smoothly, A-B-C-D, without hesitation or making a decision among alternatives, then the sequence has become a habit. James suggests that it is the sensation of the movement just finished that provides reinforcement and signals readiness for what comes next.

Reinforcement

From the discussion of behavioral concepts so far, it is evident that reinforcement comes in many forms. Early behaviorists identified reinforcement as external to the individual. Positive reinforcement is a reward, something desirable to the individual: an edible treat, a gold star, a hug, words of praise, a paycheck. In negative reinforcement, something desirable is removed: privileges, freedom, participation in a social or recreational activity, a holiday. Later behaviorists believed that reinforcement can also be internal. Bandura, a cognitive behavioral theorist, identified two kinds of internal reinforcers: vicarious and self-produced. Vicarious reinforcers are symbolic, such as a person's learned images of success and failure, or reflections of his or her values and ideals. Self-produced reinforcers come from the person's sense of competence, efficacy, and self-control. In other words, feeling good about one's self is reinforcing.

Bandura's hierarchy of reinforcement is helpful in understanding and planning learning experiences for our client groups. The levels of reinforcers progress from simple to more complex as they parallel the developmental sequence.

- Initial reinforcers refers to the external ones such as food, attention, and approval.
- Symbolic reinforcers are internal images or messages regarding probable consequences of behavior. An example of this is a child refraining from going outside his or her yard because he or she remembers how angry his or her mother got the last time he or she did it.
- Social contract refers to more complex or role dependent behavior such as performing a job or honoring one's marriage vows.
- Personal satisfaction is the best and most effective reinforcer in Bandura's opinion because it is the least dependent upon external circumstances, and therefore the least

vulnerable to extinction. When feelings of self-satisfaction or self-worth result from particular behaviors, those behaviors tend to be repeated.

Since reinforcement is what motivates learning, the occupational therapist seeking to motivate a group of clients must decide what level of reinforcement the group members can respond to. Even when treating adults, we may need to fall back on external reinforcement when motivation for therapy is found lacking.

Rehearsal and Practice

A popular technique associated with the behavioral approach is assertiveness training. This group activity requires the rehearsal and practice of newly learned assertive behaviors through group role playing, and subsequently, trying out the new behaviors in real life situations. The leader first uses self-awareness exercises to help the members analyze their own habitual responses to difficult situations as either passive, aggressive, or assertive.

- Passive: The individual does not state his or her feelings or stand up for his or her rights, and usually does not get what he or she wants.

- Aggressive: The individual insists on his or her rights, lets his or her feelings explode, and gets what he or she wants by abusing the rights and hurting the feelings of others.

- Assertive: The individual expresses his or her feelings and requests that his or her rights be honored. He or she may not always get his or her way, but his or her behavior encourages mutual respect and open communication.

Hypothetical situations may be presented by the leader, which are likely to be familiar, such as:

- Just as you reach the ticket counter at the movies after a 20-minute wait, someone cuts ahead of you in line.

- A group of friends with whom you are talking decide spontaneously to meet at an unfamiliar restaurant for coffee. You'd like to join them, but you don't know how to get there.

- You receive a credit card bill for an item you did not buy.

- While driving you to an unfamiliar doctor's office for an appointment, your friend makes a wrong turn and becomes lost. He or she refuses to stop to ask directions.

- You have made your spouse (significant other) a special birthday dinner, and he or she shows up an hour late, with no explanation or apology.

The group discusses each situation with regard to: What would I typically do? Is my response passive, aggressive, or assertive? What would be an appropriate assertive response? The exact words of an assertive response are then practiced by each member. The key is to focus on the verbal expression of feeling or statement of legitimate rights, followed by a request for change or action. Using incomplete sentences and asking each member to fill in the blanks, might be a good place to start: I feel _____ when you _____. I request that you _____. Hypothetical and real situations are rehearsed and practiced through role playing, group discussion, giving and receiving feedback, and homework. Most people have difficulty behaving assertively, and persons with disability are especially vulnerable. Assertiveness group members should be encouraged to provide one another emotional support when attempts at assertive behavior outside the group do not bring expected results. Reinforcement for assertive behavior must initially come from the group leader and members, until it is practiced often enough, and with enough success, to become a part of the individual's habitual response repertoire. (For further ideas on assertiveness groups, see Posthuma, 2002.)

Many functional skills addressed in occupational therapy require rehearsal and practice. The cognitive rehabilitation approach stresses the rehearsal of cognitive strategies in a variety of clinical contexts and practice of skills over a range of possible applications. Giving groups specific homework assignments encourages the practice of skills in real life contexts. Discussion of the results of practice allows the group leader and members to provide "reinforcement" in a controlled and predictable way.

Role Playing

According to Posthuma (2002), role playing evolved from the practice of psychodrama, in which the client (protagonist) directs his or her own real life situation by choosing other members of the group to play the roles of significant others. As a behavioral technique, the structure of role playing remains the same, but the focus is slightly different. In occupational therapy groups, playing roles provides a forum for practice and rehearsal of new behaviors within a safe and supportive therapeutic environment. Members recall or anticipate difficult situations in their own lives and bring them to the therapy setting in constructing the role play. Each role play has four parts, according to Posthuma (2002):

1. Definition of the problem
2. Assuming the roles
3. Enactment
4. Discussion

For example, a client anticipating a return to work after a long absence may choose others to play coworkers, supervisors, or clients/customers. The client (protagonist) tells each member how to play his or her role, and the furniture in the room can be rearranged to resemble the work setting for a more realistic effect. Although the protagonist may play him- or herself the first time through, it is often helpful for another member to play that role or to reverse roles. As a learning tool, role reversal has the advantage of helping the protagonist to see the situation from the other's point of view. The purpose of role playing is to practice new behaviors, develop insight to a situation, develop empathy with others, anticipate consequences, increase self-confidence, and/or decrease anxiety. A discussion of the role play allows the other members of the group to give feedback and support to the protagonist and reveals its meaning for all the group members. Role plays are also models for social learning (described later, in the section on cognitive behavioral therapies).

Systematic Desensitization and Biofeedback

These techniques have elements of both behavioral and cognitive theory. Systematic desensitization has been used successfully by clinical psychologists in interventions with phobias, such as fear of flying, and has been less successfully used to control addictions, such as drinking or smoking. The first step in desensitization is to evoke a state of relaxation, usually using some form of progressive muscle tension and release sequences combined with visualization. The "progressive" part involves the introduction of images of the feared object/situation in graded degrees of severity. For example, the person with fear of flying would begin by visualizing the drive to the airport and gradually work up to the plane taking off, while maintaining a state of relaxation. The entire process requires a series of sessions, often over a period of several months. Psychologists are required to get special training before attempting this technique. However, the same concepts form the basis of many group activities used in occupational therapy. Progressive muscle relaxation takes on many forms and may be used in occupational therapy groups dealing with stress management or

as a coping strategy when faced with any situation that tends to evoke anxiety. Guided fantasy is a form of visualization that is useful for group intervention. Although feared images should be avoided, pleasant ones may be very powerful motivators. For example, the group may begin by closing their eyes, breathing deeply, and imagining themselves lying on a sunny beach, listening to the rhythm of the ocean waves as they break along the shore. This visual image sets the stage for relaxation and prepares them for learning other useful strategies for the control of anxiety, anger, frustration, and other causes of distress.

Biofeedback refers to the monitoring of bodily functions, such as pulse, respiration rate, heart rate, and body temperature. Stein and Nikolic (1989) suggest using biofeedback in conjunction with other stress management techniques. Mechanical monitoring devices are used to give clients information about how their mental state affects them physically. Various mental strategies can then be learned to help persons gain control over their own physiological responses to stress. Biofeedback is often combined with visualization and relaxation techniques. It is also used in the biomechanical approach to monitor the effects of movement and exercise and as a safety precaution to prevent overexertion in any physically strenuous activity.

Biomechanical Approach

Note: This approach overlaps with the sensorimotor approaches covered in Chapter 9. It is included here because of its reliance on theories of learning.

This approach is primarily appropriate for clients who lack range of motion (ROM), strength, and endurance to perform daily life tasks (Trombly & Radomski, 2002). The whole is considered to be the sum of its parts: single muscles making up muscle groups or synergies, tasks divided into force and resistance, angles and directions, and rearranged into positions and movement sequences. Therefore, behavior can be broken down into its component subskills for the purpose of easier learning. The theory draws upon the kinetic principles of human movement, and its goals are to prevent injury, restore function, and/or compensate for lost function. These are some of the same principles of strength and effort that are presently associated with work hardening.

The biomechanical frame of reference is included here because it uses the behavioral principles of conditioning, habit formation, shaping and chaining, and rehearsal and practice with the goal of restoring function. Adaptation and compensation are often required when injury or illness results in chronic physical disability. Behavioral goals and objectives are set, and effects of intervention are carefully measured. Because recovery from physical loss often requires multiple repetition, building these repetitions into meaningful group activities can be helpful and motivating.

Range of Motion

The maximum motion of every joint in every possible direction is called its ROM. Average ROMs for each joint in each direction have been calculated, so that deviation from the norm, or limitation of ROM, can be determined. There are many causes of limitation in ROM; some are head injury, stroke, burns, fractures, arthritis, and peripheral nerve injury. ROM is measured with a goniometer, which, when applied to the joint, determines the angle or number of degrees the joint can move. For example, the typical ROM of the elbow joint is 0 to 150 degrees. The ROM can be measured actively— "Lift your arm high over your head" (AROM)—or passively—"Let me flex and extend your shoulder" (PROM). Specific guidelines for measuring range of motion for each joint may be found in Trombly and Radomski (2002).

In occupational therapy, activities are devised to encourage the client to increase and/or maintain range of motion. Particularly in groups of clients who are at risk, such as those with arthritis, multiple sclerosis, or post head trauma or stroke, exercise "classes" to maintain/extend range of motion are common. Crafts and games can be adapted by positioning them in a way that forces the client to reach, bend, push, pull, or grasp in order to accomplish the goal. Care should be taken to plan the right amount of movement, since overestimating it can easily cause injury. A creative activity using this approach is the "Range of Motion Dance," a supportive exercise group format for clients post-stroke to maintain their range of motion (Harlowe & Yu, 1997; Van Deusen & Harlowe, 1987).

Strength

Muscle weakness is another common problem treated in occupational therapy with physical disabilities. When illness or injury results in specific muscle weakness, or when weakness can potentially cause deformity, activities can be devised to increase muscle strength. Strength can be increased in several ways. Stress is applied to a muscle or muscle group by increase in load or weight. Lifting objects of gradually increased weight will strengthen the muscles. Duration of muscle contraction also influences strength. Holding a position or lifting and holding a heavy object for longer and longer intervals can increase strength. The rate and the frequency of contraction also affect strength; faster or more frequent exercise increases strength, even when lighter weight is used. Any combination of these parameters when applied to exercise have been found to increase strength. The challenge for the occupational therapist is to find activities that can be graded in load, duration, rate, and frequency, so that strength can be increased gradually and without injury. Craft activities, such as sanding wood or weaving on a loom, have traditionally been adapted to accomplish these goals. When treating in groups, work activities such as gardening and landscaping, cleaning and moving furniture, or stocking shelves might accomplish the goals of increasing strength.

Endurance

Endurance refers to the length of time muscles can continue to work without becoming fatigued. A person can sustain isometric contraction equivalent to 50% of maximum voluntary contraction (MVC) up to 1 minute. In normal subjects, contraction time and percentage of MVC are inversely related (Trombly & Radomski, 2002). For example, if Sally carries a 50-pound bag of dog food from her car up three flights of stairs to her apartment, she will need to sustain a 50% MVC for 2 minutes. Chances are it will be necessary for Sally to stop and rest after 1 minute before continuing. However, if she carries a 25-pound bag of dog food, she can sustain a 25% MVC for the 2 minutes it takes her to walk all the way to her apartment without resting.

In occupational therapy, endurance may be increased by using moderately fatiguing activities for progressively longer periods of time. In groups, the occupational therapist can offer activities that sustain interest over the needed increases in duration. Many active games and sports can be adapted to the goal of increasing strength and endurance. Tug of war, for example, can be timed so that the length of effort progressively increases with each round. Relay races, perhaps carrying progressively heavier items, can be graded also.

Prevention, Restoration, and Compensation

Particularly in the workplace, prevention of injury and maintenance of health are important areas for occupational therapy intervention. Insurance companies, worker's compensation, and other third-party payers are hiring occupational therapy consultants to organize educational groups in the use of correct body mechanics, positioning and seating, environmental adaptations, and energy-saving strategies to help save the cost of worker absence and medical intervention due to preventable injuries. In addition, educational groups for persons with specific injuries, such as carpal tunnel syndrome or osteoarthritis, will help them learn good health maintenance strategies.

Restoration of function is defined within the context of developing client competence in performing occupational roles. The client should identify the roles he or she will continue (e.g., worker, spouse, club member, friend). The roles played, in turn, help define the tasks the individual must learn or relearn. The goals are specific, and occupational therapy intervention centers around accomplishing those specific goals or tasks that the client has identified as his or her preferences.

The occupational therapist uses a compensation strategy for clients who need to live with a disability on a temporary or permanent basis. Using this approach, the client with physical disability uses his or her remaining abilities to perform needed tasks. Occupational therapy helps the client to develop strategies or use adaptive equipment that can compensate for the loss of physical capacities in order to accomplish activities of daily living. The occupational therapist organizes the environment, then motivates and reinforces the client toward successful completion of the task. Adaptations, compensations, and adaptive equipment may be incorporated. Competence in doing the task is achieved through repetition and practice.

Skill Acquisition—Mosey, Denton, Trombly

The above approach to the rehabilitation of physical disabilities has previously been called "acquisitional" by Mosey (1986) and others. Denton (1987) called it "functional performance," and Trombly called it simply the "rehabilitative approach" (Trombly & Radomski, 2002). This refers to the process or relearning lost skills in activities of daily living due to physical disability. Rehabilitation in occupational therapy occurs on a continuum of restoration-adaptation-compensation. That is, foundation skills of movement,

strength, endurance, and perception are remediated or brought to the highest level of recovery possible within the limitations of the illness or injury. Adaptations in everyday functioning are then made to maximize that level of recovery through use of special equipment or changes in the environment. When full recovery is not anticipated, compensatory strategies are then substituted for skills that have been lost or compromised. This practical approach to rehabilitation is so well-known in occupational therapy that it has not really needed an official "name." However, the 2002 edition of Trombly and Radomski elaborates on the approach using many names. One of these, the task-oriented OT approach, is described in Chapter 9.

Two related approaches worthy of mention here are Mosey's "role acquisition" and Fidler's "lifestyle performance profile"(Robertson, 1988).

Role Acquisition

Mosey addresses the role acquisition approach to those individuals whose disability has stabilized and who continue to have difficulty in performance of tasks of their major social roles (Robertson, 1988). She identifies the basic skills common to all social roles as task skills and interpersonal skills. These basic skills are necessary building blocks for the performance of self-care (activities of daily living), family interaction, recreation, and work. Temporal adaptation, or skill in the perception and use of time, serves to organize and balance the tasks of occupational roles on a daily basis. Table 6-2 lists task and interpersonal skills that may be helpful in setting group goals. Skills are separately defined for family interaction, activities of daily living, leisure, and work. Temporal adaptation, the ability to perceive and manage time, is defined as orientation, organization, planning, goal setting, and establishing a schedule. Mosey suggests that interventions in task skill development begin on an individual basis. Group interventions can be effective in learning the more advanced task skills and in working on interpersonal skills. She suggests topical or thematic groups be designed to address specific skills.

Velde and Fidler's Lifestyle Performance Profile

This occupational therapy model and assessment tool was developed by Beth Velde and Gail Fidler (2002). In it, skills for self-care and maintenance, self needs/intrinsic gratification, and service to others are listed and assessed within the

Table 6-2	Mosey's Role Acquisition: Task and Interpersonal Skills

Task Skills

1. Willingness to engage in tasks
2. Adequate posture for tasks
3. Physical strength and endurance
4. Gross and fine motor coordination
5. Interest in task
6. Rate of performance
7. Ability to follow oral, demonstrated pictorial, and written directions
8. Use of tools and materials
9. Acceptable level of neatness
10. Attention to detail
11. Ability to solve problems
12. Ability to organize task in logical manner
13. Ability to tolerate frustration
14. Ability to be self-directed

Interpersonal Skills

1. Initiate, respond to, and sustain verbal interactions
2. Express ideas and feelings
3. Be aware of needs and feelings of others
4. Participate in cooperative and competitive situations
5. Compromise and negotiate
6. Assert self
7. Take on appropriate group roles

Table 6-3	Fidler and Velde's Four Domains of Occupation

• Self-care and self-maintenance—Manner determined by personal needs and capacities
• Intrinsic gratification—Pursuit of pleasure and enjoyment
• Societal contribution—Contribute to need fulfillment and welfare of others
• Reciprocal interpersonal relatedness—Developing and sustaining relationships with others

framework of age, culture, and biology (Table 6-3). Fidler (1996) says:

> Each individual, over time, develops a configuration of activity patterns that can be described as a lifestyle. These patterns of doing, of being engaged, emerge through the interplay of a person's intrinsic needs, desires and capacities, and unique expectations of the environmental context of a person's living. (p. 140)

Three contributing factors to lifestyle are motivation, well-being and quality of life, and the environment. An individual's motivation is strongest when engaging in occupations that are personally and socially relevant. Success may be seen in a satisfying end product. Concepts of well-being and quality of life include the following:

- Satisfaction is one's cognitive appraisal of one's lifestyle
- Quality of life is higher when the individual can personally exert control over the environment
- Occupations that produce a sense of well-being and quality of life must be defined by the individual

The environment may be structured to respond to individual needs and interests. Elements of the environment can clarify reality and define expectations for occupational performance. An ideal environment supports autonomy, individuality, affiliation, volition, consensual validation, predictability, self-efficacy, adventure, accommodation, and reflection.

In the lifestyle performance model, intervention is required when:

- Illness or trauma affects occupation in any lifestyle domain
- Lifestyle changes become necessary
- Individuals desire to establish a more satisfying lifestyle

Figure 6-1 shows a "lifestyle web" of the interrelationship of client factors, occupational performance areas, contexts, and environments so that a complete picture of the person within his or her current or historical context can be drawn. This profile can serve as an alternative basis for grouping clients with similar lifestyles, situations, and concerns, as well as similar deficits. Lifestyle changes and adaptations may be made more easily within a supportive, therapeutic group context.

Toglia's Multicontext Treatment Approach

Self-awareness is a key in Toglia's evolving multicontext approach. Learning theory is the foundation for cognitive rehabilitation (sometimes called cognitive perceptual rehabilitation), according to Toglia and Abreu (1987). This training originally involved systematic procedures provided in each of six discrete cognitive deficit areas to assist clients in the perception of stimuli and the effective solving of problems:

1. Orientation
2. Attention
3. Visual processing
4. Motor planning
5. Cognition
6. Occupational behavior

More recently, Toglia has expanded this framework in her development of the multicontextual approach to retraining and the addition of metacognition and criteria for transfer of learning. These additions do not abandon the original delineation of cognitive deficit areas, but they do alter the approach to their treatment. Toglia's recent work acknowledges the dynamic, interactive, and holistic nature of brain functioning and maximizes the likelihood of generalization of newly learned strategies or compensatory measures in restoring occupational performance (Toglia, 2003).

Functional Brain Areas

The six basic areas of perception/cognition addressed by Toglia and Abreu (1987) are orientation, attention, visual processing, motor planning, cognition, and occupational behavior. This organization of cognitive deficit areas has its foundation in the work of the Russian physiologist Aleksandr Luria (1973, 1980). Abreu and Toglia (1987) refer to Luria's brain region classifications in their organization of perceptual and cognitive deficits. The first brain area described includes the brain stem and the old cortex, containing the midbrain, thalamus, hypothalamus, uncas, reticular formation, and cerebellum. These are the innermost portions of the brain and are responsible for attention, wakefulness, arousal, and response to stimuli. The second brain area Luria defines includes the backmost areas and is responsible for analysis, coding, and storage of information. It receives raw data from sensory systems and assigns meaning to it. Luria's third functional area includes the frontal portions of the brain and is responsible for intentions, programs, and problem solving.

A distinction is also made between the right and left hemispheres of the brain in terms of function. The right hemisphere is responsible for diffuse representation, gestalts, and organized wholes. It deals in concepts rather than specifics and processes visual-spatial data and nonverbal sounds. Body scheme and tactile, somatosensory integration are primarily attributed to the right side of the brain. The left hemisphere is analytic and sequential, concerned with language, specific details, and mathematical operations. While there are discrete characteristics for the two sides of the brain, functionally they work together to perform daily life tasks. Often, it is through clinical work with brain damaged clients that we learn what types of functions are lost when certain parts of the brain are damaged.

Accidents and illness that cause damage to discrete areas of the brain are the most likely candidates for cognitive and perceptual retraining. Abreu and Toglia (1987) have proposed an "Evaluation Model: Six Areas to Test" (Figure 6-2) as a guide in assessing the areas of dysfunction and planning strategies for retraining. Some of the theories about how cognitive rehabilitation works are outlined by Bracy (1986) as follows:

- Lower brain areas take control and compensate for lost skills at higher levels.
- Different brain areas are utilized to replace lost skills (e.g., opposite hemisphere).

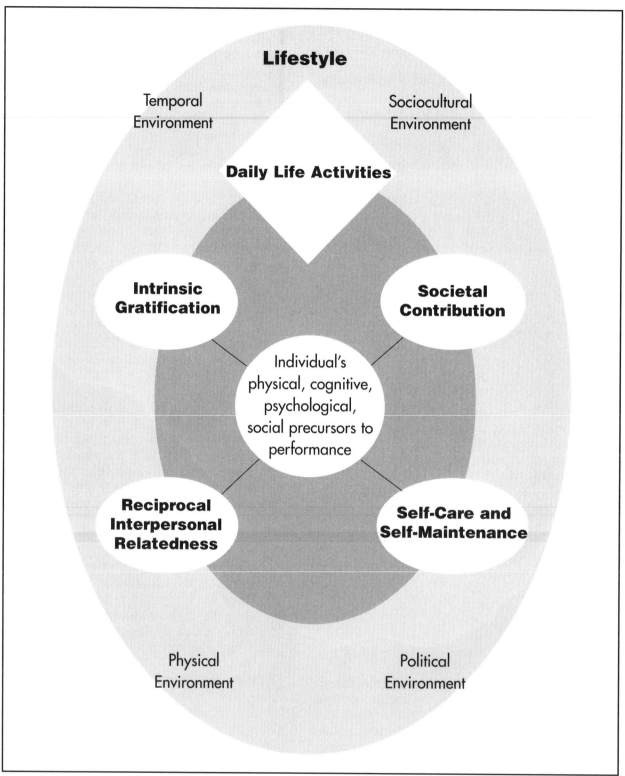

Figure 6-1. The lifestyle web. (Reprinted with permission from Velde, B., & Fidler, G. [2002]. *Lifestyle perform-ance: A model for engaging the power of occupation.* Thorofare, NJ: SLACK Incorporated.)

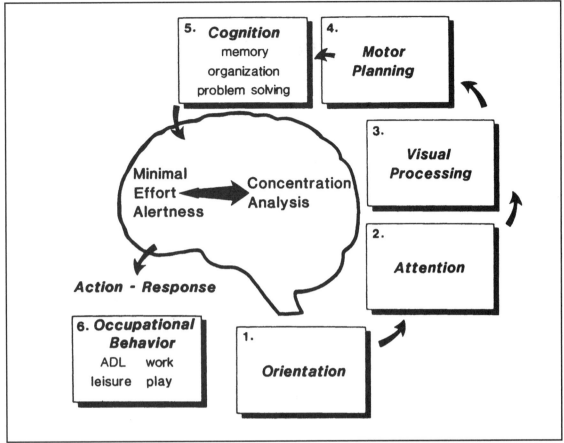

Figure 6-2. Six brain functions for cognitive rehabilitation. (Reprinted with permission from Abreu, B. C., & Toglia, J. P. [1984]. *Cognitive rehabilitation manual.* New York: Author.)

• Normal function returns as shock effect of injury subsides.

• Function is recovered through retraining.

These principles serve as the justification for the following strategies in cognitive rehabilitation.

The Multicontextual Approach

Cognitive rehabilitation with brain-injured adults involves the reorganization of functional systems so that new methods of performing old behaviors are acquired. The retraining seeks to maximize the efficiency of information processing and involves repetitive exercises that place demands on the individual to perform skills of graded difficulty. However, simply practicing each skill separately, according to Toglia (1991, 1997), does not result in the generalization of skills to life in the real world. Once cognitive strategies are relearned, they must be practiced and applied over a wide range of functional tasks, in a variety of social and situational contexts, in order to facilitate

generalization of skills. For example, a client needs to learn to monitor time during task performance so that he or she can complete tasks more quickly and be on time to appointments. He or she may begin with an individual task, writing down the time in the margin after each paragraph he or she reads in a magazine. In a group setting, he or she may complete a series of word puzzles, noting the time he or she started and completed each, and comparing with others to check for accuracy. He or she may be assigned the homework task of timing each morning task, washing, dressing, eating breakfast, shaving (or for females, applying make-up). Estimating the time it takes to get ready for an appointment may be the topic of discussion in the next occupational therapy group. In the group, time-saving ideas can be shared, and clients can learn new strategies from each other. Multiple contexts used during interventions encourage an understanding of the significance of a strategy and a recognition of properties of situations in which the strategy is applicable. The multicontextual approach does not distinguish between remediation and compensation. Rather, it focuses on a person's awareness of the need to use a selected processing strategy.

Metacognition

Toglia (1991) defines metacognition as "insight, or the degree of awareness one has regarding one's cognitive or physical capacities." Impairment in metacognition results in a misjudgment of the tasks one may attempt. This misjudgment may expose clients to significant danger, such as driving with a visual impairment, or failure to use a needed cane or walker when walking outdoors. Training increases self-awareness by a) acquiring knowledge of one's own processes and cognitive capacities and b) by developing self-monitoring strategies. Metacognitive skills include the ability to:

- Evaluate task difficulty
- Predict consequences of action
- Formulate goals
- Plan for anticipated problems
- Monitor one's own performance
- Recognize errors
- Demonstrate self-control

Toglia stresses that without metacognition, persons are unable to initiate and use either remedial or compensatory strategies. Therefore, these skills should be worked on significantly during therapy. Some suggested techniques for increasing metacognition are:

- Self-instruction—Person verbalizes plan before execution, then verbalizes speed and accuracy of performance during and afterwards.
- Self-estimation—Person rates task difficulty on a scale of 1-5 (very easy to very hard), then compares estimate to actual performance.
- Role reversal—Client watches therapist making errors while doing the task; client must identify errors and hypothesize why they occurred.
- Self-questioning—At intervals during actual performance, person stops and asks: "How am I doing? Am I using _____ (specific strategy)? Have I followed directions accurately?"
- Self-evaluation—After completion, persons asks: "Have I checked work for accuracy/completion? Have I paid attention or maintained focus? How confident do I feel about the results?"

Toglia suggests that metacognition has such a profound effect on new learning that this ability should be addressed in groups first, before attempting to teach remedial or compensatory strategies. In one experiment on memory training for persons with traumatic brain injury, group discussion and education about awareness of one's own performance increased accuracy of predictions by 50% on a recall task (Toglia, 1991). New research on the process of adaptation to disability suggests that for some clients, a series of shock waves and adjustments to the reality of chronic disability, taking several months (or years), may be necessary before the kind of insight or "metacognition" Toglia suggests is actually possible (Macdonald, 1998).

The nature of metacognitive training makes it especially well-suited to group interventions for several reasons. The obvious reason is that one's performance in a group is observed by others and has the advantage of multiple opportunities for observations and feedback. The company of others who also need to work on metacognition increases the level of support and encouragement if performance is poor, while decreasing the possibility of minimizing or denying one's difficulties. Applying the above skills to any processing task in a group context can be easily planned by the occupational therapist using Toglia's guidelines.

Generalization and Criteria for Transfer of Learning

Using Toglia's dynamic interactional model, cognitive strategies are always taught in the context of an activity. The initial demonstration of a strategy may be simple and designed for clinical use. For example, an organizational strategy might be presented to the group that involves 20 picture cards in four different categories (e.g., dishes, clothing, office supplies, and furniture). Each of the people in the group chooses one category, and takes turns picking up the cards belonging to that category. The strategy of sorting can be applied to putting away laundry (things to hang up, things for the drawer, things for the linen closet, things for long-term storage). Sorting incoming mail then follows (bills, read now, read later, throw away). Next, the group may be given a grocery list that may be sorted according to the signs in the aisles of a local grocery store, which have been photographed with a Polaroid camera. This one might be followed up with an actual trip to the grocery store to check for accuracy.

Different applications of a processing strategy represent different levels of generalization or transfer of skills. The therapist can identify a graded series of tasks that display decreasing degrees of physical and conceptual similarity to the original situation. To do this, potential tasks must be analyzed. The similarity of tasks depends on both surface characteristics and underlying concepts. Surface characteristics are as follows:

- Type of stimuli
- Presentation mode
- Variables of size, color, shape, etc.
- Stimuli arrangement
- Movement requirements
- Environmental context
- Rules or directions, number of steps

The underlying concepts of tasks are:

- Underlying skills required (eye-hand coordination)
- Nonsituational strategies (planning)
- Situational strategies (grouping, visual imagery)

Transfer of skills may be near, intermediate, far, or very far. The closer the practice task resembles the training task, the easier the transfer. Clients in the sorting group example had a fairly easy time understanding how to sort the laundry items presented as pictures. They may have more difficulty if a basket of laundry is dumped on the table in front of them because the mode of presentation and task requirement (hanging, folding) is different. The picture categories and pictures of laundry items might be considered near transfer because only two characteristics have changed (subject of pictures and categories). In intermediate transfer, three to six characteristics have changed. Actually sorting items and putting them away adds the characteristics of three dimensions—color, texture, and necessity of manipulation and movement. If the group takes a trip to the grocery store, they will be faced with a far transfer. Far transfer tasks are conceptually similar to the initial task, but the surface characteristics are either completely different or have only one surface similarity. In the grocery store exercise, the physical surroundings, number of people, number of steps, and variety of object properties makes the application of sorting by aisle and finding items on the grocery list a much more challenging task. Very far transfer refers to "generalization" or spontaneous application of what has

been learned to everyday functioning (Toglia, 1991, p. 508). After discharge from treatment, a person might be able to demonstrate the sorting strategy in cleaning out the attic or garage.

Dynamic Nature of Cognition

Grouping persons with brain dysfunction is based on Toglia's dynamic interactional assessment, which includes both the structural and functional capacity of each individual. Standardized pencil and paper or simulated tasks are not considered adequate for assessment. Processing skills in the six brain areas—orientation, attention, visual processing, motor planning, cognition (organization, memory, problem solving), and activity of daily living functions—are examined and evaluated in the context of the physical, social, and cultural environment and within the parameters and variables of everyday task performance. Often the functional capacities of brain-damaged individuals can be greater in familiar social and physical contexts than it appears in the clinic. This is because a person's capacity for cognitive functioning changes in different contexts. A person's cognitive functioning is largely dependent upon familiar cues from the environment and the expectations of one's social and cultural roles.

Therapy goals are set to match, as closely as possible, the expected roles and requirements of the discharge environments. Persons with similar learner capabilities are grouped together for learning selected strategies that are estimated to be within their capabilities. Metacognition and multi-contextual strategy training are then worked on simultaneously in these homogeneous groups. Multiple contexts for the strategy are used during interventions to encourage understanding of the significance of the strategy and a recognition of the properties of situations in which the strategy is appropriate. For example, estimating the time needed for task performance may be applied to a variety of tasks. The group might begin by estimating the time it will take them to read a one-page article, then reading the article and monitoring the time elapsed after each paragraph is completed and totaled at the end. Estimated times are compared with actual times

Cognitive Behavioral Concepts

Just as ego psychology was an outgrowth of psychoanalytic theory, cognitive behaviorism has advanced from the original behavioral theories. Cognitive behaviorists basically accept the principles of early behaviorism but have added thinking to the repertoire of human behavior that can be learned and modified. The fundamental change these psychological theories have made from their predecessors is their rejection of determinism. Behavior modification is an outdated technique by which behavior of the individual is essentially controlled by the therapist through the use of external reinforcement. This technique is seldom used nowadays, except for individuals with such a low level of self-control that self-reinforcement is not possible. Just as the concept of ego autonomy implies that man can adapt and change according to his own will, cognition in the cognitive frame allows man to regulate his own behavior. This concept has important implications for intervention.

Unlike behavior modification, which puts the control in the hands of the therapist and external forces, cognitive behavioral therapies seek to modify how a person thinks. Rather than just a stimulus and response continuum, thought processes are inserted between the two. The stimulus involves a situation and an emotion or feeling state; then an analysis of both the situation and the feeling occurs in which various response behaviors are considered and their consequences anticipated. Only after such an analysis does a behavioral response occur. Cognitive therapists seek to discover the thought processes of clients and to help clients use their own cognitive abilities to dispute thinking patterns that lead to problematic behaviors.

Cognitive behavioral therapy has become firmly planted in the field of occupational therapy, as most recently described by Duncombe (1997). In reviewing the literature, Duncombe has found that the role of occupational therapy is described by Aaron Beck and three other psychologists as follows:

> Occupational therapists who work in a psychiatric setting are primarily concerned with teaching skills to promote self-reliance and independence. These therapists have received extensive training on how to deal with actual physical, intellectual, or social deficits. In fact, they are probably better prepared than most psychiatrists, psychologists, or social workers to teach adaptive skills to persons with significant handicaps... The occupational therapist uses psychoeducational procedures, demonstrations, and in vivo rehearsal to build functional ability and self-esteem. (Duncombe & McCraith, 1997; Wright, Thase, Ludgate, & Beck, 1993)

Three major contributors to the psychological cognitive behavioral theory are identified by Bruce and Borg (2002) as Albert Bandura, Aaron Beck, and Albert Ellis.

Bandura's Social Learning Theory

Bandura's best known contribution to cognitive behavioral theory is his social learning theory (1977, p. 78). The major areas of focus in Bandura's work are:

- The role of internal and external reinforcers
- Mediating environment and person interactions
- Modeling and observation learning
- Self-control and self-regulation
- Alternative sources of motivation

Bandura's hierarchy of reinforcement, mentioned earlier, spans a range of both external and internal reinforcers. Regarding reinforcement, Bandura contends that the person as well as the environment determines behavior. A social learning interaction involves three factors: person, behavior, and environment. External reinforcers are measurable outcomes from the environment, such as getting a grade on a test. The person's interpretation and expectations are considered equally important; these are the internal reinforcers. Examples of external reinforcers are money, material goods, social approval or privileges, and penalties. Self-reinforcement develops with maturity and the enactment of internal values and self-expectations.

Person-Environment Interactions

The role of cognition in mediating environment and person interactions is another important component in social learning theory. Bandura contends that behavior is an interacting determinant of the outcome or response. For example, a group member's behavior might elicit anger in the other group members. Cognition affects the person in his or her beliefs about him- or herself and the group. Sam believes he is not an alcoholic, but that others in the group are alcoholics. This belief leads him to reflect an aloof attitude toward other members. When they ask him to participate, he refuses, and he will not respond to the comments of others. The group members interpret his behavior as critical of them—"He thinks he's better than we are." This makes them respond to Sam with anger. Sam hears their angry comments and feels rejected; he logically concludes that the group is not interested in him or able to help him. All of these processes,

beliefs, attitudes, interpretations, and logical conclusions are cognitive processes that influence the
person-environment interaction. In using this concept with clients, group leaders can design activities that facilitate an analysis of social interactions
that encourages the uncovering of underlying
beliefs and attitudes. These clients may be able to
use this process to question their own attitudes
and change beliefs that are troublesome.

Modeling and Observation Learning

Modeling and observation learning are types of
social learning that all persons engage in throughout life. Yet people do not imitate every behavior
they see. Cognition plays a major role in the analysis of observed behavior and the selection of which
behavior to model. Bandura (1977) contends that
this selection depends upon anticipated consequences. This means that individuals seek to
model behavior that they have observed to have
positive consequences. Occupational therapy group
leaders can use this process to great advantage.
Leaders can model positive responses to others,
effective interactions, and successful problem solving, for example. This technique helps clients to
increase their own interactional and problem-solving skills. An important advantage of group intervention is the learning that takes place from
watching and imitating each other.

Self-Control and Self-Regulation

Self-control and self-regulation are desired outcomes of therapy. The basic assumption is that
persons are in control of their own behavior and
can influence the outcome of their treatment.
Cognition influences their motivation, selection of
goals, and the ability to achieve them. Goals can
serve as guides for self-regulation. Persons can
measure their own progress in terms of desired
goals. Goals are always central in a cognitive
behavioral approach to group intervention. The
goals of the group are shared with clients and
agreed upon at the outset. Activities of the group
are directed toward the goal(s) and numbers often
evaluate the group in terms of progress toward the
goal. Since goals are clearly stated, progress can be
easily tested and reported by the therapist. This is
partly what makes this approach so useful in acute
care settings where gains are expected to be made
quickly and progress is evaluated on a daily basis.
This concept begins to apply at Allen's cognitive
level 4, for which goal-directed behavior is possible.

Cognition also influences the development of
insight or self-understanding. Educating clients in
how they might analyze their own attitudes,

behavior, and consequences will enhance their
ability to regulate their own behavior. When an
anxious client understands the forces in the environment and the beliefs in him- or herself that
contribute to his or her anxiety, that client can
more easily exercise self-control. He or she can
regulate the situation by reconsidering the reality
of his or her beliefs or removing him- or herself to
a less stressful environment. For example, Amy, a
college student, studies in her room where her
roommate constantly irritates her by playing loud
music. Amy believes she cannot study with loud
music playing. If she changes her attitude, she
may learn to enjoy the music or she may be able to
view it as a screen for other more distracting noises. If Amy cannot do this, she may choose to study
in the library.

Beck's Cognitive Distortions and Automatic Thoughts

Aaron Beck developed his methods of cognitive
behavioral therapy in the 1960s and 1970s
through his work with clients with depression. His
approach is founded in empirical investigation: he
treats the client's maladaptive interpretations and
conclusions about events as hypotheses to be tested. Beck collaborates with the client in conducting
behavioral experiments, verbal examinations of
alternative interpretations, reality testing, and
problem solving, with the goal of correcting cognitive distortions of reality.

From his clinical findings, Beck concludes that
psychological disturbances frequently stem from
automatic thoughts, which reflect habitual errors
in thinking (Beck, 1976). This cognitive model
does not assume that the cognitions operate exclusive of biochemistry or behavior symptomatic of
psychopathology. Cognition is considered the
problem and not the cause. The structure and
process of cognitive therapy includes setting the
agenda for the session, eliciting feedback, setting
goals for therapy, operationally defining problems,
testing hypotheses, problem-solving techniques,
and assigning homework. This structure lends
itself very well to occupational therapy groups
which can address through activities the cognitive
roadblocks to functional performance.

Ellis' Exposing Irrational Beliefs

Albert Ellis is well-known for his work in
rational emotive therapy (RET). Although Ellis and
Beck developed their techniques over approximately the same time period, each has his own
somewhat eclectic basis of which traditional
behavior therapy is only a part. Like Beck, Ellis

considered thinking to be a legitimate behavior that could be learned and modified using behavior modification techniques. A distinguishing feature of RET is its systematic exposition of irrational beliefs that result in emotional and behavioral disturbances. Ellis spends most of his energy looking for "unconditional shoulds" and "absolute musts." He contends that clients take "simple preferences" such as desire for love, approval, and success and make the mistake of thinking of them as dire needs.

Ellis's view of human nature is somewhat humanistic: he believes people have inborn tendencies toward growth and actualization. He takes for granted, however, that humans are fallible and often make mistakes resulting in "crooked thinking" and "self-defeating" behavior (Ellis, 1973). RET has developed into a kind of structured challenging and disputing of irrational beliefs. Its confrontive methodology, such as the use of exaggeration, absurdity, and humor, is not at all humanistic.

Cognitive Restructuring

Ellis suggests a philosophical restructuring process involving a series of steps (Ellis & Harper, 1975), all of which require high level thinking. This method reflects both humanistic self-determination and the supremacy of rational thinking in controlling and directing human behavior.

- Acknowledging our responsibility for creating our own problems
- Accepting our ability to change our own problems
- Seeing that emotional problems stem from irrational beliefs
- Clearly perceiving our beliefs
- Rigorously disputing beliefs
- Working hard to change beliefs resulting in disturbed emotion and behavior
- Continued cognitive monitoring and restructuring over our lifetime

Cognitive restructuring includes the process of questioning our decisions and life structures and considering alternatives. It is very much a skill development process to be used over one's lifetime. When emotional problems are identified, therapy consists of defining problems in thinking that contribute to the distressing emotions or behaviors and finding alternative, more realistic, and pragmatic ways of conceptualizing those life circumstances. The therapist acts as an educator-facilitator in collaborating with the client to achieve specific goals.

In occupational therapy groups, when we use a psychoeducational approach, our role as educator-facilitator is similar to that outlined by Ellis and Beck. Within the context of activities, occupational therapists can use cognitive restructuring principles to teach clients how to apply a scientific approach to thinking. Our goal is to teach skills that can be generalized by clients after they leave therapy groups. Groups that focus on pain management, time management, leisure planning, and health education/prevention are examples of occupational therapy groups using a cognitive behavioral approach. Discussion of the problems clients have in the performance of activities often leads to exposure of faulty thinking. In our higher functioning client groups, occupational therapist's can help the clients change their attitudes toward disability or ability as it affects performance. We can teach our group members to challenge each other and to encourage their use of rational thinking to solve problems.

Linehan's Dialectical Strategies

Dialectical behavior therapy (DBT) was developed by Dr. Marsha Linehan (1993a) over the past 15 years as an intervention specifically for borderline personality disorders (BPD). Persons with this disorder are frequently seen in hospitals (19% of mental health inpatients, 11% of mental health outpatients); they are burdensome to the health care system because there is no effective medical treatment. It is suspected that many more "undiagnosed" BPDs enter hospitals with a host of other diagnoses because of their tendency to exaggerate symptoms and their proneness to substance abuse and suicide attempts. Dr. Linehan translates the core of the disorder into cognitive behavioral terms, by emphasizing its "pattern of behavioral, emotional, and cognitive instability and dysregulation" (1993a, p. 11). Dialectic is defined by *Webster's College Dictionary* (1991) as "pertaining to logical argument" and includes "conversation revealing the truth through use of logic, juxtaposition of conflicting ideas, or forces (and) debate over a constantly changing reality." Those who are familiar with BPD will recognize immediately why this term was chosen. Hallmark symptoms of this character disorder include a tendency to distort reality, to either idolize or condemn others, to create drama and conflict in relationships, and to continually redefine their own identity. Acceptance of the nature of life as a constant struggle involving balance and imbalance of opposites is an important part of DBT. The dialectic approach to intervention meets the person with BPD on his or her own turf and teaches a logical approach to self-regulation.

Function and Dysfunction

Adaptation to the environment is the common measure across behavioral and cognitive theories. Behaviorists use the terms *adaptive behavior* and *learning* and attribute dysfunctional behavior to maladaptive learning. The emphasis is placed on concrete, observable behavior.

In the biomechanical and rehabilitation frames, a person is fully functional when he or she has no restrictions in range of motion, strength, and endurance and maintains the ability to perform the tasks necessary for work, play/leisure, self-care, and social roles. Function also includes the practice of good health maintenance habits.

Function in the cognitive rehabilitation frame of reference refers to information processing skills and their flexible use across task boundaries (generalization). Toglia and Abreu (1987) look at brain functioning as the behavior to be measured and measure this by the outward manifestations of orientation, attention, visual processing, motor planning, cognition (memory, organization, problem solving) and occupational behavior. However, Toglia rejects the notion of assessing these skills in isolation and has designed and researched several "dynamic" assessments that measure these cognitive processes during functional performance (Toglia, 1997). Dysfunction in cognitive rehabilitation is characterized by limitations in the brain's ability to process information efficiently. Symptoms of poor efficiency become obvious during the performance of everyday activities when there is a mismatch between the task and the skill level of the individual. Dysfunction in metacognition is significant in that the client's inaccurate self-perceptions cause him or her to misjudge the difficulty of tasks and the appropriateness of processing or compensatory strategies. Unawareness of one's own deficits prevents one from learning from mistakes and using feedback to modify behavior. Inefficiencies in organization, setting priorities, and shifting one's mental perspective or viewpoint are common areas of dysfunction to be treated from a cognitive rehabilitation perspective.

In cognitive behaviorism, a well-functioning individual has the ability to think logically and to form accurate perceptions of the self and the environment. He or she can use deductive reasoning to cope with problems and can logically regulate his or her own thoughts, feelings, and behavior. Dysfunction may be defined as faulty thinking, inaccurate self-perception, and the inability to handle one's affairs competently. Failure to adapt to the environment and to function independently in society in this frame of reference is seen as a product of cognitive disability. Therefore, it is cognitive impairments in attention, sensory awareness, perception, memory, and other thought processes that prevent efficient problem solving, interfere with learning and application of new coping strategies, and cause problems in doing functional activities. These cognitive functions, therefore, should be the focus of intervention in occupational therapy.

In designing groups with persons of similar cognitive ability, many assessments are available to use as guidelines. Claudia Allen (1997, workshop materials) has prepared a comparison chart of some of the most commonly used assessment scales, which may be helpful in selecting group membership (Table 6-4). Allen's Cognitive Levels scales are further defined in Chapter 7. The Medicare Physical Assistance and Cognitive Assistance Scales are taken from Medicare Part B Guidelines. Global Assessment of Functioning (GAF) comes from American Psychiatric Association (APA) (2000). For other scales, readers can refer to Katz (1997).

Change and Motivation

Following the guidelines of learning theory, the basic strategy for change is reinforcement. Change occurs when behavior is reinforced in some way. In behavior modification, behavior may be controlled and shaped by the therapist (or other person) using external reinforcement. The type of reinforcement that can be effective will vary from client to client. Some clients do not seem to have the internal motivation to learn new skills. For these clients, external reward is most appropriate. This can be anything the client is willing to work for, such as praise, extra attention, candy, cigarettes, or privileges. Bandura expanded the definition of reinforcement to include a range of internalized reinforcements. Some clients respond to social reinforcement, such as the praise and acceptance of their peers, family, or friends. At a higher level, clients will strive to learn skills or improve functioning in order to gain the approval

Table 6-4   Comparison of Various Medical Scales

Allen Cognitive Level	Medicare Cog. Assist. %	Medicare Physical Assist. %	Rancho Head Trauma	Global Deterioration Scale	Global Assess Scale	GAF DSM-IV Axis V	Age (Bayley Maturational) *approx.
0.8	100	100	I				
1.0	99		II				0 to 1 mo.
1.2	98		III				1 to 5 mo.
1.4	96	75					4 to 8 mo.
1.6	92						4 to 10 mo.
1.8	88	50		Severe			6 to 12 mo.
2.0	84	25	IV	7			9 to 17 mo.
2.2	82	15					10 to 20 mo.
2.4	78	10			1 to 10		
2.6	75						12 to 23 mo.
2.8	70					1 to 10	
3.0	64		V	Moderately	11 to 20	11 to 20	18 to -24 mo.
3.2	60			severe	21 to 30		
3.4	54			6	31 to 40	21 to 30	
3.6	50				41 to 50		3 yr.
3.8	46			Moderate		31 to 40	
4.0	42	8	VI	5	51 to 60		4 yr.
4.2	38						5 yr.
4.4	34			Mild	61 to 70		6 yr.
4.6	30		VII	4		41 to 50	
4.8	25				71 to 80		
5.0	22	6					7 to 10 yr.
5.2	18	4			81 to 90		11 to 13 yr.
5.4	14	2		3		51 to 60	14 to 16 yr.
5.6	10	0	VIII	2	91 to 100	61 to 80	17 yr.
5.8	6			No deficits		81 to 90	
6.0	0			1		91 to 100	18 to 21 yr.

of society or meet the expectations of their cultural group. The highest form, self-reinforcement, spontaneously emerges as the individual strives to measure up to his or her own internal standards. In occupational therapy, simple skills are mastered before more difficult ones are attempted. Thus the clients can develop a feeling of competence as each new skill is mastered. The feeling of competence gained from successful occupational performance, in itself, provides reinforcement. This is known as self-reinforcement, the highest form of motivation clients can achieve.

In the cognitive behavioral approaches, people change by changing the way they think. For adults with acquired brain injury, cognitive rehabilitation produces change by training in the use of remedial or compensatory processing strategies in the context of a broad range of tasks. To the extent that they are capable, persons use metacognitive strategies, increasing awareness, and monitoring of their own cognitive capacities and limitations. The occupational therapist can use a psychoeducational approach to teach clients to apply logic to produce adaptive change in persons with intact processing skills (e.g., persons with disorders of substance use, eating disorders, obsessive compulsive disorders, or personality disorders). In DBT, becoming aware of beliefs and attitudes that result in problem emotions and behaviors is the first step. Clients are sometimes asked to sign a contract, agreeing to try out new thinking and self-regulation strategies for a defined period of time. Challenging their "faulty thoughts" can often convince clients to change or replace them, and this will lead to a change in behavior.

Current cognitive approaches assume that people have a natural drive toward competence and mastery and to achieve a better position in life. People wish to be self-directed and to have an effect on others and on the environment. To achieve these goals, most people are willing to learn and try new coping strategies for problem solving and for self-improvement/regulation. A difficulty with this approach may be to find effective reinforcements for those clients who do not seem to be motivated or are unaware of a social pressure to improve their status.

Group Interventions

Groups are homogeneous in this frame of reference. This does not mean, however, that all the members have the same diagnosis. Since a broad range of functional levels, verbal and reasoning abilities, and diagnostic categories is being addressed, assessment of the critical abilities for group involvement is an important prerequisite. In planning group intervention, clients with similar needs or deficits are usually grouped together, and goals are set to address their common issues. Groups of no more than eight members focus on learning specific skills or strategies. Members should be at approximately the same cognitive level so that they will be able to learn at the same pace and through similar modes of presentation. Groups working on perception and memory skills in cognitive rehabilitation, for example, might be given several memory games during a therapy session. All the members should be able to understand the verbal directions if the activity is to be successful in accomplishing its goal. In a psychoeducational problem-solving group, the goals might be to master each step in the problem-solving process. Clients will be able to:

- Clearly state the desired outcome of the problem
- Gather relevant information
- Analyze and interpret the data
- Devise a plan to solve the problem (describe actions and sequence of steps)
- Implement the plan
- Evaluate the outcome

The goals in the behavioral-cognitive frames of reference are always very specific, observable, and measurable. This is because the intervention approach is very goal directed. Problems are generally addressed narrowly and specifically, and the learning, rehearsal, and practice of specific skills is usually the goal. The most closely aligned to behavioral theory is the biomechanical/rehabilitative frame of reference. When planning groups in this model, exercises to increase range of motion, strength, and endurance are demonstrated, imitated, and practiced in the groups within the context of functional activities. Groups may be designed around the need for training in the use of adaptive equipment or in techniques of energy conservation. Biofeedback and monitoring techniques during exercise groups allow individual members to participate at different levels, while having the advantage of group support and socialization. For the sake of clarity, any group examples that include elements of physical rehabilitation or the monitoring of physical attributes, such as relaxation, will be called biomechanical/rehabilitative, even though it may also draw upon behavioral techniques.

In cognitive rehabilitation, Toglia and Abreu's six cognitive areas—orientation, attention, visual processing, motor planning, cognition, and occupational behavior—may be used as guidelines for the selection of group activities. Persons who share similar functional problems may be treated in groups of three to six, or up to eight with a co-leader. The group should be structured so that several different contexts are presented for using the same strategy. For example, attention-sustaining strategies may be practiced with pencil and paper tasks, like alternating numbers and letters in a sequence when connecting dots on a page. Done in a group, partners can take turns monitoring and giving each other cues. Attention must be used when playing group board games, card games, or word games. Likewise, many visual processing, motor planning, memory, and problem-solving strategies may be learned and practiced in the context of group activities. There are numerous workbooks and collections of exercises that exist in the literature that are most helpful in planning groups (Dougherty & Radomski, 1987; Toglia & Abreu, 1987). Some of the advantages of working on cognitive strategies in groups are:

- Group "games" can be motivating and fun.
- Groups provide a real-life context for the use of skills.
- Therapeutic groups allow practice with guidance and safety.
- Feedback on performance from others increases self-awareness.
- Observation of a variety of group responses encourages generalization of skills.
- Possible applications of skills can be discussed and explored.

Psychoeducational groups, based on behavioral and cognitive-behavioral principles, may be designed for skill training, such as assertiveness, social skills, or stress management. Occupational therapists often use a psychoeducational approach involving the imparting of information and the use of structured learning exercises. In DBT, Dr. Linehan has identified specific issues that need to be addressed by persons with BPD, which she defines as a "disorder of self-regulation" (1993a). These are dysregulation of:

- Emotion
- Interpersonal relationships
- Behavior
- Cognition
- Sense of self

Group intervention has traditionally been the treatment of choice for individuals with BPD because of their difficulty with authority, their need for peer feedback, and the desirability of avoiding the power struggles that are inevitable in one-on-one relationships, therapeutic or otherwise. Linehan (1993b) has designed a workbook for psychosocial skills training, which outlines specific group exercises in four major categories:

1. Core mindfulness
2. Interpersonal effectiveness
3. Emotion regulation
4. Distress tolerance

Core Mindfulness

This teaches the mind to focus on one thing at a time, to pay attention to all the information available in a situation, and to refrain from quick judgments, jumping to conclusions, or acting on the basis of emotional responses. A useful technique is writing; taking time to describe conflict situations in words delays the response and leads away from the emotional and into the rational, analytical mind. Awareness of beliefs and attitudes one typically uses and analyzing these applying logic, labeling behaviors, and emotions as harmful and destructive or helpful and productive in accomplishing one's objectives in the conflict situation are also a focus of group exercises in the mindfulness category.

Interpersonal Effectiveness

Skills for achieving specific objectives in relationships, getting and keeping good relationships, and maintaining self-respect in relationships are learned and practiced in these group exercises. Recognition of the factors that interfere with relationships, strategies for challenging these negative factors, and self-reinforcing positive responses are also included. Exercises for expression of feelings and opinions, negotiating, reciprocating, and making specific requests help to build a repertoire of skills for building and maintaining healthy interpersonal relationships.

Emotion Regulation

This series of exercises begins with challenging beliefs about emotions and their importance. Describing and naming the emotions (love, joy, shame, fear, sadness, and anger are major categories) becomes the first step toward a rational approach, reducing vulnerability to the negative effects of emotions. Exercises in effective self-interventions when emotions threaten to overwhelm or take over include strategies for evoking positive emotion, building positive experiences, and steps to reduce painful emotions.

Distress Tolerance

These exercises for groups teach techniques for crisis survival. The goal is to stop the negative behavioral responses typical of BPD, such as substance abuse and self-destructive or suicidal acts. Strategies for distracting, self-soothing, and improving the moment (prayer, relaxation, deep breathing, brief escape) allow time for reason to gain control. Attitude change from "This is awful" to "I can survive this" is practiced. This is followed by exercises in the application of logic: listing the pros and cons for tolerating the distress and directing "willfulness" (imposing one's will on reality) toward what works, and not what interferes with survival. Developing an awareness of the pleasures of ordinary tasks and cultivation a "half-smile" of acceptance leads group members toward the expectation that it is OK for life to be ordinary and that life circumstances are not always going to be ideal.

Care is taken to address each of these psychosocial skill areas in positive terms, avoiding the least hint of criticism (which commonly evokes anger and thus interferes with learning). The exercises use a variety of cognitive restructuring techniques to modify dysfunctional assumptions and beliefs and other behavioral and cognitive techniques mentioned earlier, including practice and rehearsal, therapist reinforcement, feedback and coaching, modeling and role playing. Groups of six to eight members are suggested for skill training, and these are offered in 8-week modules, complete with worksheets, handouts, and homework. Linehan offers workshops for training in DBT, which are open to occupational therapists as well as other professionals. Her *Skills Training Manual for Treating Borderline Personality Disorder* includes handouts that may be photocopied for use with client groups (Linehan, 1993b).

Role of the Leader

The occupational therapist's role is more directive in this frame of reference than it is in most others. In a hospital setting, the focus is often on evaluation. The therapist typically chooses the activity or task and structures the group for concentrated work toward a specific goal. Efficiency in goal attainment is all important, and the occupa-

tional therapist structures the group and the environment with this in mind. The therapist's role is active during the group, giving assistance, providing cues, and asking questions that will guide group members to improve their performance. Discussion may require frequent redirection to remain focused, with the guiding principle of reinforcing the learning of specific skills and achievement of specific goals. The occupational therapist should carefully monitor interaction to make sure the feedback given by members to each other is of a therapeutic nature.

Goals of the Group

Goals are behaviorally defined, specific, observable, and measurable. Occupational therapy goals are practical in nature, focusing on increasing functional performance. This fact alone makes the behavioral cognitive approach the best fit in the current health care atmosphere. Measurable goals are easy to document and justify the need for intervention. In working with the physical or cognitive perceptual dysfunction, the therapist sets goals for the group based on his or her best assessment of the client's potential. Norms are helpful in setting goals in the biomechanical areas (e.g., "resume normal strength in the injured right leg," "increase range of motion from 160 to 180 degrees in a spastic elbow"). In clients with temporary cognitive impairment, Allen's Cognitive Level 6 or Rancho Los Amigo's head trauma level VII may be an appropriate goal. For clients with the capacity for rational thought, the goal is insight. Only when a client understands the impact of his or her cognitive distortions and irrational beliefs is he or she able or willing to change them. It is assumed that a change in thinking will produce a change in behavior. Therefore, goals will generally address the thought processes rather than the affective or overt behavioral components.

Current literature in occupational therapy has emphasized the importance of culture and individual values in goal selection. For this reason, the client's own preference and social expectations may play a part in determining the goals. Research has shown that a meaningful task increases motivation and elicits a client's best effort. Long-term goals may be set collaboratively with each client, based on his or her expected environment, culture, and social roles. Within the group, limited choices can be offered, so that individual interests and preferences may become incorporated into the group experience.

Activity Examples

In psychoeducational groups, occupational therapists use and adapt many specific behavioral techniques to enhance group learning. Some of these techniques should be recognized as very powerful and therefore dangerous to use without specific training. Some of the techniques occupational therapists should avoid unless specifically trained are flooding, paradoxical intention, and systematic desensitization. These techniques involve vivid imaging of much-feared and disturbing situations, and the management of clients who have been so aroused requires more advanced therapeutic skills.

However, in moderation, imaging and visualization may be incorporated into a structured activity or may be expanded into drawing, sculpture, or dramatic role play. The use of images or visualization is a technique many occupational therapists have found helpful. For example, the guided fantasy can enhance relaxation and foster creativity and self-awareness. Once goals are set, visualizing images of their successful achievement is often motivating. Drawing images of various kinds is one way to structure our groups to work on specific goals.

The concepts of group problem solving, keeping journals, and giving homework are also useful ideas in occupational therapy groups. Behavior rehearsal may be useful in the learning and practice of social skills. Some other techniques are contracts with one's self or with the group to change certain thoughts and behavior, self-reward or self-punishment, writing beliefs in words and then deciding if the statements are true or false and positive or negative labeling of thoughts, feelings, and behavior. The reader is referred to McMullin's *Handbook of Cognitive Therapy Techniques* (1986), Linehan's *Skills Training Manual for Treating Borderline Personality Disorder* (1993b), Moyers' *Substance Abuse: A Multi-Dimensional Assessment and Treatment Approach* (1992), and Precin's *Living Skills Recovery Workbook* (1996) for more ideas.

At the end of the chapter are some examples of cognitive behavioral groups (Activity Examples 6-1 through 6-8). They will be identified as belonging to one of the following categories: biomechanical/rehabilitative, cognitive rehabilitative, or psychoeducational. All of these categories use behavioral and cognitive principles, techniques, and strategies.

Group Leadership

The seven-step group format is not changed in structure. If anything, in this frame of reference, groups become even more structured. The beginning of the group places an emphasis on defining specific problems and collaborative goal setting. The therapist may do this individually before the group begins.

Introduction

This kind of group will dispense with the warm-up and get right down to business. A more complete explanation of the goals and purpose will substitute. Expectations are spelled out in behavioral terms, and the group is told how their progress will be evaluated. The time frame of the group should coincide with the members' level of cognitive functioning.

Activity

Cognitive behavioral groups focus on learning coping skills and improving task performance. There is usually didactic instruction given in the form of short lectures or demonstrations of the steps in doing a task. The activities are learning experiences and opportunities for practice. In a leisure skills group, for example, members learn to do a series of specific activities: how to knit, how to cook, how to catch a fish, how to play card games. In a stress management group, the occupational therapist gives mini-lessons in cardiovascular fitness, high nutrition diets, and progressive relaxation in conjunction with activities. The experience may take longer, up to two-thirds of the session, leaving the rest for discussion/demonstration.

Sharing

If members have done an individual activity, such as a worksheet, this is the time for reading it aloud or holding it up for the group to see. The leader should give recognition and feedback and encourage other group members to do the same. In the cognitive rehabilitation groups, this is an opportunity to discuss self-evaluations and compare results. Leaders should be cautious not to encourage competition, but to place emphasis on how well each member was able to predict and monitor his or her own performance. For cognitive behavioral and psychoeducational groups, feedback from others is an important social reinforcement to learning and should be offered to all members. Feedback comes mostly from the therapist in the lower level groups and from fellow members in higher level groups.

Processing

Discussion of the underlying dynamics of the group is also not an area of focus. Most of the interaction should be between the leader and each member, just as a teacher interacts with a class. However, when the feelings or the implicit forces of the group begin to interfere with group learning, then the therapist must temporarily make group process the focus. This is not to say, however, that feelings about the activity should be ignored. This part of the discussion should invite honest expression of emotions, both positive and negative, as they pertain to the issues addressed by the activity. The group energy may be rallied in support of members who are discouraged with their progress or having difficulty adapting to residual or permanent dysfunction. Group leaders need to beware of the offering of false hope or flattery by members, and discussion should be kept focused and controlled.

Generalizing

Inductive reasoning is encouraged in the members to come up with general principles to be learned from the experience. Inductive reasoning involves collecting evidence from many specific examples to build a general principle or theory. Members can do this best when they have heard several responses to the experience from other members, which has hopefully been done in the sharing and processing steps. In a well-planned group, the general principles suggested by the members will coincide with group goals. If this does not happen spontaneously, the therapist should help the group to make the connections. In cognitive rehabilitation groups, for example, members may take this opportunity to verbalize the specific strategies on which they have worked, take note of what they learned about their own ability to process information, and summarize insight they have gained.

Application

There is more emphasis here than in any other part of the discussion. An effective group will include a carry-over of behavior change from the clinic to the community environment. An open group discussion of how newly learned strategies may be concretely applied in everyday life will increase the likelihood of carry-over. Members should know before they leave the group exactly how they will apply their new knowledge or skill. Application requires deductive reasoning, the application of theoretical ideas to specific, individual situations. Often the therapist must structure this reasoning with thought-provoking discussion questions and concrete examples. Members may then share ideas on how to do this. The activities done by the group are usually planned to address specific problems, so the application is generally built into the group experience at the outset. If clients leave the group consciously aware of the usefulness of certain skills, they may communicate this to family members and caretakers, and they may initiate the process of self-reinforcement. Homework may be given by the therapist to support the application of what is learned. When homework is given, a time frame should be included, and members should know when and where they will be asked to report on the results of the homework activity.

Summary

A verbal summary by the therapist is a tradition to be continued throughout the frames of reference. In this one, its major purpose is to reinforce learning. It is best done by the therapist in most cases. Emphasizing the important points of the session and giving positive feedback to members are the important elements. The few minutes it takes to summarize may make the difference between forgetting and remembering what was learned. Reminders about homework and announcements about what is planned next are also appropriate.

Bibliography

Abreu, B., & Toglia, J. (1987). Cognitive rehabilitation: A model for occupational therapy. *American Journal of Occupational Therapy, 41,* 439-448.

American Occupational Therapy Association. (2002). Occupational therapy practice framework: Domain and process. *American Journal of Occupational Therapy, 56,* 609-629.

American Psychiatric Association. (2000). *Diagnostic and statistical manual* (4th ed., revised). Washington DC: Author.

Bandura, A. (1977). *Social learning theory.* Englewood Cliffs, NJ: Prentice-Hall.

Beck, A. (1976). *Cognitive therapy and emotional disorders.* New York: International University Press.

Bracy, O. (1986). Cognitive rehabilitation: A process approach. *Journal of Cognitive Rehabilitation, Mar/Apr,* 10-17.

Bruce, M., & Borg, B. (2002). *Psychosocial frames of reference: Core for occupation-based practice.* Thorofare, NJ: SLACK Incorporated.

Corey, G. (1996). *Theory and practice of counseling and psychotherapy* (5th ed.). Monterrey, CA: Brooks/Cole.

Denton, P. L. (1987). *Psychiatric occupational therapy: A workbook of practical skills.* Boston: Little, Brown, & Co.

Dougherty, P., & Radomski, M. V. (1987). *The cognitive rehabilitation workbook.* Rockville, MD: Aspen.

Duncombe, L. (1997). Cognitive behavioral model in mental health. In N. Katz (Ed.), *Cognition and occupation in rehabilitation: Cognitive models for intervention in occupational therapy.* Bethesda, MD: American Occupational Therapy Association.

Duncombe, L., & McCraith, D. (1997). *Cognitive approaches for psychosocial evaluation and intervention, AOTA, SIS Practice.* Phoenix: Paper Presentation.

Ellis, A. (1973). *Humanistic psychology: The rational emotive approach.* New York: McGraw-Hill.

Ellis, A., & Harper, R. (1975). *A new guide to rational living.* North Hollywood, CA: Wilshire Book Co.

Fidler, G. (1996). Lifestyle performance: From profile to conceptual model. *American Journal of Occupational Therapy, 50,* 139-147.

Greenfield, J. M., & Godinez, M. (1989). *Stroke patients learn independence by leading their own therapy group.* Bethesda, MD: American Occupational Therapy Association.

Harlowe, D., & Yu, P. (1997). *The ROM dance: A range of motion exercise and relaxation program.* Madison, WI: Uncharted Country Publishing.

James, W. (1985). Habit: Its importance for psychology. *OT in Mental Health, 5*(3), 55-67.

Katz, N. (1997). *Cognition and occupation in rehabilitation: Cognitive models for intervention in occupational therapy.* Bethesda, MD: American Occupational Therapy Association.

Linehan, M. (1993a). *Cognitive-behavioral treatment of borderline personality disorder.* New York: The Guilford Press.

Linehan, M. (1993b). *Skills training manual for treating borderline personality disorder.* New York: The Guilford Press.

Luria, A. (1973). *The working brain.* New York: Basic Books.

Luria, A. (1980). *Higher cortical functions in man.* New York: Basic Books.

Macdonald, K. (1998). Adaptation. In *Disseration Abstracts.* New York: New York University.

McMullin, R. E. (1986). *Handbook of cognitive behavioral techniques.* New York: Norton.

Mosey, A. (1986). *Psychosocial components of occupational therapy.* New York: Raven.

Moyers, P. (1992). *Substance abuse: A multi-dimensional assessment and treatment approach.* Thorofare, NJ: SLACK Incorporated.

Posthuma, B. (2002). *Small groups in counseling and therapy: Process and leadership* (4th ed.). Boston: Little, Brown & Co.

Precin, P. (1996). *Living skills recovery workbook.* Boston: Butterworth Heinemann.

Robertson, S. (1988). *Mental health focus.* Rockville, MD: American Occupational Therapy Association.

Skinner, B. F. (1953). *Science and human behavior.* New York: Macmillan Co.

Stein, F., & Nikolic, S. (1989). Teaching stress management techniques to a schizophrenic patient. *American Journal of Occupational Therapy, 43,* 162-169.

Toglia, J. (1991). Generalization of treatment: A multi-context approach to cognitive perceptual impairment in adults with brain injury. *American Journal of Occupational Therapy, 45,* 505-516.

Toglia, J. (1997). A dynamic interactional approach to cognitive rehabilitation. In N. Katz (Ed.), *Cognition and occupation in rehabilitation: Cognitive models for intervention in occupational therapy.* Bethesda, MD: American Occupational Therapy Association.

Toglia, J. (2003). Multicontext treatment approach. In E. Crepeau, E. Cohn, & B. Boyt Schell (Eds.), *Willard & Spackman's occupational therapy.* Philadelphia: Lippincott, Williams & Wilkins.

Toglia, J., & Abreu, B. (1987). *Cognitive rehabilitation.* New York: Authors.

Trombly, C., & Radomski, M. V. (Eds.). (2002). *Occupational therapy for physical dysfunction* (5th ed.). Philadelphia: Lippincott, Williams & Wilkins.

Van Deusen, J., & Harlowe, D. (1987). The efficacy of the ROM dance program for adults with rheumatoid arthritis. *American Journal of Occupational Therapy, 41*(2), 90-95.

Velde, B., & Fidler, G. (2002). *Lifestyle performance: A model for engaging the power of occupation.* Thorofare, NJ: SLACK Incorporated.

Webster's College Dictionary. (1991). New York: Random House.

White, R. H. (1967). Competence and the growth of personality. In *Science and Psychoanalysis, Vol. XI, The Ego.* New York: Grune and Stratton.

Wright, J., Thase, M., Ludgate, J., & Beck, A. (1993). *The cognitive milieu: Structure and process in cognitive therapy with inpatients.* New York: Guilford.

Behavioral Cognitive

Activity Example 6-1

I Can Remember (Cognitive Rehabilitation)

Materials: Twenty objects on a tray, selected from three different categories (e.g., things normally found in the kitchen, things normally found in an office, and grooming items normally found in a bathroom cabinet), towel to cover items from sight, pencils and paper for each member, and a printed list of 10 commonly known names of objects (e.g., telephone, ruler, picture frame, mailbox, baseball, lamp, pitcher, teddy bear, stool, boat) for each member.

Strategies: Repetition and rehearsal, grouping and counting.

Directions: There are many reasons why we might need to be able to remember things. What are some things that are important for you to remember? Today we will practice two strategies to assist you in remembering things.

Repetition and Rehearsal

When you encounter something you want to remember, say it over and over to yourself. For example, when you meet someone new, say the person's name to yourself four or five times. Look at the person as you are doing this so that the name and the face will be connected in your brain. To practice this, turn to the person next to you and introduce yourself. (If they already know each other, making up a new name or using their middle names may suffice.) Using his name in the next sentence of conversation is another way to practice: "Nice to meet you, Henry" or "Henry, how are you feeling today?"

Next, we will use the same strategy to memorize a list of words. (Give out printed list.) You will note that the worksheet lists common objects numbered 1 to 10. Before we start, I would like you each to predict how many of these items you think you will be able to remember after 1 minute of practice. Write this number down on the top of your paper. Now begin memorizing, using repetition and rehearsal, repeating the words over and over. (Time for 1 minute.) Time is up. Please turn you paper over and write on the back as many words as you can remember. No looking at each other's papers is allowed. How does the result compare with your prediction? Look back at the list and correct your errors. This can be repeated if desired.

Next, we will practice remembering objects that we see. I will show you a tray full of objects, and you will have 1 minute to look at them. During that minute, you should say the name of each object to yourself. When I cover the tray of objects, you will write down as many names of objects as you can remember, so get your pencils out. Paper will be given out as soon as the objects are covered. No note-taking is allowed. (Place the tray in the center of the table, uncover it for 1 minute, then re-cover it.) How did everyone do? How many objects did you list? How many were there all together? Did anyone count?

Behavioral Cognitive

Activity Example 6-1

I Can Remember (Cognitive Rehabilitation) (continued)

Grouping and Counting

The second strategy we will use is counting the items you wish to remember and then grouping them into categories. When we try this again, count the objects first, then try to remember items together that are associated in some way. This strategy is used in addition to the repetition and rehearsal we have already practiced. There are objects from three categories on this tray. Did anyone notice what those might be? (Discuss and clarify the strategy as needed. Give out blank paper.) Before we begin, we will predict how many items we can remember this time, and write that number down in the corner of your paper. Now we will begin. (Uncover tray and time for 1 minute, then re-cover.) Write down as many as you can remember. (Pause.) How many items were there? (20) How many were in each category? Let's make a master list. (Have someone volunteer.) Write the three categories, then have group list the items. When finished, uncover tray once again to self-correct errors. How did people do in comparison with last time? Did the grouping help you to remember more items? Now compare with your predictions. Application discussion follows, in which members discuss two or three ways they can use these strategies during the next week. Homework may be given as needed.

Behavioral Cognitive
Activity Example 6-2
Setting Priorities (Psychoeducational)

This activity has been used as the first session of a time management workshop for clients with substance abuse. It serves as an ice breaker for clients who do not know each other well, and also helps the therapist to formulate goals for the group.

Materials: Values Survey Worksheets (p. 168) and pencils.

Directions: Often the things we spend our time doing are not the things we want most to do. Setting priorities means deciding what is important to us and doing that first. As a first step in helping to plan our time better, we will look at what we value.

(Pass out Values Survey Worksheet.) Take the next 10 minutes to think about the values listed, and number them according to their order of importance to you. Put number 1 next to the most important item, number 2 for the next level of importance, and so forth, up to number 8 for the least important. Do not use the same number more than once.

(Ask each member to share their top three values and discuss in what way these values are a part of his or her life right now.)

Write your top three values on the lower section of the Values Survey Worksheet, and below each write one specific goal that reflects that value. For example, if "freedom to do what I want" is one of your values, your goal might be to move out of your parents' house and get your own apartment. You have 5 minutes for this part.

Looking at your goals, choose one to work on this weekend. At the bottom of the worksheet, write down one activity that you can plan this weekend to help you accomplish the goal.

From Cole, M. B. *Group dynamics in occupational therapy: The theoretical basis and practice application of group intervention* (3rd ed.). Thorofare, NJ: SLACK Incorporated. © 2005 SLACK Incorporated.

Values Survey Worksheet

Directions: Eight commonly held values are listed here. Think about your own life in relation to these values. Then give each a number, beginning with number 1 for the most important to you, number 2 for the second most important, and so forth, up to number 8 for the least important. Do not use any number more than once.

_____ A good love relationship
_____ Financial security
_____ A satisfying religious faith
_____ Freedom to do what I want
_____ Meaningful family life
_____ Success at my chosen career
_____ Excitement and adventure
_____ Making lots of money

First most important value:

Goal:

Second most important value:

Goal:

Third most important value:

Goal:

Planned activity to work on goal:

From Cole, M. B. *Group dynamics in occupational therapy: The theoretical basis and practice application of group intervention* (3rd ed.). Thorofare, NJ: SLACK Incorporated. © 2005 SLACK Incorporated.

Behavioral Cognitive

Activity Example 6-3

Telling Others About Your Illness (Psychoeducational)

This behavioral cognitive activity has been part of a client group on coping with illness. The group is given short lectures each week on a different aspect of coping with illness, followed by participation in a related activity. This one uses role playing and behavioral rehearsal, and the support of the group serves as social reinforcement.

Materials: Two chairs placed in the center of the group.

Directions: Each patient will take a turn sitting in the chair in the center. First, the client will tell the group what his or her illness is, and why it is difficult to talk to others about it. Then the client will choose another member to play the part of a relative or friend. The therapist is the "director" and directs as follows:

Friend or relative: Ask how the patient is and ask follow-up questions.

Client: Answer him or her as if it were a real conversation.

Client: Now change places with your friend and respond for him or her. Now change places again and be yourself again. Try to tell your friend how you "feel" about being ill. Try to keep each conversation going for about 5 minutes. Members should volunteer for this and no one should be forced.

After each discussion, the group is asked to respond and to discuss the role play. Were the players being "genuine?" Were feelings being expressed freely? What are other ways to make the discussion helpful?

Behavioral Cognitive

Activity Example 6-4

Relaxation Fantasy Activity (Biomechanical/Rehabilitative)

This activity has been a part of a stress management group in which members use the techniques of visualization and guided fantasy to control their state of tension.

Materials: Carpeted open space, patients wearing sweatsuits and sneakers or other comfortable clothing, and pillows for each person.

Directions: Members sit in a circle on the floor, pillows in their laps. They should be far enough apart that all can lie down and reach out their arms without touching one another.

1. Introduction—Relaxation is as much in your mind as in your body. Therefore, if you want to be relaxed and free your body from stress, your mind must take the lead. It is very difficult to feel relaxed when your mind is preoccupied with worry. As you do this exercise, try to concentrate on the visual images that come into your head. Instructions will be given for you to move your physical position as well as parts of your body. Try to do these with your eyes closed, so you will not lose the mental images created.

2. You are about to take a 30-minute relaxation break from your busy, stressful, or boring day. Maybe you have a lot of work to do or a difficult situation to face. Put that out of your mind for the next 30 minutes. Afterward, when you are relaxed, you will have more energy to cope with life's hassles.

3. Begin by reaching both arms up over your head in a big stretch. Open your mouth wide and yawn. Now place the pillow behind your hips and lean back on your elbows. Close your eyes and imagine a door far across the room in front of you. Without moving your position, imagine yourself walking toward the door. Move your feet, your ankles, your knees, and your hips as if you were walking. When the right leg is tense, allow the left one to relax. Now point your toes each time you take a "step." Slow down your steps and inhale as you tense your right leg, then exhale as you tense your left leg. As you approach the door, your steps become slower and slower (2 minutes). When you reach the door, stand in front of it and continue breathing slowly.

4. Push yourself up with your arms to a sitting position. With your eyes still closed, lean forward and peek through a small hole in the door. You see a welcome view. It is a lovely, sunny patio with a sparkling in-ground pool. It is surrounded by clean, comfortable lounge chairs. Keep your hands behind you on the floor as you lean forward to get a better view. Stretch your back and push yourself forward with your arms until you feel the stretch behind your thighs. Keep breathing slowly.

5. With eyes still closed, bend your knees up to your chest. With one hand gripping each knee, imagine that your knees are the handles of the door. Pull gently on the "handles," straightening your back as you pull. Then let go as the door opens wide. As you pass through the door, you leave behind all the worries of the day. On the other side of the door there are no worries, no stress, so let them all go.

6. Without opening your eyes, straighten your legs and move the pillow under your head as you lie down on one of the comfortable lounge chairs. The sun feels good as it warms you. Imagine you are wearing a bathing suit under your sweatshirt. While still lying down, pretend to take the sweatshirt off. First, put hands near hips and push down on elbows to raise hips slightly off the floor. Then raise hands up to chest level, elbows still on the floor. Push head back into the pillow as you raise shoulders slightly off the floor. Pause here and breathe. Now raise your head off the pillow as you pretend to lift the sweatshirt off over your head and let it drop to the ground behind your pillow. This done, slowly return arms to your sides while breathing out slowly. Just lie there breathing slowly, enjoying the warm sun (2 minutes).

Behavioral Cognitive

Activity Example 6-4

Relaxation Fantasy Activity
(Biomechanical/Rehabilitative) (continued)

7. Check your body to be sure it is relaxed. Wiggle your fingers and your toes. Roll your head to the right, then roll your head to the left. If there is tension anywhere, shake it out. Put your hand behind your neck and massage your neck muscles. Keep breathing slowly. It feels so relaxing to lie here in the warm sun (2 minutes).

8. The sun is getting hot now. Maybe it is time to go for a swim. Raise yourself up to a sitting position again and bring your knees up to your chest. Now imagine you are sitting on the edge of the pool. Dangle your legs into the pleasantly cool water. Turn around to the left and look behind you; turn around to the right and look behind you. The signs say "Good Swimming Today," so turn over slowly onto your stomach as you lower your self into the water.

9. As you float on your stomach, your pillow has become a life preserver. Hold onto the pillow as you kick your legs slowly, floating around the pool. Your feet need not even leave the floor. It takes almost no effort at all to move you through the water. Your body does not feel heavy. Now inhale as you kick your right leg, exhale as you kick your left leg. As you reach the edge of the pool, push away again, continuing to hold onto the life preserver with one hand, then the other.

10. Now lift up on your elbows and push the pillow down under your ribcage, so it supports your chest as you lean on your elbows. Continue to breathe slowly. Shrug your shoulders up toward your ears, then release. Shrug away your last bit of tension. Now you are relaxed, refreshed, and energetic. Now you are capable of resuming your day without feeling tension and stress. Miraculously, you are out of the pool, dry and dressed again, standing in front of the door. Now you feel prepared to go back through that door and take on the world. When you are ready, open your eyes.

From Cole, M. B. *Group dynamics in occupational therapy: The theoretical basis and practice application of group intervention* (3rd ed.). Thorofare, NJ: SLACK Incorporated. © 2005 SLACK Incorporated.

Behavioral Cognitive
Activity Example 6-5
Building Our Community (Psychoeducational)

This activity is part of a psychoeducational group focusing on independent living skills with clients who have mental health issues. The goal of this session is to help the group become aware of community resources. My thanks to D. M. Hancock, occupational therapy student at Quinnipiac College, for this creative idea.

Materials: One square of 1/4-inch plywood, approximately 30 x 30 inches, a variety of small blocks of scrap wood with rough edges and splinters sanded off, jars of poster paint in several colors, brushes, and wood glue. This project may take two sessions to complete.

Directions: The group begins by discussing the communities in which they live and what services and resources are available there. The occupational therapist helps the group develop a list of services members need to have available in their community. A typical list includes a hospital, grocery store, department store, drug store, police department, fire department, school, and movie theater. Why they need each one and how they would use it is discussed.

Next, the group members build from the blocks a community they would like to live in. Each member chooses one or more community resources to build, and constructs a school, a movie theater, etc. by gluing blocks together. The "buildings" are then painted and colored signs are painted on to label them. Buildings are then placed and glued onto the plywood square, something like an architect's model city. Streets, parking lots, parks, or bodies of water may be painted directly on the plywood if desired (Figure 6-3).

Discussion/Summary: Sharing has already been done during the activity. Members are asked how they felt about doing the activity and about the result. Some generalization was done earlier, in the choices of structures and organizations to be included in the community, and their uses and importance. This may be reinforced and elaborated here, with an emphasis on how to contact and use community resources appropriately to meet one's needs. Each member then compares the "model" they have built to his or her own neighborhood or community. Application includes each member's plans for using his or her own community resources, now and in the future.

Figure 6-3. Our community.

From Cole, M. B. *Group dynamics in occupational therapy: The theoretical basis and practice application of group intervention* (3rd ed.). Thorofare, NJ: SLACK Incorporated. © 2005 SLACK Incorporated.

Behavioral Cognitive
Activity Example 6-6
Exercise Groups (Biomechanical/Rehabilitative)

Exercise to music or dance activities have good potential as therapeutic tools. Circle or group dancing is usually best suited to our purpose in occupational therapy. In physical disability areas where goals involve maintaining and increasing strength and ROM, group activities that accomplish these goals are more enjoyable and motivating than individual exercise programs. A good example of this type of group is the "Range of Motion Dance," an exercise program for patients with rheumatoid arthritis developed by Diane Harlowe and Patricia Yu at St. Mary's Hospital Medical Center in Madison, Wisconsin (Van Deusen & Harlowe, 1987). This is a guided fantasy done with groups of arthritis clients seated in chairs. The exercises, while following the story, go systematically through the ROM for nearly every joint in the body. Once the sequence of motions is learned, it can be repeated by the patients at home by listening to the story on an audiotape.

Greenfield and Godinez have introduced a similar group for persons recovering from stroke, called "Self Range of Motion Exercises" (1989). They have defined eight skill levels for these exercises, ranging from complete dependence on the therapist leader to independence in performing the exercises.

In doing such groups, it is important to use the potential of the group to provide mutual support, encouragement, and feedback. Do not let the activity speak for itself; combine it with verbal reinforcement, progress checks, and education about how and why it is helping. It is generally the social and emotional aspects of a group that keep members coming back.

Behavioral Cognitive
Activity Example 6-7
Map Reading (Cognitive Rehabilitation)

A group of clients with cognitive impairments has the goal of improving skills in visual processing and verbal communication. They are given a map of their community, and a worksheet with a list of 10 locations. The following are examples of their tasks:

1. Write directions from Merritt Park Way to the Trumbull Shopping Mall on Main Street.
2. Write directions from the corner of Madison and Stonehouse Roads to Trumbull High School on Stroebel and Daniels Farms Roads.
3. Describe two alternate routes to get from the golf course on Tashua Road to Main Street at the Bridgeport line.
4. Direct someone from Teller and Whitney to the dog pound on Church Street.
5. Plan a route to pick up three friends, on Indian Ledge Road, Brittany Road, and Autumn Ridge Road, and take them to the Town Hall meeting room on Quality Street.

To change the context, other maps or diagrams can be introduced and directions given verbally or in writing. Each client in the group should have at least one location to find on his own, and then communicate the directions to the rest of the group. The therapist should encourage members to give each other feedback about the accuracy of the directions and clarity of communication.

From Cole, M. B. *Group dynamics in occupational therapy: The theoretical basis and practice application of group intervention* (3rd ed.). Thorofare, NJ: SLACK Incorporated. © 2005 SLACK Incorporated.

Behavioral Cognitive

Activity Example 6-8

Design Duplication (Cognitive Rehabilitation)

This activity appears in *The Cognitive Rehabilitation Workbook* by Dougherty and Radomski (1987). The goals are to give and follow verbal directions. The objectives are to develop vocabulary to give precise directions, increase accuracy in conveying detailed information, and develop a tolerance for the pitfalls in making one's self understood. Followers of directions are expected to increase their accuracy, develop skills in clarification and confirmation, and increase speed of processing verbal directions.

A group of six is divided into pairs. One from each pair acts as the direction giver and holds a line drawing of several lines and shapes. The other half of each pair sits with his or her back to his or her partner and holds a clipboard with blank paper and a pencil with an eraser. Both partners are provided with rulers. Partner 1 must verbally describe the line drawing so that Partner 2 can draw an exact duplicate of the drawing being described. Attention must be paid to shapes, spacing, and dimensions. The pair has 20 minutes to accomplish the task. Then, a new drawing is given to each pair and roles are reversed.

It is very important that a feedback session follows each trial. The pairs should discuss the results and analyze any errors in communication in order to correct these on the next trial. This activity can be fun as well as useful, and the therapist should try to create a relaxed atmosphere for the group.

Chapter 7

Allen's Cognitive Disabilities Group

The group approach discussed here is the cognitive disabilities theory of Claudia Allen. Allen has been developing this theory since the early 1970s. Her basic premise is that functional behavior is based on cognition, and that in order to produce a more functional behavior, the thinking process must change. Group activities combine assessment and intervention in this approach, and these usually occur concurrently. Therapist observation of behavior during group activities leads to new assumptions about how information is being perceived and processed. Allen has developed a hierarchy of six cognitive levels and has described typical behaviors of each based on clinical observation. Using her guidelines, we can easily evaluate our clients and place them in activity groups that are appropriate for their cognitive level.

Many of the clients we will treat in occupational therapy are cognitively disabled. Examples of some disorders that involve a cognitive disability are stroke, traumatic brain injury, schizophrenia and other psychotic disorders, anxiety and substance abuse disorders, personality disorders, Alzheimer's and other dementias, mental retardation, autism, and learning disability. Some of these disorders can be successfully treated. For those cases, Allen groups provide one of the most accurate measures we have for documenting progress. However, for many persons with these disorders, a plateau will be reached beyond which no further cognitive development is possible. These clients need ongoing care, protection from danger, and assistance with many activities of daily living. For these clients, an assessment of cognitive level during a group activity will provide useful guidelines for the level of assistance that will be needed after discharge.

Framework Focus

The cognitive disabilities theory is broadly applicable for both chronic and acute care settings. This theory is best applied when there is a need to measure and monitor a client's problem-solving ability and safety while performing daily activities in any of the "areas of occupation" listed in the *Occupational Therapy Practice Framework* (American Occupational Therapy Association [AOTA], 2002). Clients with health conditions that affect their cognition may be grouped together according to the Allen levels and may be re-evaluated and monitored as a group, saving valuable time for the occupational therapist. Caregiver groups or "families with dementia/traumatic brain injury, etc." may be guided to facilitate the client's best ability to function using Allen principles. Guidelines for assistance at various cognitive levels fit the *Occupational Therapy Practice Framework's* definition of "facilitating engagement in occupation." Adaptation of the "physical" and "social contexts" are a focus in the Allen approach as the occupational therapy structures the materials, assistance, and "activity demands" to provide a "just-right challenge." Allen's task analysis considers all aspects of "activity demands" listed in the *Occupational Therapy Practice Framework*. Routines of daily occupation may be equated to "performance patterns" in the *Occupational Therapy Practice Framework* domain (AOTA, 2002).

Allen provides a pragmatic approach to living with the consequences of illness or injury. Some theorists have been critical of the Allen approach because it focuses on "disability" and seems to emphasize weaknesses rather than strengths. This is a misinterpretation. In fact, it is by acknowledging and understanding disability that Allen gives us the profession's most precise guidelines for utilizing a client's remaining ability to maximize function. "Therapists should identify the person's best ability to function and select intervention goals that maximize these abilities" (Allen, Blue, & Earhart, 1995, p. 1). The focus of therapy is on assessment and enabling best ability to function.

Assessment

Perhaps Allen is best known for the Allen's Cognitive Levels Screen (ACLS), which uses leather lacing to assess the precise cognitive level of the client (from 3.0 to 5.8). This test has become increasingly standardized over the past decade and is widely used by occupational therapists as a screening tool. It gives a quick estimate of the client's current capacity to learn (Allen, 1999). Other standardized tests of cognitive level developed by Allen are the Routine Task Inventory (RTI) and the Cognitive Performance Test (CPT) (Allen & Earhart, 1992). These assessments use everyday activities to determine the cognitive level. The Allen Diagnostic Module (ADM), the most recently developed test, takes motivation and socialization into account and uses a dynamic approach to assessment of cognitive level. (The latest updates of these assessments may be obtained from S & S Worldwide at 1-800-243-9232.) The ADM uses a group format to observe performance while doing a variety of standardized craft activities. Crafts make an effective evaluation at levels 3.0 to 5.8 and are motivating because they are meaningful across the spectrum of cultures. Observation of an individual's response to instructions and sensory cues from the materials and tools of the craft provide the basis for predictions about many other aspects of human performance. Examples of these crafts are given later in the chapter in the section on activities.

In the past few decades, science has dictated a standardized, rigid approach to assessment. In this context, neither crafts nor routine daily activities have face validity. There are too many variables and too many individual differences for scientific accuracy to be applied. Therefore, therapists should use caution in making judgments about cognitive level based on the observation of these activities. Allen's levels and modes should never be considered labels, which prejudice others and limit the person's options or autonomy. Rather,

they should be used as guidelines, upon which to plan initial activities, or make tentative discharge arrangements, which will only become valid when the person with cognitive disability has an opportunity to demonstrate his or her best ability to function.

Since the Allen approach advocates that clients be treated in groups of similar cognitive level, the initial screening becomes an important part of group planning. The approximate cognitive level must be determined in order to place clients appropriately in occupational therapy intervention groups.

Enabling Best Ability to Function

Once the client's best ability to function (ACL) has been determined, decisions about lifestyle and discharge placement need to be made. The occupational therapist's role is to make recommendations about the level of assistance the client will need in the immediate future. Enabling a client's best ability to function involves two aspects: 1) assistance from caregivers and 2) adaptation of the environment. The guiding principles for management come from the cognitive modes of functioning within each level. Goals for expected behaviors in activities of daily living are defined, along with the amount of physical and cognitive assistance needed at each mode/level (Allen et al., 1995).

Environmental adaptation flows from the amount of conscious awareness the client has at his or her disposal. To elicit his or her best effort in doing a task, the usable task environment must be defined. Supplies needed for a task to be done must be placed within the limits of conscious awareness, for example, within arm's reach at Level 3. Concurrently, all distractions and unsafe items should be removed. Think about how hard it is to get anything done when your desk is piled high with junk mail or your kitchen is stacked with dirty dishes. Our clients need our help to remove the clutter and help them focus on what is necessary to perform essential tasks.

Another essential component of client management is providing needed assistance. Allen also builds into the cognitive levels and modes the quality and quantity of assistance needed. To elicit the client's best performance, the caregiver must first observe the client's response to the task environment and then intervene as needed in a variety of ways. Four of the possible ways to give cognitive assistance suggested by Allen are:

Table 7-1	Allen's Cognitive Assistance for Levels 1 Through 6	
Level	Cognitive Assistance Needed	Compensation Provided for the Following Cognitive Functions, Which Are Lacking
1	Total	Sensory stimulation (and 2 to 6)
2	Maximum	Prevent getting lost or into unsafe areas (and 3 to 6)
3	Moderate	Help with self-care (and 4 to 6)
4	Minimum	Maintaining the home (and 5 and 6)
5	Standby	Planning, advising, supervision
6	None necessary	None

© Claudia Allen, conference materials, 1997. Adapted with permission.

1. Facilitate—Give sensory cues appropriate to the level.
2. Probe—Ask focused questions to encourage problem solving.
3. Observe—Allow client time to process cues and questions and try out new behaviors.
4. Rescue—When frustration arises, correct error or do a step for the client.

The experienced therapist should never do for clients what they can do for themselves. For example, the person at Level 3 responds best to tactile cues. The caregiver, therefore, facilitates by using touch to get the client's attention and demonstrates the use of necessary objects. To assist with dressing, the caregiver hands the client a shirt and touches the right hand to be inserted in the sleeve. Probing or asking questions that suggest the next step might then be tried (e.g., "How can you get your arm in the sleeve?"). Observing the response determines if more assistance is needed. If the response is unproductive, a third attempt might be a direct verbal instruction, accompanying the demonstration, "Hold it by the collar with this hand, and put the other arm in here." The "rescue" is always a last resort; if the client shows significant signs of frustration, put the arm in the shirt for him or her.

In general, the amount of assistance needed to do a task decreases as the cognitive level increases. Table 7-1 is a general guideline for the amount of cognitive assistance needed at each level.

Basic Assumptions

Cognitive Disability Defined

Allen (1987a) defines cognitive disability as "a limitation in sensorimotor actions originating in the physical or chemical structures of the brain and producing observable and assessable limitations in routine task behavior." Allen accepts the concept that a person's cognitive level has biological and chemical determinants resulting from one or more health conditions. However, she maintains that engagement in activities and participation can be maximized by assessing activity limitations and adapting both task demand and contextual factors. Applying the framework of the *International Classification of Functioning, Disability, and Health* (World Health Organization [WHO], 2001), assessment and enabling best function in occupational therapy involve assessing the cognitive impairment, using assistance and environmental adaptation to compensate for activity limitations, and promoting routines that allow continued participation in the occupations of daily life (Table 7-2). Allen's theory provides a way for occupational therapists to predict the activities clients with cognitive disabilities will be able to participate in competently and safely.

Being unable to work, care for others, and maintain a home are some of the roles that are commonly lost as a result of cognitive disability. However, there are other roles that may be acquired, such as volunteer, hobbyist, family help-

Table 7-2	International Classification of Functioning, Disability, and Health Overview of ICF Components (2001)

- Body functions: Physiological functions of body systems, including psychological function
- Body structures: Anatomical parts of the body, such as organs, limbs, and their components
- Impairments: Problems in body function or structure, such as significant deviation or loss
- Activity: Execution of a task or action by an individual
- Participation: Involvement of a life situation
- Activity limitations: Difficulties an individual may have in executing activities
- Participation restrictions: Problems individuals experience in life situations
- Environmental factors: Physical, social, and attitudinal contexts in which people live

er, and organization participant, with the appropriate cognitive assistance.

Allen's Task Analysis

Task analysis is defined as a method of determining the functional complexity of an activity by separating the activity into steps and determining the physical and cognitive functional abilities required to do each step. In recent years, Allen has developed a more dynamic approach to task analysis, which includes factors like culture, motivation, and situational context, as well as the basic ability to process information. This approach is visually outlined in Figure 7-1, and this serves as the basis for planning and interpreting craft activities such as those used in the ADM. In 1999, Allen updated her information processing theory by making a distinction between working memory and procedural memory. Working memory is what we use when we are actively processing information. It is necessary for the continual orientation to time and social context as well as new learning. Procedural memory is what we use for our habitual actions done without conscious awareness (Allen, 1999, p. 5). This type of memory may be useful when well-learned self-care habits and routines remain in memory even when new learning and problem-solving ability is impaired.

Cues

Cues consist of the environment itself; the materials needed for a task; and all forms of verbal, written, or demonstrated instruction. In normal everyday activity, when we find ourselves in a kitchen at mealtime, the cues we use are the food in the refrigerator or cabinets, the recipe or preparation we have in mind, and the equipment avail-

able for preparing a meal (e.g., bowls, baking pans, dishes, knives). Visual, olfactory, and gustatory memories may guide and motivate us.

Attention

Attention to cues is necessary for functional activity to occur. How our brain receives or screens out cues may depend on many psychological, physiological, social, and cultural factors. In cognitive disability, the limitations of attention and sensory screening need to be evaluated in order to plan appropriate intervention. When using cues in intervention, Allen advocates carefully planning of the environment (clinic or home setting), thoughtfully selecting and placing supplies and equipment to be used for a task, and varying the amount and type of assistance given, according to the specific guidelines at each cognitive level or mode.

Action/Activity

The combination of cues and a person's ability to attend and focus will hopefully result in an action or response (the performance of functional activity). Continuing the kitchen analogy, when I go home to my kitchen after a hard day's work, my meal preparation task will be greatly enhanced by how well I have prepared ahead. If I bought the right ingredients at the grocery store, if the pots and pans and dishes are clean and ready to be used, and if I remember or have easy access to the recipe or procedure to be used, the meal will be prepared correctly and in a timely manner. All sorts of things can go wrong, even in the absence of disability... telephone calls, unexpected company, key ingredients being eaten by another family member, the right size baking pan borrowed and not returned. Problem solving is needed to cope with unexpected obstacles.

Figure 7-1. Allen's functional information processing system.

When therapists select tasks to be performed by clients in the clinical setting, the client's problem-solving ability may be observed and evaluated. Allen has given us specific guidelines for making these observations and for interpreting them. The six cognitive levels are based on compiling typical behaviors at each cognitive level (and subsequently, each mode) in response to a variety of tasks (cues). From these sample behaviors, cognitive disability theory makes inferences about the thinking processes that produced them. These inferences explain how the person's brain processes the information being presented.

Speed

The speed of response depends upon the speed with which the brain processes information. Biological factors, such as brain chemicals, are responsible for setting the rate of thinking and

behavior. Persons functioning below Level 5 generally have a difficult time adjusting the speed of their performance.

Underlying Mental Processes

Information processing involves visual spatial components (right hemisphere), in conjunction with short- and long-term memory, and verbal-propositional components (left hemisphere), in conjunction with short- and long-term memory. Allen has analyzed these components for each cognitive level and mode. While these differences are too detailed to describe here, their contribution to the functional performance we observe in our clients during group activities should not be underestimated. In activity selection, a therapist should consider the client's prior knowledge, experience, and preferences, as well as sensorimotor and verbal abilities.

Table 7-3	Allen's Cognitive Levels 1 Through 6					
	1. Automatic Actions	2. Postural Actions	3. Manual Actions	4. Goal-Directed Actions	5. Exploratory Actions	6. Planned Actions
Attention to Sensory Cues	Subliminal	Proprioceptive	Tactile	Visible cues	Related cues (all senses)	Symbolic cues
Motor Actions						
Spontaneous Imitated	Automatic None	Postural Approx- imations	Manual Manipu- lations	Goal-directed Replications	Exploratory Novelty	Planned Unnecessary
Conscious Awareness						
Purpose Experience	Arousal Indistinct	Comfort Moving	Interest Touching	Compliance Seeing	Self-control Inductive reasoning	Reflection Deductive reasoning
Process	Habitual or reflexive	Effect on body	Effect on environment	Several actions	Overt trial and error	Covert trial and error
Time (Attention Span)	Seconds	Minutes	Half hours	Hours	Weeks	Past/future
Occupational Therapy Activities	Sensory stimulation	Gross motor, games, dance	Simple, repetitive tasks	Several-step tasks	Concrete tasks	Conceptual tasks

© Claudia Allen, conference materials, 1997. Adapted with permission.

Six Cognitive Levels

Allen divides cognitive disabilities into six well-defined cognitive levels and provides several assessment tools to help occupational therapists evaluate the cognitive level. Assessment and intervention are based on how the client learns and performs tasks. Originally, the six levels were derived from Piaget's work on intellectual development. However, based on Allen's clinical observation, the cognitive levels are largely presented as descriptions of typical behaviors at each level.

For the purposes of understanding how cognition impacts task performance, three dimensions of task performance are outlined at each level:

1. Attention
2. Motor actions
3. Conscious awareness

Attention

In observing people interacting with their environment, the first thing noted is what sensory stimuli capture their interest. The sensory systems most utilized at each cognitive level seem to more or less follow a developmental sequence, beginning with body sensation (position and movement); proceeding to incorporate touch and vision; and then integrating these and using them together.

Motor Actions

Secondly, motor actions are observed in the context of task performance. The therapist uses observations of a person's movements and verbalizations to make some assumptions about his or her perception, understanding, and intention, all a part of cognition.

Conscious Awareness

Finally, conscious awareness of the surroundings is observed. The scope or range of awareness and the ability to use that awareness to determine appropriate action increases with each level. Table 7-3 describes a simplified description of attention, motor actions, and conscious awareness at each of the six levels. For a more complete understanding of these levels and their assessment, the reader is referred to Allen's books (Allen, 1985; Allen & Earhart, 1992).

Level 1—Automatic Actions

In most cases, clients at Level 1 are bedridden. They are conscious but respond mainly to internal or subliminal cues (sensations from within the body), such as hunger or pain. Behavior is largely habitual or reflexive. Arousal and response to others may be elicited for a few seconds at a time. Most daily needs (dressing, grooming, feeding) have to be done by caregivers. Occupational therapists at this level are most helpful in providing appropriate sensory stimulation and attempting to elicit motor responses of any kind.

Level 2—Postural Actions

At Level 2, clients can be stimulated to perform postural actions (changes in position) in response to proprioceptive (sense of motion and position) cues. Clients can imitate gross motor actions and can assist a caregiver in bathing, dressing, and grooming. Usually clients at Level 2 can feed themselves, although this may be messy. Twenty-four-hour nursing care is required. Engaging the client in any self-care tasks is an appropriate intervention at this level. Movement or exercise groups using imitation of position can be done. However, clients cannot benefit from interactive group intervention until they are at Level 3. A good quick test to determine whether a client is a Level 2 or 3 is to administer the Lower Cognitive Level (LCL) test. Ask the client to watch you while you clap your hands three times loudly (approximately one clap per second). If the client starts before you finish three, stop him or her and ask him or her to watch you first. If the client is able to imitate three claps, he or she is probably a Level 3, and therefore should be considered for group intervention.

Level 3—Manual Actions

At this level, clients perform manual actions (movements with their hands) in response to tactile cues (touch). Actions based on interest in objects found within arm's reach may be repeated many times. Attention can be maintained up to 30 minutes. Basic daily grooming tasks may be done independently with reminders; clients can walk to familiar places but get easily lost in new surroundings. Repetitive work tasks can be done at Level 3. Some of the tasks requiring supervision are care of

belongings and clothing, money management, preparing meals, following a schedule, and use of a telephone. Care should be taken to place potentially dangerous items out of reach or locked away, as a person at Level 3 cannot discriminate items by their intended use (e.g., paper napkins in the toaster). Tool use must be supervised, as it may be inappropriate (e.g., using a hammer to shut a window). However, with proper instruction, familiar repetitive actions can be fairly skilled, such as using a peeler to peel a potato or a paring knife to cut an apple. Tools that are an "extension of the hand," such a fork, paintbrush, or nail file, are usually safe to use with supervision at Level 3. Steps in a task can be imitated one at a time, when demonstrated.

Level 4—Goal-Directed Actions

Becoming goal directed represents a major step toward independent functioning. It is goal directedness that makes activity purposeful; therefore, actions below this level are generally random or habitual. At Level 4, basic living skills are intact: grooming, dressing, toileting, bathing, and feeding. In addition, clients at Level 4 perform goal-directed actions in response to visual cues. In other words, if they see a toothbrush, toothpaste, and a cup next to the bathroom sink, this visible cue will remind them to brush their teeth. These clients are able to complete short tasks such as making a sandwich or washing the dishes. Attention is up to 1 hour and steps toward a goal can be imitated in short sequences. Clients perform most daily self-care activities but need assistance in coping with new events, anticipating needs, and managing money. Visual stimuli are the focus, but nonvisible properties in the environment, like heat and electricity (e.g., a hair dryer near the bathtub or paper towels near a hot stove), may pose a danger. Directions for getting places or doing tasks must be demonstrated visually, since verbal and written directions are not followed. Familiar routine tasks should be reinforced as new routines are established only by repetitive "drilling." Because persons at Level 4 are aware of the goal, they are able to ask for assistance, and this plays a major role in keeping them safe and functional.

Level 5—Exploratory Actions/Independent Learning

Use of trial and error is the hallmark of Level 5. Here, for the first time, persons use inductive reasoning and are capable of new learning. Clients at

Level 5 can imitate new procedures and remember several steps at a time. In task performance, novelty is sought and variation explored. In choosing group projects, this is the first level at which choices may be given.

Deficits at Level 5 are in functions that require anticipation and planning. Persons at Level 5 are concrete thinkers primarily and have trouble imagining the long-term consequences of their actions or inactions. Hence, preventative measures are often not taken. In the home, for example, needed repairs may be neglected (a broken step is neglected until someone trips and falls). Cooking presents a problem when timing is involved (e.g., burning is not anticipated). Money management is a major problem since clients at Level 5 seldom save for emergencies or anticipate future expenses. Also neglected are purchasing needed items for a meal, cleaning or laundering clothing, and getting prescriptions refilled. The lack of abstract thinking prevents these clients from understanding the nature of their illness or the effects of medication. Jobs and social relationships may suffer because of failure to anticipate the consequences of self-centered behavior. Positive interventions at this level are activities that increase social awareness, reciprocation in relationships, and accepting the supervision of others in helping to avoid negative consequences.

Level 6—Planned Actions

This is the highest level and represents the absence of disability. The main distinguishing characteristic is the ability to use deductive reasoning and to plan ahead. Future events are anticipated and behavior is organized. Verbal and written directions can be followed without demonstration, and the person is able to use symbolic cues (Allen, 1988).

The Principle of Brain Conservation

It is natural to think of ourselves as Level 6, which is Allen's representation of "normal." However, everyone has a flow of effort within the entire range of cognitive levels over the course of the day. We may indeed be functioning at Level 6 when we are listening to a lecture and rapidly taking notes in class. But there are many tasks we engage in that do not require that much effort. Bathing and dressing for the day are routine activities that may only require a Level 3 effort. Jogging around a track for exercise allows our brain to take a break and sink to a Level 2. Our brains have a tendency to conserve energy whenever possible. The difference between "normal" and "disabled" is that in disability, no amount of effort can evoke a higher level of cognitive functioning. This limitation is what puts cognitively disabled persons at great risk when they encounter unexpected problems in everyday life. For example, Margaret, at Level 4, can drive a car from her home to a familiar nearby grocery store. But when road construction necessitated a detour, she ended up lost. She was unable to alter her usual route or to locate the necessary resources to find her way home. She wandered around on unfamiliar streets until someone noticed and called a policeman to escort her back home.

The Usable Task Environment

Allen's theory tells us that as the cognitive level increases, awareness of the environment also increases. Specific guidelines are included in Figure 7-2.

For example, a new client, Sam, is being observed eating a meal. If he is being fed by an aide at his hospital bed, most likely he is at Level 1. If a piece of bread is placed in his hand and he brings it to his mouth and takes a bite, he is at least a Level 2 because he is able to use movement functionally. If Sam reaches for the pitcher of juice in the center of the table, an Allen therapist knows he is at least a Level 3 because his attention extends to everything within arm's reach. If Sam asks that the catsup on the opposite side of the table be passed, the therapist will know immediately that Sam is at least a Level 4. He is using his visual system to look for what he wants, and his attention is projected beyond arm's reach. If he likes barbeque sauce, and he gets up and goes to get it out of the refrigerator, he is probably at least a Level 5. He looks for items he cannot see in places where they are typically kept, an action that integrates sensation, perception, and memory. At Level 6, Sam may remember he is out of milk, and go to buy some next time he's out shopping. At each level, Sam's usable task environment has expanded.

Principle of Task Equivalence

Many people wonder why Allen uses crafts in her group assessment activities (ADM). The answer lies in the principle of task equivalence. The cognitive processing necessary in doing a craft activity is presumed to be equivalent to a variety of

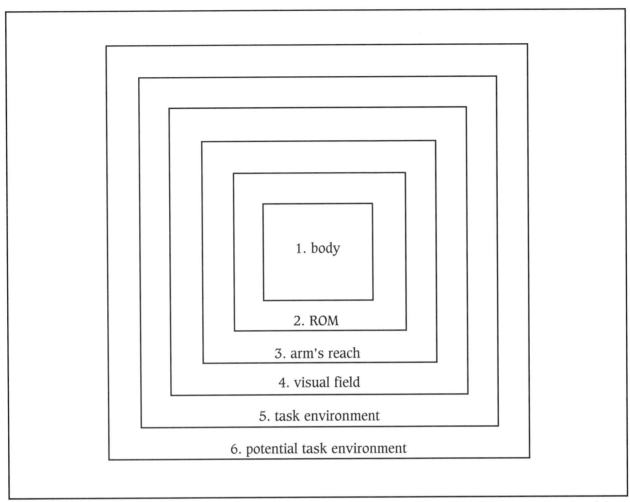

Figure 7-2. The usable task environment. (Adapted with permission from Allen, C. K. [1985]. *Occupational therapy for psychiatric diseases: Measurement and management of cognitive disabilities.* Boston: Little, Brown and Co.)

everyday tasks that a client will choose to participate in after discharge from an acute setting. The careful observation of the client doing a craft activity in a group allows the trained occupational therapist to determine the client's level of cognitive processing. A client who paints a wooden box on the top and three sides, but does not turn the project to paint the back, the bottom, or the inside, is showing some important limitations in his or her ability to process information and apply it to task performance. This client is only attending to what is immediately visible. Before he or she goes home, the therapist will be able to predict equivalent tasks that are likely to be problems for him or her there, such as personal grooming, keeping clothing clean, appropriate food preparation and storage, and many other aspects of home safety and maintenance. Because of task equivalence, recommen-

dations for the level of assistance, supervision, and environmental adaptation needed for the best function and safety of the individual at home can be made more accurately. The usefulness of task equivalence, however, depends on the accuracy of the therapist's task analysis, using Allen's principles.

Function and Dysfunction

Allen gives the profession its best defined system for measuring the impact of cognitive dysfunction. Not only are there six levels, ranging from comatose (1) to highly functional (6), but there are 52 modes of performance in between. Modes are identified by the decimal points after the level. Scores on the ACL Test are expressed as 3.0,

Table 7-4	Quick Overview of the Allen Cognitive Modes

ACL	Common Behavioral Descriptions
1.0 to 1.4	Bedridden; stimulus/response of head
1.6 to 1.8	Sits with support; moves trunk/limbs; says "no"
2.0 to 2.4	Stands, righting actions, walks; names body parts, bed, toilet
2.6 to 2.8	Steps up/over; pushes/pulls; holds for support; sings; names target of action
3.0 to 3.4	Spontaneous grasp/release; repetitive actions; speaks in short phrases
3.6 to 3.8	Looks at effects of actions and follows cues to do the next step in self-care; understands waiting a minute, being done (finished with activity)
4.0 to 4.4	Independent in doing routine activities; identifies and sustains goals for 1 hour; speaks in sentences
4.6 to 4.8	Looks around and gets supplies; learns new procedure inflexibly; "Is this right?"—needs help now!
5.0 to 5.2	Discovers how to improve actions through overt trial and error; normal intonation and expression in speech; impulsive and poor judgment
5.6 to 5.8	Understands safety precautions; uses information gained by reading Compares hypothetical plans, anticipates consequences

© Claudia Allen, conference materials, 1997. Adapted with permission.

4.4, 5.8, etc. Each mode has implications that guide the occupational therapist in observing a progression of cognitive skills from one level to the next. A recent Allen publication, *Structures of the Cognitive Performance Modes* (1999), describes each mode from 1.0 to 6.0 with regard to expected cognitive abilities, functional goals, intervention methods, and safety. This text incorporates the most current research on cognition and provides excellent guidelines for accurate assessment, caregiver education, and discharge planning or placement. It requires some training and experience to learn to use the modes in assessment, intervention, and documentation.

For the purposes of students and therapists who are not previously familiar with cognitive disabilities theory, just identifying the low and high end of each level makes a good starting point for placing clients in groups. Table 7-4 outlines some simple behavioral observations that can be used to approximate the cognitive level for the purposes of group placement and initial activity selection. The level can then be confirmed by observation of task behaviors during the group itself.

The function-dysfunction continuum of cognitive abilities fluctuates in every individual, including those without a diagnosed disability. For this reason, intervention in the cognitive disabilities frame of reference cannot really be separated from ongoing evaluation. Intervention groups are primarily used, not so much for cognitive skill training, but as an opportunity for the client and therapist to discover the optimal environmental conditions necessary for the client to safely engage in purposeful activity. The client's response to a group activity may be understood as one example of the way he or she will respond to similar activity situations outside the intervention environment. The observation of group behaviors, together with Allen's modes of performance, allows the occupational therapist to make reasonable predictions about the difficulties clients are likely to encounter in everyday activities. This information is invaluable to medical teams who must document the need for services, as well as to families who must take appropriate safety precautions and provide needed guidance. In this regard, Allen uses group intervention as an ongoing evaluation.

Allen has been concerned with competence, which legally means the ability to handle one's own affairs. There is no cut-off cognitive level for defining competence. Determination of competence or incompetence is generally based on the ability to make sound judgments and reasonable decisions about those activities that the individual intends to do.

Change and Motivation

Cognitive change occurs when the brain physiology or chemistry changes. We see an increase in cognitive level through activity when 1) the brain recovers from acute illness, or 2) the brain chemistry is affected by a change in activity level, hormones, diet, or medication. Using Allen's cognitive levels, the therapist verifies the presence or absence of a functional disability. If a client's cognitive ability stabilizes below Level 6 ("normal"), the occupational therapist assists the client and caregivers in making the necessary adjustments in daily living required by a residual cognitive disability. However, even when cognitive processes are irreversibly damaged by trauma or disease, Allen suggests that we can still produce changes in adaptive functioning by manipulating the environment. Allen's updated writings and presentations acknowledge the importance of culture and context in motivating a client to put forth his or her best effort. Offering a choice of craft projects, as well as including socialization in the selection of activities, helps to engage clients in group intervention. In doing a task, there are several factors to be manipulated. The task environment includes the placement and storage of materials, lighting, seating, facilities available, and assistance available. The task demand is the supplies, steps and instructions, and physical and cognitive abilities necessary to complete the task. Allen suggests that both the task environment and the task demand can be altered in ways that allow the client to perform more independently within his or her cognitive level. In planning activities, therapists should give group members a "just-right challenge" (i.e., the task should match, but not exceed, the members' capabilities). For example, clients at Level 4 can reach their maximum adaptive functioning when presented with a three- or four-step task, setting out all the necessary materials within their visual field, demonstrating the instructions, and providing a completed sample for them to copy. Successful performance of a task that is perceived as socially positive will reinforce the client's sense of well-being and increase motivation. Clients at Level 4 will be motivated to perform most self-care tasks at home with appropriate assistance and a suitable and safe environment.

Cognitive Disabilities Group Intervention

Intervention group membership in occupational therapy is based on cognitive level. Clients are treated in homogeneous groups of similar cognitive level. Level 2 is the lowest that can be treated effectively within a group. Level 3 is the lowest level at which group interaction can be expected. Earhart (Allen, 1985) suggests that in a large facility a variety of groups should be offered for Levels 2 through 6. Some clients will move up a level or two as their acute symptoms remit. Others will stabilize at a lower level and will require a variety of tasks within that level. Activities appropriate for each level are suggested. Table 7-5, which describes the cognitive abilities of clients at each of the six levels, can serve as a guide for planning activities. The table is based on an earlier chart by Allen, revised by Mary Brinson and Mary Ann Mayer.

Role of the Leader

The leader must be more directive in this approach than in most others. In a hospital setting, the focus is often on evaluation. The therapist typically chooses the activity or task or limits choices. The occupational therapist must use expertise in activity analysis, controlling or adapting the environment, and instructing the group members in the procedures of the task. The therapist's role requires skill in assisting clients in acquiring/demonstrating cognitive skills at increasing cognitive levels. The size of groups should not exceed eight members when led by one occupational therapist. However, when assisted by one or more occupational therapy assistants, groups of up to 12 members can still be effective. One occupational therapist assisted by one or more occupational therapy assistants may be ideal in using the Allen approach, since skilled observations of task performance are necessary for ongoing assessment. The most significant factor in determining group size is the members' need for assistance. The lower the cognitive level, the more frequently members need assistance with the task. However, at Levels 4 and 5, verbal interaction consumes a larger portion of group time, and more individual attention is needed for social and emotional support. For higher cognitive levels, groups should be limited to

Table 7-5	Task Analysis for Cognitive Disabilities		
	Level 1: Automatic Actions	Level 2: Postural Actions	Level 3: Manual Actions
Setting	Reduce the number of stimuli when possible. Patients do not screen out external stimuli.	Open space. Patients enjoy planned gross motor actions.	Clutter free. Patients are engaged in doing simple tasks that have repetitive actions.
The Therapist's Directions			
Demonstrations	Looks at demonstrated directions but does not imitate them.	The therapist may need to physically guide the action.	Patients will follow a demonstration of a familiar action on an object.
Verbalizations	Verbs, introjections.	Pronouns, names of body parts, simple verbs reinforce demonstration.	Names of material objects, repeated simple nouns and verbs.
Number of directions	One action or direction, repeated.	One action or direction, repeated.	One action or direction, repeated.
Task Selection			
Structure of the activity	Alerting stimuli. The most important tasks are eating and drinking.	Familiar, repetitive gross body movements.	An activity that has one step or scheme repeated.
Choice and sample provided		The therapist plans movements and demonstrates actions. The therapist may respond to patient's suggestions or actions.	Activity is preplanned by therapist. Choices limited to two or three material items/objects.
Tools	Stimulated use of body parts.	Spontaneous use of body parts. Objects that are associated with gross body movement (e.g., softballs, jump ropes).	Hands: Some use of familiar tools.
Storage of materials/ projects	Taken care of by the therapist.	Taken care of by the therapist.	Taken care of by the therapist.
Preparation by the therapist		Play movements and obtain any needed equipment.	Supplies are laid out in advance. Do any preliminary or finishing steps that are not repetitive or familiar.

(continued)

Table 7-5	Task Analysis for Cognitive Disabilities (continued)		
	Level 4: *Goal-Directed Actions*	*Level 5:* *Exploratory Actions*	*Level 6:* *Planned Actions*
Setting	Other patients working on the same task, a shared goal. Setting conducive to production of immediate end product.	Clutter can be present, and other performing variations on similar tasks. Setting fosters exploration, trial and error.	Free access to materials and supplies to stimulate covert problem solving, sharing of plans with others.
The Therapist's Directions			
Demonstrations	Patients will imitate single steps in a series and moderately novel actions that expand familiar schemes.	Patients can learn through serial imitation, so a number of steps may be demonstrated. Unfamiliar steps assimilated.	Not required. Patients learn through serial limitations so directions may be retained.
Verbalizations	Simple adjectives, adverbs, nouns, and verbs; avoiding open-ended questions or discussions.	Adjectives and prepositions may be used in explaining variations.	Conjunctions, conjectures, images.
Number of directions	One step at a time.	Several steps at a time.	Unlimited. Images, diagrams, written directions may be followed.
Task Selection			
Structure of the activity	Simple quick tasks with a tangible end product. Avoid childish connotations.	An activity that permits variation, and that allows results to be easily seen and corrected.	An activity that permits variation in the selection and planning of steps.
Choice and sample provided	Avoid confusion by limiting the decisions and materials. The opportunity for exact replication of a sample is present.	Several choices in materials, tools, and activity selection. Demonstrate and clarify tangible possibilities.	Several choices in materials, tools, and activity selection. Discuss the hypothetical possibilities.
Tools	Hand tools limited to familiar objects. No power tools.	Simple tools that are linear extensions of the hand and arm.	Patients learn how to use unfamiliar machines and tools.
Storage of materials/ projects	Patients will place and/or find supplies when clearly visible or very familiar.	The patient will search for things in probable locations and can place/find things in labeled drawers or cabinets.	The patient will follow verbal directions to place or find materials.
Preparation by the therapist	Supplies are laid out in advance. Provide an exact sample of the end product. Do those steps that require unfamiliar tools or schemes.	The sample of the finished product need not be exact. Patterns and procedures are supplied by the therapist.	Materials, designs, and/or pictures are provided to assist covert problem solving.

© Mary Ann Mayer and Mary H. Brinson. Information gathered from Claudia Allen's 1988 ACL workshop at the Institute of Living, Hartford, Connecticut.

eight members so that group leaders can facilitate group discussion to reinforce learning. Therefore, the occupational therapist needs to weigh several factors before deciding on the size of an Allen group.

Structure and Goals

Allen's goals for clients have to do with function and adaptation. Specific goals might be set to encourage a client to progress to a higher level or to provide the ideal environmental support and assistance so that a client can maximize function within a given cognitive level. Allen has designed several excellent evaluation tools and specified many behaviors that indicate progress toward higher cognitive levels.

The structure and goals for an Allen group are different for each level. For this reason, groups at each level will be discussed separately, with examples of appropriate activities.

Level 2 Groups

Movement activities are suggested to meet the needs of clients at Level 2 clients (clients at Level 3 may also be included). Activities consist of imitation of gross body movement, such as clapping, bending over to touch toes, and passing or tossing a large, soft ball. Simple movement games such as bean bag toss or Nerf basketball may be useful, although clients at Level 2 are apt to disregard directionality. Setting limits in Level 2 groups may be difficult because disruptive behaviors of clients at Level 2 or 3 are oblivious to verbal direction (but often responsive to demonstrated direction). Movement at this level provides a pleasurable sensory experience, as well as needed stimulation and exercise. However, motor skill is likely to be limited.

Level 3 Groups

The guiding principles in choosing appropriate activities for Level 3 are repetition and manipulation. Persons at this cognitive level are not goal directed. The process must interest them in order for them to be drawn to participate in an activity. Therapists should think of activities that focus on these attributes as strengths.

Many of our daily activities have the attributes of manipulation and repetition. Washing the dishes, sewing a button, clipping fingernails, and eating a bowl of cereal are examples. It is timing that is difficult for Level 3s, knowing when to begin

and when to end. For example, in doing a woodworking project, clients at Level 3 may keep on sanding long after the wood is smooth. They will apply much more glue than is necessary. They will string beads until they get to the end or all the beads are used up. They may place tiles in a row along the edge of a frame, without regard for color or spacing. The therapist must be responsible for structuring the activity into steps and keeping track of time to move the group along.

The ADM identifies a variety of craft projects that are appropriate for Level 3 groups. Some of them are tile trivets, ribbon mugs, sticker cards, canvas placemats, bargello bookmarks, whale note holders, and recessed tile boxes. (All of these projects have standardized materials, which are available from S&S Healthcare, and a free catalog may be obtained by calling them at 1-800-243-9232.) Standardized materials are desirable to increase reliability of the therapist's observations in assessing the mode of performance within each cognitive level. The ADM is recommended for groups in acute care or other settings in which the accuracy of assessment is important in planning for discharge.

However, in chronic care settings, such as group homes or skilled nursing facilities, where functional maintenance programs are needed, more interactive group activities can be planned using Allen's guidelines. When selecting activities for Level 3 groups, repetition and manipulation should be the guiding principles. For example, one therapist who works with clients at Level 3 with dementia may have them make long chains with yarn with crochet hooks and attach balloons to decorate for a party or string popcorn and cranberries for a Christmas tree. An occupational therapy aide or recreation aide may be taught to use Allen principles in executing such activities.

The timing of a Level 3 group should not exceed 30 minutes, as that is the limit of their attention according to Allen. Many work tasks are ideal for Level 3, for example, stuffing envelopes, attaching labels and stamps, or collating multiple-page documents. Such tasks have successfully been assigned to sheltered workshops. The workshop might be contracted to assemble packets of plastic utensils, napkins, salt, pepper, sugar, and powdered creamer in plastic bags for serving meals on airlines. In a hospital or day treatment setting, a Level 3 group might be assigned the task of copying and distributing an in-house newsletter or invitations to an event. Again, the principles of repetition and manipulation should guide selection of appropriate work tasks. All materials should be within arm's reach for each Level 3 participant, and the task should be structured so that one step at a time can be performed repeatedly.

Activity Examples

Two examples of activities are included here. First, the "Recessed Tile Box" (Activity Example 7-2), a standardized craft activity selected from the ADM (Earhart, Allen, & Blue, 1993), is described. Although this craft is also used to assess clients at Level 4, only instructions for Level 3 have been given here. An ADM craft activity should be used for groups when assessment of the level and mode of functioning is desired. Activity Example 7-3 is an interactive skill maintenance activity called "Summer Salad," which uses the same Allen Level 3 principles, but is not set up as a standardized assessment.

Level 4 Groups

At Level 4, activities are goal directed. Sequences of steps toward a goal are now possible. Having a goal in mind represents an important step toward problem solving. However, attention is still limited, and group activities should not be planned to last for more than 1 hour. Projects are either completed in one session, or separate steps may be done in two sessions. For example, the wooden tile trivet may be sanded and painted in the first session, and tiles selected and glued in a second session.

Craft projects are ideal experiments in problem solving. A woodworking kit with three pieces, such as a napkin holder, can be structured into a simple sequence: 1) sanding, 2) painting, and 3) gluing. A finished sample must be available to represent the goal. This takes advantage of Level 4s' tendency to attend to visual cues. Some ADM crafts suggested for Level 4 are tile trivets, Indian key fobs, ribbon cards, Hug-a-bear, and various bear clothes. Many other crafts may be structured in a more group interactive way, using similar Allen Level 4 principles of goal orientation, several step sequences, and visually stimulating colors and contrasts.

The environment is of special concern to Level 4 groups because their usable task environment now extends beyond arm's reach to the entire visual field. Items necessary for the task to be accomplished should now be placed in plain view. But more importantly, all irrelevant items should be placed out of sight or they will cause major distraction. If a workroom is small, lacking in storage space, and/or has multiple uses, getting rid of

visual "clutter" is easier said than done. Considerable preparation time must be spent setting up the room before a Level 4 group begins. Likewise, the storage of objects is guided by the principle of visibility. What cannot be seen, for all intents and purposes, does not exist. Once this is understood by the therapist, it is clear what must be done. Clients at Level 4 will not go searching in cabinets and drawers. The same principle holds true for the home environment.

Assistance needed at Level 4 will be with processes that are not visible, such as the drying of paint or the changing of color or glaze as it dries. Although many food preparation tasks are ideal for this level, processes that involve heating or cooling are not understood or considered. Verbal direction alone is not enough when giving instructions for a task; demonstration should accompany verbal instruction. Written instruction is not at all useful, but sometimes pictures or diagrams can assist the client in progressing through the steps of a task that is familiar. Clients at Level 4 have a tendency to come to the end of a step and then ask, "What do I do now?" They know there is a goal they are working on, a completed project or a meal on the table, but they are not sure how to get there. Probing or asking leading questions can encourage the client to think about the sequence and use available cues, such as the sample or the work of other members, to learn to problem solve at a higher level. If the task is too difficult, or the client's cognitive abilities are lower than what is required, the therapist may need to "rescue" by correcting an error or completing a step for the client. The information gathered from client-therapist interactions is then used for selecting a more appropriate activity for the next session.

Level 5 Groups

At this level, the focus is on safety. The difficulties requiring intervention usually involve impulsivity and a lack of planning or anticipation. For this reason, clients at Level 5 are introduced to more complex tasks in groups. Some activities suggested are clay and mosaics, cooking, and advanced crafts. While one-step, demonstrated directions are not necessary, the safe use of tools and procedures must still be demonstrated at Level 5. Several steps can be taught at one time, and clients are capable of selecting projects and varying colors and designs. Planning is involved and projects may continue for more than one session. The occupational therapist still needs to monitor safety and check understanding of directions, especially with regard to the intangible variables of time and temperature.

The ADM includes the following activities for Level 5: sewing Raggedy Ann and Andy dolls and doll clothes, constructing and stenciling of multiple piece woodworking projects, and an assortment of projects using stenciled designs or iron-on decals. The cautious use of hot irons, power tools, ovens, or hot plates under supervision is suggested so that the occupational therapist might observe the client's knowledge and use of caution when handling these items. Group projects involving cooking, grilling outdoors, or participating in recreational activities, such as hiking, swimming, boating, or fishing, can also be used therapeutically to learn/evaluate safety in Level 5 groups.

Persons functioning at Allen's Level 6 may be placed in craft groups for assessment purposes or included in Level 5 groups if possible decline is suspected.

Cognitive Disabilities Group Leadership

Introduction

Names are mentioned around the table for acknowledgment, and the therapists introduce themselves. The leader explains the purpose of the project in concrete terms. Each member has materials for the activity set up at his or her place in advance. The purpose of the group is different from its goals. Because each member's mode of functioning is different, the goals for each member are individual. But the goal of the group is to provide a practical example in problem solving, which serves as both practice for the members and ongoing assessment for the therapist.

The purpose should be stated so as to elicit each member's best effort. The therapist should use concrete terms in explaining the purpose, the structure, and the procedure, in language known to be understood by the members at their cognitive level. Projects are to be kept by the clients once completed. The usefulness and desirability of the project should be emphasized, and this can be individualized. Social recognition is an important component when motivating clients to select and begin to work on a project. For example, the tile box may be a gift for someone special, so "you should do your best to make it look nice." Timing is mentioned for Level 4 and higher, and it should

be stressed that anyone needing assistance may signal one of the therapists at any time during the group.

Activity

The structure of groups described by Allen resemble Mosey's "Project Groups" (see Appendix A). Interaction occurs mainly between therapist and each member. Doing the activity really takes the entire session. Demonstration will be given according to the cognitive level, and the project sample can be referred to as the goal. Even for those not yet goal oriented (Level 3s), the sample is an important learning tool to use for error recognition and correction, imitation, and encouragement of higher level thinking. Cleaning up, as appropriate to the task, may take up the last 5 or 10 minutes of the session. Assistance given by the occupational therapist enables engagement in the activity, and this assistance changes with each cognitive level.

Sharing

No formal sharing takes place in Allen groups. However, informal comments about the projects of others by group members can provide needed social recognition for members.

Processing

A brief discussion at the end may focus on processing. Persons at all levels should have an opportunity to express their feelings about doing the task. The concrete end product is usually the focus of this discussion. Leaders should be careful not to give false praise, but limit comments to appropriate, reality-based feedback.

Generalization

Generalization by clients is really not possible until Level 5. For lower levels, therapist comments reflecting the purpose and the goal can be made when appropriate. Level 5 groups should be encouraged to find meaning in the activity at hand, and appropriate discussion questions by the leader will elicit this response.

Application

Applying new learning to everyday life can be reviewed at the end of the session. The therapist is directive in individualizing application. However, no individual feedback is given during the session regarding problem behaviors. The occupational therapist may choose to give feedback to clients individually after having an opportunity to score the activity (using ADM worksheets) or to determine the most useful response to specific situations.

At Level 5, application focuses on task equivalence and discussion of safety issues in the home or work environment. The use of peer discussion may help group members to accept critical feedback or the need for change. In terms of the *Occupational Therapy Practice Framework*, the occupational therapist facilitates an awareness of possible barriers to participation presented by safety issues of members.

Summary

The therapist ends with instructions about the project itself, that it may be taken (if completed) or that it may be picked up later (e.g., after paint is dry). Names on projects should be dealt with if projects are to be left. More interpersonal issues are mentioned as the level of the group increases.

Bibliography

Allen, C. K. (1982). Independence through activity: The practice of occupational therapy (psychiatry). *American Journal of Occupational Therapy, 36*, 731-739.

Allen, C. K (1985). *Occupational therapy for psychiatric diseases: Measurement and management of cognitive disabilities.* Boston/Toronto: Little, Brown & Co.

Allen, C. K. (1987a). Measuring the severity of mental disorders. *Hospital & Community Psychiatry, 38*, 140-142.

Allen, C. K. (1987b). Eleanor Clarke Slagle Lectureship-1987: Activity, occupational therapy's treatment method. *American Journal of Occupational Therapy, 41*, 563-575.

Allen, C. K. (1988). Cognitive disabilities. In S. C. Robertson (Ed.), *Focus: Skills for assessment and treatment.* Rockville, MD: American Occupational Therapy Association.

Allen, C. K. (1991). Cognitive disability and reimbursement for rehabilitation and psychiatry. *Journal of Insurance Medicine, 23*, 245-247.

Allen, C. K. (1994). Creating a need-satisfying, safe environment: Management and maintenance approaches. In C. B. Royeen (Ed.), *AOTA self-study series: Cognitive rehabilitation.* Bethesda, MD: American Occupational Therapy Association.

Allen, C. K. (1997). Cognitive disabilities: How to make clinical judgments. In N. Katz (Ed.), *Cognitive rehabilitation: Models for intervention in occupational therapy.* Rockville, MD: American Occupational Therapy Association.

Allen, C. K. (1999). *Structures of the cognitive performance modes.* Ormond Beach, FL: Allen Conferences, Inc.

Allen, C. K., & Allen, R. (1987). Cognitive disabilities: Measuring the social consequences of mental disorders. *Journal of Clinical Psychiatry, 48*(5), 185-190.

Allen, C. K., Blue, T., & Earhart, C. A. (1995). *Understanding cognitive performance modes.* Ormond Beach, FL: Allen Conferences, Inc.

Allen, C. K., & Earhart, C. (1992). *Occupational therapy treatment goals for the physically and cognitively disabled.* Bethesda, MD: American Occupational Therapy Association.

American Occupational Therapy Association. (2002). *Occupational therapy practice framework: Domain and process.* Bethesda, MD: Author.

David, S. (1988). Allen cognitive level and sensorimotor treatment in acute care. *Sensory Integration SIS Newsletter, 11*(1), 1-3.

Earhart, C. A., Allen, C. K., & Blue, T. (1993). *Allen diagnostic module instruction manual.* Colchester, CT: S & S Worldwide.

Heinmann, N. E., Allen, C. K., & Yerxa, E. J. (1989). The routine task inventory: A tool for describing the functional behavior of the cognitively disabled. *Occupational Therapy Practice, 1*, 67-74.

Josman, N., & Katz, N. (1991). Problem-solving version of the Allen Cognitive Level (ACL) test. *American Journal of Occupational Therapy, 45*, 331-338.

Levy, L. L. (1997). The use of the cognitive disability frame of reference in rehabilitation of cognitively disabled older adults. In N. Katz (Ed.), *Cognitive rehabilitation: Models for intervention in occupational Therapy.* Bethesda, MD: American Occupational Therapy Association.

World Health Organization. (2001). *International classification of functioning, disability, and health.* Geneva, Switzerland: Author.

Cognitive Disabilities
Activity Example 7-1
Rope Dancing (Level 2)

Materials: 12-foot-long piece of white nylon rope, 1-inch thick, with ends tied in a overhand knot; and a cassette player with instrumental music in a variety of rhythms (e.g., John Philip Sousa marches, Strauss waltzes, the overture from "The King & I").

Participants: Six maximum.

Directions: Start the music to alert members and get their attention. Therapist stands inside the rope circle and motions members to come toward him or her. Therapist greets each member and places each member's hand or elbow around the rope, approximately 2 feet apart. Begin by walking in a circle to the right, marching to the rhythm of the music. Turn to face the rope and hold with both hands or elbows. Therapist leads group in raising rope up high, then down low, to the rhythm of the music. Group imitates the therapist in doing a variety of in/out motions with arms and legs, while holding the rope. Have members take turns ducking under the rope and standing inside the circle. Two members can hold the rope bending over so that rope is 1 foot high, while therapist leads other members in stepping over it. Teams of three then take each end and pull each other back and forth slowly, changing their force when pulled or pushed gently by the therapist. Action ceases when the music ends (approximately 20 minutes). Therapist says "goodbye" to each member by shaking hands, saluting, or other gesture of recognition and farewell.

No verbalizations are needed to direct this group. However, proprioceptive cues are used as needed to direct the actions of the group and to recapture attention of straying members.

From Cole, M. B. *Group dynamics in occupational therapy: The theoretical basis and practice application of group intervention* (3rd ed.). Thorofare, NJ: SLACK Incorporated. © 2005 SLACK Incorporated.

Cognitive Disabilities
Activity Example 7-2
Recessed Tile Box (Levels 3 and 4)

Materials: Box with lid; 3/8-inch tiles, two colors separated into bins; sandpaper; brown wood stain; brush; rag; glue; and one completed sample for every two patients (checkerboard pattern in two contrasting colors). See Figures 7-3a and 7-3b. Access to a sink and water for clean-up is preferred. Glue bottles should be opened, and stain uncovered and stirred.

Participants: Six to eight members. Seat persons at table, each with individual set of supplies. Figures 7-3c and 7-3d depict the standardized set-up for evaluation.

Figure 7-3a. Key for supplies needed. (© Claudia Allen, Allen Diagnostic Model. Reprinted with permission.)

Figure 7-3b. Sample designs. (© Claudia Allen, Allen Diagnostic Model. Reprinted with permission.)

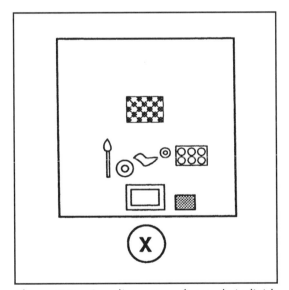

Figure 7-3c. Supplies set-up for each individual. (© Claudia Allen, Allen Diagnostic Model. Reprinted with permission.)

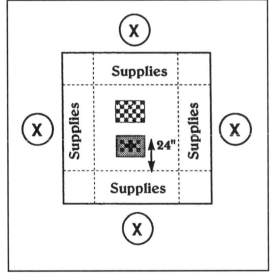

Figure 7-3d. Table set-up for four individuals. (© Claudia Allen, Allen Diagnostic Model. Reprinted with permission.)

From Cole, M. B. *Group dynamics in occupational therapy: The theoretical basis and practice application of group intervention* (3rd ed.). Thorofare, NJ: SLACK Incorporated. © 2005 SLACK Incorporated.

Cognitive Disabilities

Activity Example 7-2

Recessed Tile Box (Levels 3 and 4) (continued)

Timing: Introduction and purpose—5 minutes

Sanding, staining, and gluing tiles—20 to 30 minutes

Processing and summary—5 minutes (does not include clean-up)

Since the maximum attention span for Level 3 is 30 minutes, progress must be monitored and timing adjusted accordingly. If more than half the group has not finished staining at the end of 15 minutes, it is recommended that gluing the tiles be done in a second session.

Directions: Introduce group and explain purpose of the activity. Instructions are taken from the ADM (1993, pp. B2-5). "This is a tiled box which can be used to store jewelry, medicine, change, or other small items. All the supplies needed to complete it are in front of you. In order for me to see how you are doing today, it is important for you to try to make your box look as much like... the sample as possible."

Provide steps as indicated below as needed. Observe performance, provide appropriate prompts or assistance, and rate behavior for each step (see rating criteria). Move to the next step when the last one has been abandoned, or when a person says "I'm done" or requests next step.

Step 1: Sanding—"The first step is to sand the wood on all sides until it is smooth." Pick up sandpaper and demonstrate sanding with the grain and feeling for smoothness.

Step 2: Staining—"This is stain. It may need to be stirred. It is painted on with the brush and then wiped off with the rag like this." Demonstrate painting and wiping one side. "Do all the sides."

Step 3: Gluing tiles—"The tiles are glued on in rows like this." Demonstrate placing glue on the back of a red tile and placing it in the corner of recess in lid. Repeat with a white tile along short side. Space the tile but do not comment on this. "Try to make a pattern like... this sample." Critical observations of each member's sanding, staining, wiping, gluing, and placing tiles are given, and rating is done by the therapist to assess the mode of functioning for each member according to the rating criteria. The critical observations for sanding are feeling/looking for smoothness, altering pressure and direction, turning box to access all surfaces, altering the shape of the sandpaper, and noting effects.

Rating Criteria: The ADM specifies detailed rating criteria for each step: sanding, staining, and gluing tiles. Table 7-6 shows behaviors expected at each cognitive mode (3.0 through 4.8) for the first step (sanding). Refer to Allen (1993) for ADM criteria for this and other steps of the craft.

From Cole, M. B. *Group dynamics in occupational therapy: The theoretical basis and practice application of group intervention* (3rd ed.). Thorofare, NJ: SLACK Incorporated. © 2005 SLACK Incorporated.

Recessed Tile Box (Levels 3 and 4) (continued)

Table 7-6	Sanding
3.0	Reaches for and grasps object; holds, feels, may name object
3.2	Sands randomly; may not look at box while working; stops and starts on command; may comment with short phrases
3.4	May begin before instructions given, fail to stop when asked; actions sustained 1 minute or longer, may change suddenly; looks at object inconsistently, does not note effects
3.6	Begins before instructions are given, stops when told; copies demonstration one step at a time; notes effects, moves location; may miss all/part of visible surface
3.8	Stops between steps after visible surfaces are sanded and says "I'm done"; sands all visible surfaces but misses inside surfaces
4.0	Does not spontaneously refer to sample within 24"; sands all large visible surfaces; may miss or refuse to sand small or hidden surfaces
4.2	Refers to sample when only cued; may miss hidden surfaces or ask if inside/bottom should be done
4.4	Refers to and compares work to sample; may ask for verification before going on to next step; bends over box to reach back, still misses small edges
4.6	Scans environment to locate sample or supplies in plain sight; varies pressure/force/duration for better effects; may attempt to fold/tear sandpaper to do inside of box
	Rotates/examines all surfaces after sanding is completed; may not note grain of wood; may ask for help for best way to access small edges

© Claudia Allen, conference materials, 1997. Adapted with permission.

Processing and Summary: A brief discussion about how members liked the activity follows. All generalizations must be done by the therapist. Members may be asked questions about possible uses for their box—a gift, to keep jewelry, to store coins, etc. In summarizing, feedback from the therapist about the strengths of each member in following directions, responding to cues, and general workmanship is often helpful and appreciated, and ends the session on a positive note.

Cognitive Disabilities
Activity Example 7-3
Summer Salad (Level 3)

This Level 3 group activity represents a functional maintenance activity that uses the same Allen guidelines as the standardized craft previously described but is more interactive. Up to eight members whose functioning has stabilized at Allen's Level 3 may be placed in groups like this, which are designed by a registered occupational therapist or certified occupational therapist assistant using the principles of repetition and manipulation. Other staff members may be instructed by the registered occupational therapist or certified occupational therapist assistant in leading these groups. The activity should not exceed 30 minutes, and sharing of tools and materials should not be required at this level.

Materials: One serrated plastic knife, one heavy plastic fork, and one cutting board or thick paper plate for each member. One big bowl in the center of the table is filled with as many pieces of fruit as there are members. Good choices are apples, pears, bananas, oranges, peaches, cantaloupe halves (wrapped in plastic), and pineapple slices (wrapped in plastic).

Participants: Six to eight members are ideal, with a cotherapist. Members should wash their hands before starting this group.

Directions: The therapist explains that the group will make a delicious fruit salad. The ground rules are that no one eats anything until all the fruit is cut, put back in the bowl, and mixed with a coconut-and-yogurt dressing. Each member introduces self and selects a piece of fruit from the bowl. Covering eyes and identifying fruit by touch may be an interesting variation. Members should be reminded not to eat the fruit, but to wait for a therapist to demonstrate to each member how their specific fruit should be prepared and cut into bite-size pieces. Approximately 15 minutes are spent cutting and trimming. A plastic-lined trashcan is passed around to throw away cores, pits, and peels with the help of the therapist. A volunteer mixes one pint of plain yogurt, one scoop of brown sugar, and half a cup of coconut flakes. Other volunteers take turns stirring the dressing into the fruit. Other volunteers scoop the fruit salad into bowls and pass them out to the members. Eating the fruit is a well-deserved reward for their hard work.

From Cole, M. B. *Group dynamics in occupational therapy: The theoretical basis and practice application of group intervention* (3rd ed.). Thorofare, NJ: SLACK Incorporated. © 2005 SLACK Incorporated.

Cognitive Disabilities
Activity Example 7-4
Falling Leaves (Level 4)

This is a basic craft group for Level 4 patients. It is a group project following the guidelines of goal orientation, visual cues (colors and shapes), and short sequences of steps, in this case, leading to a common end product.

Materials: The table is set up by the therapist for six to 10 patients. Half of the patients have a sheet of colored paper, a pencil, a pair of paper scissors, and a cardboard pattern of a leaf. Leaf shapes used are maple, elm, oak, ash, tulip, and birch. Real leaves can be traced to produce these patterns; however, this is done by the therapist. The other half of the patients have a piece of white posterboard with a tree trunk and branches traced in black magic marker and the name of the tree outlined in black. Chunky capital letters are best, saying OAK, MAPLE, etc. with the centers to be colored in. Patients with the tree trunks also have two wide-tip markers, brown or gray and another color, and a small bottle of glue.

Directions: The therapist should demonstrate the processes.
1. Leaves. Place the leaf pattern on the colored paper and trace around it with the pencil. Fit as many as you can on the paper without overlapping any lines. When finished cut out each leaf along the lines you have traced.
2. Tree trunks. Color in the tree trunk with the appropriate color. Then color in the letters with another color. When finished, glue the appropriate leaves on the tree branches. Patients may work in pairs, so that maple leaves are glued to the maple tree trunk, etc. Colors of the leaves should be appropriate for autumn. For variation, two autumn shades may be used for each leaf to create a more interesting pattern.

Processing and Summary: Feelings about the craft activity and its end result are then elicited. Generalization discussion will center around the autumn season, what happens in the fall, and what kinds of tasks must be done to prepare for the autumn/winter season. Application can concretely be interpreted in discussing where to display the posters, and what other decorations might be desired. Therapist feedback may be given in summary. The tree posters make a good decoration for the ward.

From Cole, M. B. *Group dynamics in occupational therapy: The theoretical basis and practice application of group intervention* (3rd ed.). Thorofare, NJ: SLACK Incorporated. © 2005 SLACK Incorporated.

Cognitive Disabilities
Activity Example 7-5
Straw Hats with Potpourri (Level 5)

This is an appropriate activity for spring, and utilizes the strengths of Level 5, trial and error exploration in creating a pleasing result with the materials provided, utilizing more than one sensory system (visual and olfactory). It also includes a safety check, as members are supervised in the use of the hot glue gun and advised of the need for caution as needed.

Materials: 6-inch straw hats for each member, four rolls of thin satin ribbon (one each in pink, baby blue, red, and white), a variety of 1/2-inch silk flowers (daisies, roses, etc.), scissors, a glue gun with glue sticks, bags of potpourri in floral and herbal scents, nylon netting, spool of thread, and several colorful samples of finished hats.

Timing: Introduction—5 minutes
Activity—30 minutes
Processing/summary—20 minutes
Clean-up—5 minutes

Directions: The leader introduces members, and explains the project and its purpose. It could be a door decoration, a gift, or a preparation for the Easter holiday. Doing the craft will be a way to monitor the skill level of members and to observe how they deal with limited choices, verbal instructions, and safety precautions. The goal is for each member to design and decorate one straw hat.

Step 1: Potpourri—Cut a circle of nylon netting about 6 inches in diameter. Fill this with enough potpourri to fill the interior portion of the straw hat. Gather in the edges of the netting and tie it with a piece of string. Set this aside to be glued in later.

Step 2: Decoration—Choose ribbons to tie around the center portion of the hat. Ribbons may be tied with bows or knotted with streamers hanging down. Each member may choose two to four flowers to glue around the ribbon cluster. One piece of ribbon should be cut about 10 inches long, with the ends tied in an overhand knot to serve as a hanger.

Step 3: Gluing—The therapist should have the glue gun plugged in and heated to the correct temperature. A separated area with a fireproof surface and nothing flammable nearby should be maintained for gluing. Members can approach the gluing area several times during the session. First, the ribbons should be stabilized with a blob of glue right under the bow or knot. Next, the silk flowers are attached with glue. The nylon packet of potpourri is glued with the "tail" tucked inside the hat. Finally, the ribbon hanger loop is glued on the back, so that the hat may be hung from a hook on the door or wall.

Discussion and Summary: Feelings about the craft are elicited, followed by generalization of what other spring tasks around the house have similar attributes (i.e., getting out spring clothes, fixing up the house, making it smell nice). Discussing the use of the glue gun may be a good lead-in for reinforcing safety precautions around their homes. Other tasks involving heat and electricity (e.g., cooking, ironing, or using hair dryers, curling irons, or electric razors) should be discussed with each individual member with regard to safety. The straw hat activity may also trigger discussion of planning ahead for spring, the importance of spring cleaning, storage of winter clothes, care of lawns and gardens, or other tasks requiring anticipation, a typical problem area for Level 5. Summary should include feedback from the therapist. Hats are kept by the members to use however they like.

Chapter 8

Developmental Approaches

In the temporal context, a client's developmental stage gives occupational therapists important guidelines for exploring client occupational concerns. For example, social interactions and dating might be primary concerns for young adults, while productivity and caregiving might be more central concerns for the middle adult. Clients at midlife may have little interest in leisure occupations, while retired older clients may struggle with filling their leisure time with meaningful activities. The guiding principle of all developmental theories is that there is a developmental sequence from birth to maturity and throughout life to death. This sequence is determined by both biological and environmental forces. This development occurs in stages that are specific, progressive, and hierarchical. Development is divided into stages for the benefit of our understanding. In reality, the transition from one stage to the next is gradual. Each stage, however, is subdivided into specific skills, issues, or conflicts and each has characteristics that distinguish it from other stages.

Progressive stages refer to the idea that each stage increases in complexity and represents, in some way, progress toward maturity. It is assumed that maturity is the highest stage, and therefore the goal. Bigsby (2003) discusses some current challenges to theories of ages and stages. She points out the importance of both environment and experience in explaining the variability of skills and behaviors in the development of children. Hierarchical stages mean that each stage builds on the previous one. It reinforces the idea that there are foundation skills upon which higher level skills are built. In applying developmental theory to rehabilitation, skills that are deficient must be relearned in the same sequence in which they normally develop. This idea seems common to all the theorists reviewed here.

Framework Focus

Developmental stage is a part of each client's "personal context" as implied by the *Occupational Therapy Practice Framework* (American Occupational Therapy Association [AOTA], 2002). Developmental tasks at different stages of development are defined according to each theorist's unique focus. As one progresses developmentally, one's priorities in life will change, and one's occupational "performance patterns" are likely to reflect this. Illness and disability can disrupt the normal developmental progression, requiring a restructuring of the client's lifestyle. Occupational therapy may need to assist clients in exploring their priorities with regard to occupation and in changing or developing new habits, routines, and roles (AOTA, 2002).

The developmental frames of reference are best used as a guidepost by which to measure the effects of illness, and thereby set realistic goals for recovery. Age is never a true measure of development. However, by viewing persons with disability through the perspective of developmental stages, discrepancies between developmental and chronological age can help the therapist to appreciate the true impact of disability on a person's life.

Most developmental theories define points of change, crises, or conflicts to be resolved before the person moves up to the next stage or level. These points of stress may be instrumental in bringing about the onset or exacerbation of illness. If the occupational therapist pays attention to developmental theory, he or she can take advantage of the knowledge that specific tasks need to be mastered in order to resolve the conflict or crisis that is really a normal part of development. These life tasks can form the basis for therapeutic groups in occupational therapy.

Basic Assumptions

There are many different theories of human development, some ending with adolescence (Freud) and others continuing right through old age (Erikson, Jung). Those discussed here are chosen because they help clarify our thinking about occupational therapy groups. Included are Jung, Erikson, Levinson, Kohlberg and Wilcox, and Gilligan. Some of the theories of physiological and cognitive development, such as Ayres and Piaget, have been eliminated here and are covered instead in the next chapter on the neurodevelopmental frame of reference.

Jung

Jung, who wrote in the 1940s and 1950s, might be considered the father of adult development theory. He differed from Freud in extending the developmental process throughout life and in acknowledging the contribution of external factors to growth and adaptation. Jung divided life into four basic stages:

1. Childhood
2. Youth
3. Mid-life
4. Old age

In Jung's view, childhood is spent in blissful ignorance. Although influenced by many inherited predispositions, children develop with no doubts, unaware of their own growth processes. Youth is marked by the onset of consciousness, of doubts, problems, contradictions, and responsibilities. Jung described the second half of life as beginning between ages 35 and 40, when the essential character of life changes and energy becomes rechanneled. Before age 40, the individual has put his or her energy into external events such as establishing occupation, community position, marriage, and family. After age 40, Jung believes the individual turns inward, focusing more on the spiritual (Schultz, 1976).

Middle age is described by Jung as the "afternoon of life." Polarities are opposite tendencies of the self present in an individual, such as introversion vs. extroversion, rationality vs. intuitiveness, aggressiveness vs. sensitivity, and action vs. contemplation. At mid-life, Jung contends that whatever sides of the self were expressed in the person's youth, the opposite sides will prevail in midlife. It was Jung who identified individuation as the true goal of life, a concept much in question in the 1980s. Individuation is a kind of enhancement of identity that involves further definition of the self. Individuation continues through each of the stages in greater depths and in different ways. The end result of individuation was thought to be integration, a uniting of all parts of the self into a qualified whole.

Old age is the final stage. As a person ages, he or she faces physical decline, removes him- or herself from positions of authority and responsibility, and faces the inevitability of his or her own death. Jung assumed a belief in the presence of an afterlife and began the idea that all individuals ultimately contribute to a "collective unconscious," and so live on through others (Table 8-1).

Erikson

Erikson also built on Freud's psychosexual stages and extended his theory to include adolescence and adulthood. His ideas are compatible with Jung's, but more social in nature and based on the central issues of each stage as conflicts to be resolved. The stages that most impact our adult client groups are:

- Identity vs. role confusion-Ages 13 to 22
- Intimacy vs. isolation-Ages 23 to 35
- Generativity vs. stagnation-Ages 36 to 50
- Integrity vs. despair-Ages 50 to death

Erikson's stages are well-known and referred to often in occupational therapy literature. The conflict areas can guide our choice of activities in occupational therapy and can serve as a basis for setting goals at the various age levels. For example, trust issues can be worked on through movement activities, such as "Falling" and "Being Caught," or through verbal activities, such as giving and receiving emotional support (Table 8-2).

Levinson

Levinson (1978) has published the most extensive (although admittedly controversial) research

Table 8-1	Jung's Stages of Development (Spiritual)

Age	Stage
Birth to puberty (childhood)	Blissful ignorance, inherited predispositions
Puberty to age 35 (Youth)	Conscious and doubting, taking on responsibility
Age 35 to old age (Mid-life)	Change in direction to express latent parts of self-individuation and integration
Infirmity and death (Old age)	Infirmity, acceptance of death, afterlife, and collective unconscious

Table 8-2	Erikson's Eight Stages of Development (Psychosocial)

Age	Stage
Birth to infancy	Trust vs. Mistrust
2 to 4 Toddlerhood	Autonomy vs. Shame and Doubt
5 to 7 Early childhood	Initiative vs. Guilt
8 to 12 Middle childhood	Industry vs. Inferiority
13 to 22 Adolescence	Identity vs. Role Confusion
23 to 35 Young adult	Intimacy vs. Isolation
35 to 50 Adulthood	Generativity vs. Stagnation
50 to Death	Integrity vs. Despair

study to date on the developmental stages of adulthood. He based his findings on a longevity study of 40 men. Levinson presents adulthood as periods of stability alternating with periods of transition. The three life transitions he identifies are:

1. Early adult—Ages 17 to 22
2. Mid-life—Ages 40 to 45
3. Late adult—Age 60 to 65

These periods of conflict are interspersed with periods of relative stability in which the individual lives within an established life structure and stays more or less on course (Table 8-3).

Levinson contends that each transition period occurs during specific age ranges and each transition has its own developmental tasks. Like Erikson, he saw each transition as requiring the resolution of conflicts before the person can move on to the next stage.

Primarily the tasks of each transition period are to re-evaluate the existing life structure, explore the possibilities of change, and make choices that will restructure life in the next era. Eras are in between stages of stability described as young, middle, and late adulthood. In the Levinson study of 40 men, work was considered to be a "base for life in society," giving the man his life structure in a cultural, class, and social sense as well as occupational sense (Levinson, 1978, p. 9). Since the thrust of the study was to examine the mid-life transition, subjects selected were age 35, from four different occupational groups, and were followed

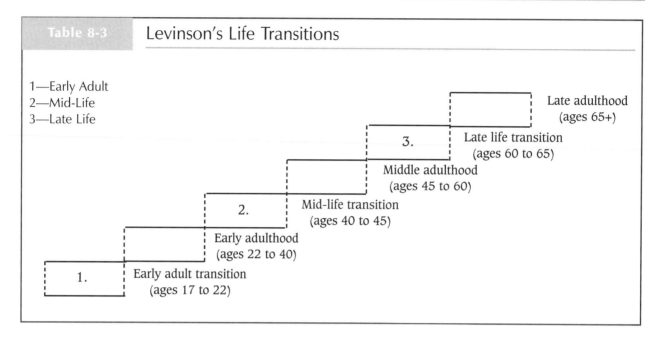

Table 8-3 Levinson's Life Transitions

1—Early Adult
2—Mid-Life
3—Late Life

Late adulthood
(ages 65+)

3.

Late life transition
(ages 60 to 65)

Middle adulthood
(ages 45 to 60)

Mid-life transition
(ages 40 to 45)

2.

Early adulthood
(ages 22 to 40)

1.

Early adult transition
(ages 17 to 22)

to age 45. Biographical information collected from these subjects forms the basis of the young adult transition. The late adult transition is only briefly covered by Levinson and is considered to parallel the preceding transition.

Levinson's theory has been selected for focus because it presents a good structure around which to understand life problems of clients and to plan occupational therapy groups.

The Early Adult Transition

The essence of this transition is the separation from the family of origin in order to establish a new home base. The separation is both geographical and emotional and generally creates a sense of loss. Yet the excitement involved in establishing one's self in the adult world provides a sense of satisfaction. Exploration in the early adult transition quickly pushes toward commitment as the young man is required to take on adult responsibilities. Balancing exploration with the need for structure is an ongoing struggle. The major tasks of the early adult transition are forming the dream, finding a mentor, forming an occupation, and starting a marriage and family.

Forming the Dream

The first task that plays a powerful role in early adulthood is called forming a dream. Levinson states that the dream emerges during the early adult transition where the boy/man imagines himself settled in the adult world. This may be con-

nected with concrete reality or far removed from his actual world. The ability to play make-believe in early childhood is the forerunner of this imagining in early adulthood. The dream is a vehicle for exploring his image, and "provides a source of hope, self-esteem, and personal integrity" (Levinson, 1978, p. 93). The young adult's task includes forming relationships with others who can facilitate his work on the dream and find ways of living it out in his life. If the dream is unconnected with choices made in this stage, it will resurface during the mid-life transition and demand a place for self-expression then.

The Mentor Relationship

According to Levinson, the mentor relationship is very complex and extremely significant for a man during early adulthood. The mentor is a transitional figure in a person's life, serving as a teacher, sponsor, guide, and adviser. The most important function of the mentor is "to support and facilitate the realization of the dream" (Levinson, 1978, p. 98). Offering expertise and counseling to a young man, yet not being parental, the mentor is usually older than his protégé by a half-generation. All men in the study had male mentors, although Levinson's own mentor was a female, and it is expected that as more women enter currently male-dominated fields, they too will serve as mentors to both men and women.

In a study made by Margaret Hennig of 25 high-level women executives, it was shown that all had found male mentors early in their careers (Sheehy,

1976). Interestingly, these successful women chose careers rather than marriage in their 20s, yet realized around age 35 that something was missing and began to explore their feminine sides. Levinson reports a similar happenstance for men who become less involved with their mentors by age 40, and face the task of reintegrating the feminine side of their personality.

Choosing an Occupation

The process of choosing an occupation extends throughout the entire life cycle, beginning in childhood with make-believe games like "doctor" or "teacher." As Levinson remarks about other important life choices, "The great paradox of human development is that we are required to make crucial choices before we have the knowledge, judgment, and self-understanding to choose wisely" (1978, p. 162). Transforming one's early interests into an occupational choice during young adulthood is a complex psychosocial process, and a pattern usually emerges with some definition by the early 30s. An occupation often serves as an index of an individual's worth in society, both economically and socially, and defines his role in the community. For many of the men in Levinson's study, establishing an occupational identity is often tied up with parental expectations, and the nurturing given to the dream concept with or without the presence of a mentor. There are enormous differences between individuals regarding the meaning of success and failure, and concepts around these values change as growth occurs throughout their lifespan.

This stage has important implications for occupational therapy. Because illness almost always interrupts the work role of the client, values around self and work need to be reconsidered. Group activities dealing with values around the work role and the exploration of alternate roles in the home and community are appropriate for a wide variety of client populations.

Marriage and Family

The developmental task of forming a marriage and family also involves making premature choices. It is unusual to have integrated the many components of a stable adult relationship in the early adulthood stage. Sexuality, dependency, emotional intimacy, friendship, and the capability for commitment are but a few of the issues that extend beyond this phase. Actually, the ability to relate to the feminine or masculine aspects of self is a lifetime task, one of the many polarities that both Levinson and Jung give importance to in adult development. Undertaking the obligation to marry and have children does not necessarily mean one is prepared for the responsibilities and commitments. Often this step is intricately bound up with the other tasks of early adulthood, such as separating from parents and finding support for the dream pursuit. Levinson describes a "special woman" (1978, p. 109) who facilitates a man's entry into the adult world by providing boundaries within which his aspirations can be realized and giving nourishment to his occupational journey. If the marital choice is made in such a way as to be antithetical to the dream, the relationship may suffer conflicts at a later date. Obviously, the relationship will be modified over time to accommodate the dreams of both the man and woman, and there are endless possibilities for creating a family pattern that is suitable for both. The importance of fatherhood and motherhood may not emerge until the individual has outgrown his occupational mentor and is prepared to provide those types of functions himself to his younger associates and to his own offspring.

The Mid-Life Transition

This period is said to provide the bridge from early to middle adulthood. It brings a man to question, search, and re-examine his life and his values. For the great majority of men in the Levinson study (80% of subjects), this great struggle within the self and the external world may reach crisis proportions. Often several years are needed to go through the process and come to some resolution. A culminating event often signifies success or failure in the man's fantasy, and this self-judgment may be all encompassing. If he fails to get a promotion, he may regard himself as a failure in other aspects of his life as well. This transition period begins when a man realizes that he cannot go on as before, that he cannot "become his own man" under his existing life structure, and that changes will be necessary in order to advance sufficiently in any chosen direction. Three main tasks are defined by Levinson for this stage of development:

1. To terminate the era of early adulthood (reappraising the past)
2. To take the first steps toward middle adulthood (modifying the life structure)
3. To deal with the polarities that are the sources of deep division in his life (individuation at mid-life)

Each of these broadly defined tasks has many specific aspects to consider.

Reappraising the Past

Recognition of his own mortality gives a man a renewed sense of urgency about the use of his remaining time. He examines his accomplishments in relation to earlier hopes, values, and expectations, asking "Have I accomplished all that I set out to do?" Because of the nature of a dream, which is essentially fantasy, many ideas, assumptions, and beliefs associated with the dream do not withstand the comparison with actual experience. Levinson defines "de-illusionment" as "a recognition that long-held assumptions and beliefs about self and the world are not true" (1978, p. 192). The process of de-illusionment is accompanied by emotions of disappointment, joy, relief, bitterness, grief, wonder, freedom, and pain. At this stage a man may ask: "What have I done with my life? Is what I'm doing now what I want to be doing in the future? Have I reached success at my job? Am I fulfilled by my marital relationship? What are my present values and priorities? Am I spending my time on the things I really value? Is what I have done really meaningful? How have I been fooling myself? (and/or) What is my true worth in my eyes and society's?" Occupational therapy groups can focus on some of these issues to help clients who are facing a mid-life transition to answer some of these questions.

Modifying the Life Structure

Having taken stock of the past, man now begins to plan for the next phase: exploration of new patterns for living occurs. Some changes are externally motivated. The realities of growing families, aging parents, and changes in spouse and the marriage require certain changes in role and point of view. Experience of world politics, economy, cultural, and social values also influence the planning of man's new life structure. But whether or not visible change occurs, one's outlook, values, and expectations of life are essentially different as a result of the developmental tasks of the mid-life transition. Questions to be asked are: "What do I want to change in my life? What are my options for change in occupation, marriage and family roles, roles in the community? What are the external changes in my life that put pressure on me to change? What pressures do I feel from society, friends, associates, and family, either to change or to remain the same? How can I feel more fulfilled? What parts of myself have gone undeveloped that I would now like to give expression? What faults do I see that I would like to eliminate? What new character traits can I work on developing? How can

I set a more realistic goal for the future? What new beliefs can be adopted to replace the delusions of the past?" The possibilities of occupational therapy activities to help with the planning process are endless. Furthermore, the potential for self-discovery and exploration of options are maximized in group intervention.

Individuation at Mid-Life

At mid-life, individuation is a continuation of past processes. An increasingly separate existence has been evolving since birth, gradually forming clearer boundaries between the self and the outside world. This individuation plays a part at each transition. Levinson takes his cue from Jung in describing the mid-life individuation tasks as resolving four polarities:

1. Young/old
2. Destruction/creation
3. Masculine/feminine
4. Attachment/separateness

Every life structure necessitates giving high priority to certain aspects of the self while minimizing others. In young adulthood, youth, creativity, masculinity, and attachment often outweigh their counterparts. At mid-life, neglected parts urgently seek expression.

1. The Young/Old Polarity: Young and old are viewed as relative terms, not specifically tied with any age. Young takes on such meanings as birth, growth, possibility, initiation, openness, energy, potential, promise of spring, fertility, and vision of things to come. Conversely, old represents termination, fruition, stability, rigidity, completion, impotence, senility, and death.

   The issues of the young/old dichotomy at mid-life are realization of one's own death, fear of loss of youth, decline in bodily and psychological powers, realization that one's time is limited, wish for immortality and fear that man is not immortal, loss of omnipotence, and acceptance of limitation. Out of the recognition of one's own mortality comes the imagery of the legacy, or what a man will pass on to future generations. Among possible legacies are children, teachings or discoveries, concrete and social structures, objects of lasting value, written documents, and artistic works.

2. The Destruction/Creation Polarity: A new awareness of the destruction as a universal process takes on several forms in the mid-life

transition. A man must come to an understanding of his grievances toward others for their destructiveness toward him. This typically results in anger toward loved ones: parents, wife, mentors, and friends whom he sees as having hurt him. He must also look at his own destructiveness in terms of how he has hurt others. It is necessary for him to accept destructiveness as a natural part of life and to take responsibility for it. Taking action in any direction always has consequences, some creative and some destructive. "If he is forced to maintain the illusion that destructiveness does not exist, he will also be impaired in his capacity for creating, loving, and affirming life" (Levinson, 1978, p. 224).

3. The Masculine/Feminine Polarity: Levinson refers to the terms masculine and feminine as going beyond the biological and social differentiation. Masculinity refers to bodily prowess and toughness, homosexuality, rationality, achievement and ambition, and an intolerance of weakness. Femininity refers to motherhood, caring and emotionality, artistic creativity, softness, and lack of strength and stamina. The masculine and feminine are really both aspects of the same person and are seen as poorly integrated in early adulthood, due to immaturity, cultural tradition, and the necessity for aggressive pursuit of one's occupation and social position. In middle adulthood, however, man comes to new terms with this polarity, seeing masculine and feminine as less rigidly divided within the self and combining them more creatively in work, personal relationships, and acceptance of self. Aggressiveness may give way to a more nurturing and sensitive side of the personality without really injuring the masculine role identity. The resolution of the masculine/feminine dichotomy opens new possibilities for the man in both love relationships with peer women and mentor relationships.

In occupational therapy, we are constantly faced with the masculine and feminine identities of our clients. In doing activity groups with male and female clients, it is important to consider their values and expectations. For example, male clients may refuse to do activities like cooking or sewing, which they consider to be "women's work." Female clients may have negative feelings about doing money management or using power tools. In using developmental theory, the age and gender of our clients as well as their disability will determine what activities they are willing to try.

4. The Attachment/Separateness Polarity: Attachment is defined by Levinson as "to be engaged, involved, needy, plugged in, seeking, and rooted" (1978, p. 239). Separateness is distinguished from isolation and loneliness in that it refers to a person's involvement in his inner world, his fantasies. In early adulthood, with marriage and mentor relationships, typically attachment takes precedence at the expense of separateness. At mid-life, developmentally a more equal balance between the two must be achieved. This generally means the man at mid-life moves further into himself, and through this process is able to examine his own feelings, values, and goals apart from external and social expectations.

The Late Life Transition

Levinson (1978) positions the late adult transition at ages 60 to 65. The tasks of this period are to reappraise the past, create a new life structure, and make choices that are relevant to the final stage of life. Levinson's study does not extend beyond mid-life and must be viewed as speculation. The issues facing the older adult are physical decline, loss of a productive role, and coming to terms with death, both of self and loved ones. According to some theorists, changes in perception of time begin at mid-life, from "time since birth" to "time left to live." In the late adult transition, the approach of death can no longer be ignored. The limited time remaining must be devoted to resolving old conflicts, finishing unfinished business, deepening important relationships, and arranging to leave one's legacy. These life tasks lend themselves very nicely to group activities in occupational therapy. Life review groups are one example of how occupational therapy can address these issues.

Physical Decline

By the year 2020, the average life expectancy will be 77 years and 20% of the population in the United States will be over age 65. As people live longer, the effects of normal physical decline become more prominent. At the most basic level, aging cells begin to degenerate and die. Loss of neurons in the brain are the cause of senility and occur naturally but more rapidly in degenerative diseases like Alzheimer's. Brain cell loss causes functional loss of memory and personality changes as well. Functioning of vital organs, including heart and lungs, slows down. Anatomic changes result in loss of hearing, decline in eyesight, loss of height, and lower muscle mass and tone. Most people are familiar with the graying of hair and the general loss of strength and endurance. Osteoporosis (brittle bones) and osteoarthritis (painful joints) are common.

Changes in the immune system often make older persons more susceptible to disease. Longevity has been shown to be related most closely to heredity. However, regular medical check-ups and a healthy lifestyle are still the best preventive measures. Vulnerability to stress also increases with age. Despite the skills accumulated over a lifetime, change at older ages is still more difficult and more stressful.

Coping with bodily decline requires an acceptance of a more passive role with respect to the environment. Changes in lifestyle that limit physical demands while providing a sense of worth and satisfaction are preferable. Occupational therapy groups can center around energy conservation, setting goals and priorities, exercise and fitness, health education and maintenance, and exploring activities that encourage continued use of skills and maintenance of self-esteem and social recognition.

Loss of Productive Role

Retirement may be voluntary or mandatory between ages 60 and 65. Either way, the changes produced by it are many, and the responses shown by individuals are mixed. For some, the increased time to relax and pursue leisure interests is welcome. But for many, retirement is a negative experience that lowers self-worth and leaves them socially isolated. The economic impact of retirement is very real, and those without pensions or retirement plans may find themselves having to accept a lower income and lower socioeconomic status. Retired persons need to find a new structure to replace the worker role and new interests to give them a sense of self-worth. Occupational therapy groups dealing with retirement issues can address time management, financial management, leisure planning, community involvement, volunteering, socialization, new skill development, and many others.

Coming to Terms With Death

Loss is a predominant theme in the lives of older people. Erikson's view of the final conflict to be resolved may be helpful in understanding how loss can be accepted. His eighth stage, integrity vs. despair, suggests that contentment in old age results from the view of a life productively lived (Kaplan & Sadock, 2003). The late adult transition necessarily includes reviewing one's life experiences and reappraising them to sum up their worth. The results of this reappraisal may determine how an individual copes with the later years. At best, in later life, grandparents enjoy spoiling their grandchildren, and retired workers enjoy knowing that the younger generations will benefit from their life's work. Teachers may enjoy watching the success of their students, for example. According to Erikson, peace and contentment in old age occurs only if one has previously achieved intimacy and generativity. An older person needs to know that his or her life has been productive and that he or she has passed on his or her wisdom to others in some way. Without this belief, there is only despair. Despair, according to Erikson, is indicated by a fear of death and the realization that it is too late to start over.

Preparation for death is another necessary prerequisite for integrity in old age. As life is reappraised, old conflicts and unfinished business may be recalled. It is not unusual to wish for reconciliations with estranged friends or relatives. Often there are old wrongs to forgive, apologies to make, and unkept promises to reconsider. These are important emotional concerns of the elderly and should not be prematurely dismissed. Those who are physically or cognitively impaired may need help in dealing with these issues. Even when actual reconciliations are not feasible, a great deal can be done through group experiences incorporating role play and other creative activities. Developing a point of view about death is a spiritual and philosophical concern. Carl Rogers, psychotherapist and major spokesman for humanistic psychology, described a new interest in his 70s as he explored the world of the paranormal with his wife. His experiences changed his understanding of death. Whereas in his 50s and 60s he regarded death to be the end of the individual, he now considers it possible that the spiritual essence of man continues to live after death. He mentions the views of Arthur Koestler about each individual's consciousness being a part of the "cosmic consciousness" (Rogers, 1980, p. 88), a view that echoes Jung's ideas regarding the collective unconscious. Zemke and Gratz (1982) point out that for the aged, illness and disability tend to renew earlier crises:

> The (occupational) therapist must acknowledge and work toward resolution of these just as she would with any other disabled adult. Only then can the ego integrity crisis be faced. Techniques such as remotivation or life review provide a basis for the thoughtful review and acceptance of life experience necessary for resolution at this final stage of life. (p. 61)

Table 8-4	Kohlberg and Wilcox Development of Moral Reasoning

Age	Stage
2 to 4	Preconventional level: decisions made on the basis of punishment and reward Stage 1: person is egocentric no ability to empathize Stage 2: reciprocity makes deals with authority
6+	Conventional level: decisions based on pleasing others Stage 3: confirms identity as good authority is fair good people get best treatment Stage 4: law and order orientation rules necessary to maintain social structure only one system is "right"
11 to 12	Postconventional level: fairness is free standing logic Stage 5: individual rights and human dignity can override rules empathy influences decisions right and wrong are separate from rules Stage 6: ideal stage, rarely encountered in reality unconditional value of rights of humanity empathizes with all participants in a moral dilemma creatively resolves polarities and contradictions

Kohlberg and Wilcox

Kohlberg and Wilcox built on the work of Piaget, who developed stages of intellectual development. They looked at the way logic was used in the development of moral reasoning (Wilcox, 1979). How people get along in society, their view of themselves, and the social structure depend on how they make decisions about right and wrong. Kohlberg and Wilcox suggest three levels and six stages of moral development (Table 8-4). This perspective is useful in planning groups with clients who are not psychotic but have problems with society or in dealing with authority figures or rules. Motivation to move up to the next level is having experiences that contradict one's former beliefs and cause one to question his or her own reasoning. According to Kohlberg, all of the stages can be brought into adulthood. Many adults have been found to operate at the preconventional and conventional levels. Therapists should look for lags in moral reasoning as a possible explanation of behavior in clients.

Bruce and Borg (1993) suggest that occupational therapy group leaders encourage growth in moral reasoning by creating dissonance. Therapists do this by exposing the group members to reasoning at a slightly higher level and encouraging role taking and role reversal. Introducing moral dilemmas for a group to discuss and solve might provide an appropriate setting for this kind of developmental learning.

Gilligan-"A Different Voice"

Gilligan (1982) challenges previous theories of development in two respects. She sheds doubt on the "age and stage" concept of development, and she suggests that women have a different way of thinking about life than men do and that their developmental stages may also be fundamentally different. Gilligan points out that prior theorists, including Erikson, Kohlberg, and Levinson, have based their beliefs primarily on observations of men. A professor at Harvard, Gilligan performed her own research regarding men and women from childhood through maturity, regarding their identity and moral development, rights and responsibilities, and the role of conflict in development.

In relation to Kohlberg, Gilligan (1982) suggests that these stages relate more to men than women and do not consider the variables of culture, time, occasion, and gender. She observes that events of women's lives and of history promote the view that concern with individual survival is "selfish" or "bad," as opposed to the "responsibility" of a life lived in relationships. For women, life is caring in relationships. When the focus on individuation and individual achievement extends into adulthood and maturity is equated with personal autonomy, concern with relationships appears as a weakness of women rather than a human strength.

The stereotypes of adulthood or maturity suggested by Levinson and Erikson favor separateness or self-sufficiency over connection to others. This is primarily a "male" point of view, according to Gilligan (1982). According to these theorists, young adulthood is characterized by a conflict of commitment in which either identity or intimacy wins out. The male believes that separation empowers the self and permits full self-expression, and intimacy, the choice of women, represents immaturity and impedes expression of the self. Gilligan states that "the silence of women in the narrative of adult development distorts the conception of its stages and sequence" (Gilligan, 1982, p. 156).

Gilligan does not suggest an alternative sequence of developmental stages, nor does she describe how pre-established stages are different for women. Yet her points are well taken and encourage us, in using this frame of reference, not to accept the proposed ages and stages as absolute reality.

In considering Gilligan's message for occupational therapy groups, we need to consider more carefully the role of relationships for our clients. There is no better place than a group to explore and work on the skills that affect relationships.

Function and Dysfunction

If one uses an age and stage theory, then healthy functioning is having achieved appropriate developmental tasks for his or her age. For example, a 23-year-old will have separated from his or her parents, chosen a career, and if not married, at least developed a support system of peers with whom to identify. Conversely, dysfunction may be looked at as failure to develop age-appropriate skills or failure to achieve the tasks of an age-appropriate stage. The stages of childhood and adolescence have been studied historically in much greater detail than those of adulthood. So as Gilligan (1982) implies, it is better to use the ages given for developmental tasks as approximate guidelines. Furthermore, as illness interferes with normal development, the discrepancy between age and developmental level may become so great that the term "age-appropriate" becomes meaningless. It is the developmental stage that we as occupational therapists are concerned with, since that is what determines the level of function and adaptation to the environment. Dysfunction can be seen as a lack of adaptive skills necessary for effective and satisfying interaction with one's environment. It can be caused by a failure to develop these skills (developmental delay), a loss of these skills (e.g., due to brain trauma), or a regression to an earlier stage of development (such as that caused by depression or schizophrenia).

In adult development theory, just the normal tasks at each transitional stage may be enough to cause a crisis situation. If Levinson (1978) speaks of the mid-life transition as a potential crisis for 80% of the population, think of the impact it must have on those with physical or mental disability. If Levinson is right, the stress produced by this kind of crisis is likely to contribute to physical and mental breakdown, even in those without previous illness.

Development is almost always affected by illness. As clients with disability are referred to occupational therapy, the assessment process is likely to uncover missing skills that clients have failed to learn in earlier stages of development. The difficulty in coping with illness in the present is often due to the inadequacy of earlier skill development. Because the stages of development are hierarchical, occupational therapy cannot address issues of the client's current age until earlier skills are learned. For example, a 20-year-old may not be expected to work on career choice and separation from parents if his or her illness has resulted in a lack of ability to form peer relationships and his or her own identity is not developed. Because of discrepancies between chronological and developmental age in persons with illness and disability, groups in occupational therapy often include clients of varying ages. Occupational therapists organize group interventions by developmental levels (not age levels) so that members can work together on similar skills.

Change and Motivation

Motivation comes from an individual's natural desire for mastery of age-appropriate skills. The drive toward mastery is, at least in part, biologically determined. However, as a person matures, the environment plays a greater part in motivation. If a person's attempts to progress developmentally are met with success, motivation will likely remain intact. Repeated failures to keep up with peers, on the other hand, may discourage a person from continuing to try. Occupational therapy may encourage the rediscovery of the drive toward mastery by creating a "just-right challenge." This is a task or situation that encourages a client to use higher level skills, but one that is not beyond his or her reach.

When there is a developmental lag or loss of skills, they must be learned or relearned in the correct developmental sequence. Mosey (1970) called this "recapitulation of ontogeny." If the client is more than one level behind, the change process may be slow, but it follows a more or less predictable pattern. Since developmental stages are hierarchical, the earlier skills must be mastered before the learning of later developing skills is possible.

Consider a group of individuals with chronic mental illness. The age of onset for several chronic mental illnesses is the early 20s. Often clients have achieved at least some of the developmental tasks of the young adult transition before becoming ill. Many have vocational or educational training in a chosen career, some have begun working and have moved out of their parents' homes, and some have married and had one or two children. These are accomplishments beyond the capacity of most clients with chronic mental illness. One might see these clients as regressed. Because of their illness, they have gone backward to an earlier, less mature stage of development. In treating these clients, the occupational therapist needs to determine the correct level at which to begin. This will be the level at which mastery is possible and growth and change can be motivated.

Mosey's concept of the six adaptive skills is helpful in identifying a client's correct developmental level, as well as determining which skills need work. These skills are:
1. Perceptual motor
2. Cognitive
3. Dyadic interaction
4. Group interaction
5. Self-identity
6. Sexual identity skills

Each adaptive skill has several subskills whose typical ages of development are identified. These are described fully in Appendix C (Mosey, 1986).

Change occurs through the learning of new skills. This can be encouraged by setting up a growth-facilitating environment. The occupational therapist looks carefully at the physical environment in terms of safety. The emotional environment may best be set through the client-therapist relationship and through the use of groups. Mosey's (1970) concept of developmental groups is useful here. The hierarchy of group structure and leadership requirements in these groups can help occupational therapists to plan group interventions for clients that are appropriate to their level of development (see Appendix B).

However, the benefits of group intervention go beyond the learning or relearning of group interaction skills. All six adaptive skills identified by Mosey may be effectively learned in a group context through occupational therapy activity. At the higher developmental levels, the tasks of adult development may be facilitated through group activities in occupational therapy.

Group Intervention

It has been implied that groups in this frame of reference are best organized along the lines of developmental level. Occupational therapy groups would be primarily homogeneous. At lower levels, clients in a parallel group may be participating in activities that promote sensorimotor or cognitive skill development. At higher levels, groups may use interaction skills to work on career choice in the young adult transition, re-examine their values in the mid-life transition, or participate in retirement planning in the late-life transition. The structure of occupational therapy group intervention is organized according to the developmental level, and this guides the occupational therapist's choice of activity as well.

The limitations for use of this frame of reference are minimal. Clients of every age and almost any type of disability are appropriately treated within its bounds. The theories of adult development described in this chapter, however, are most helpful in planning groups for the later stages of development. Guidelines for the earlier stages, dealing with sensorimotor and cognitive development, are described in Chapters 6 and 9.

Role of the Leader

In developmental groups, the occupational therapist takes a directive role. Knowledge of the predictable conflicts and skills in each developmental stage guides the use of activities and setting of group goals. He or she evaluates clients' skills to determine their developmental levels and attempts to predict their potential for further development. When placed in appropriate groups, clients can work together on their mutual tasks with the leader's guidance. Because the sequence of learned tasks is hierarchical, the occupational therapist cannot give too many choices to the group. If the groups are planned appropriately, their area of interest should coincide with the developmental tasks of their level. Occupational therapists need to challenge their groups to develop further by consistently introducing higher level activities at appropriate times.

It is also the responsibility of the leader to create and maintain a growth-facilitating environment (Mosey, 1970). In the intervention setting, clients should be supported and rewarded for growth, not discouraged. If a group is ready to take on more responsibility, this should be allowed. If growing requires a stage of upset and turmoil, and it has to get worse before it gets better, this should also be met with patience and support.

The occupational therapist should be on the lookout for signs of developmental transitions in clients with physical disability as well as mental illness. Even when the illness is physical, addressing developmental issues can be the most beneficial in helping the client to cope. Coping with illness or developmental crises often requires the learning of enabling skills. These are specific cognitive, psychosocial, or sensorimotor learned behaviors that make it possible for the individual to meet his or her developmental needs (Bruce and Borg, 1993). Examples are reading and writing, communication skills, or the ability to empathize with others. Mosey's adaptive skills might be used as a guide.

Examples of Activities

The chosen activities should address issues to be resolved or specific skills appropriate to the developmental level of the client group. The theorist, the specific stage to be addressed, and the specific task or skill within that stage should be identified. Since most of the theorists have an identified hierarchy of issues, tasks, or skills to be learned at each level, these can easily serve as guidelines for activity choice. See Activity Examples 8-1 through 8-10. Most of the group activities at the end of this chapter originally appeared in Cole and Gross (1982).

Group Leadership

The seven steps of group leadership can remain intact when working with most adult groups in this frame of reference. The introduction is done according to the guidelines offered in Chapter 1.

Activity

Activities and goals are chosen using specific guidelines from the ages and stages of development. The learning exercise in Worksheet 8-1 may be helpful in identifying the theory and stage that is appropriate for your particular clients. Fill in the chart by writing under the various chronological ages the appropriate information from the theories reviewed at the beginning of this chapter.

It is especially important to plan an environment that incorporates safety, support, and challenge. The goals for these groups are to help members progress to higher levels of development. The timing of groups may be altered to suit the group, the activity, and the goal. Many of the tasks of adult development are quite complex, and there are many aspects to be explored. Activities such as those listed above may take several sessions, depending on how they are planned and how much discussion seems appropriate. If clients are motivated by a particular activity, it may be desirable to give homework. Clients may be asked to think about the issues discussed between sessions, to explore options for change, or to try out new behaviors with family and friends.

A good resource for the late life developmental tasks is the AOTA publication, *Lifestyle Redesign: Implementing the Well Elderly Program* (Mandel, Jackson, Zemke, Nelson, & Clark, 1999). This manual provides many prevention activities dealing with transitions of older adulthood.

Sharing and Processing

Sharing, including self-expression and feedback, is an important part of the developmental group. However, while members are working on similar tasks, there is no expectation that they will produce similar results, since each person must

Worksheet 8-1
Developmental Theories
Comparative Chart

Directions: Using information from this text and others, fill in the developmental stages for each of the theorists. Estimate the chronological age range for each stage and fill in on the chart below.

Chronological Age	0-1	2	5	Years 10	15	20	
Jung (Spiritual Stages)							
Erikson (Psychosocial Stages)							
Levinson (Life Transitions)							
Kohlberg (Moral Development)							
Mosey (Appendix C) (Adaptive Skills)							
Perceptual-Motor, Cognitive							
Dyadic Interaction, Group Interaction							
Self-Identity, Sexual Identity							
Physical Milestones/ Attributes Typical of Age							

Worksheet 8-1
Developmental Theories
Comparative Chart (continued)

Chronological Age	25	30	40	Years 45	50	60	65
Jung (Spiritual Stages)							
Erikson (Psychosocial Stages)							
Levinson (Life Transitions)							
Kohlberg (Moral Development)							
Mosey (Appendix C) (Adaptive Skills)							
Perceptual-Motor, Cognitive							
Dyadic Interaction, Group Interaction							
Self-Identity, Sexual Identity							
Physical Milestones/ Attributes Typical of Age							

From Cole, M. B. *Group dynamics in occupational therapy: The theoretical basis and practice application of group intervention* (3rd ed.). Thorofare, NJ: SLACK Incorporated. © 2005 SLACK Incorporated.

complete a developmental task in his or her own way. This expectation is consistent with the concepts of client-centered practice (AOTA, 2002). Processing the group may uncover many feelings about both past and present experiences. This is one frame of reference in which talking about past events is not discouraged. Relationships among members evidenced during processing can be helpful in supporting clients through many traumatic memories as well as stressful present day realities. Group cohesiveness in this frame is desirable and encouraged.

Generalizing and Application

Generalizing an experience should be somewhat predictable, since most of the activities will address specific developmental issues. The therapist really has to take the lead to guide the discussion of general principles along developmental lines.

Application is a particularly important aspect of developmental groups, since the group experiences are designed to have a specific impact on development. If there is a focus to the discussion of developmental groups, it should be the application of learning to each individual's everyday life. The summary can be shared by members and the leader, depending on the ability of the group, and this should also stress application of learning.

Bibliography

American Occupational Therapy Association. (2002). Occupational therapy practice framework: Domain and process. *American Journal of Occupational Therapy, 56,* 609-639.

Bigsby, R. (2003). Developmental and neurological perspectives. In E. Crepeau, E. Cohn, & B. Boyt Schell (Eds.), *Willard & Spackman's occupational therapy* (10th ed., pp. 243-245). Philadelphia: Lippincott, Williams & Wilkins.

Bruce, M. A., & Borg, B. (1993). *Frames of reference in psychosocial occupational therapy* (2nd ed.). Thorofare, NJ: SLACK Incorporated.

Cole, M., & Gross, M. (1982). *Structured group experiences for life's adult transitions.* Unpublished manuscript.

Gilligan, C. (1982). *A different voice.* Cambridge, MA: Harvard University Press.

Kaplan, H., & Sadock, B. (2003). *Synopsis of psychiatry* (9th ed.). Baltimore: Williams & Wilkins.

Levinson, D. (1978). *The seasons of a man's life.* New York: Ballentine Books.

Mandel, D., Jackson, J., Zemke, R., Nelson, L., & Clark, F. (1999). *Lifestyle redesign: Implementing the well elderly program.* Bethesda, MD: American Occupational Therapy Association.

Mosey, A. C. (1970). *Three frames of reference for mental health.* Thorofare, NJ: SLACK Incorporated.

Mosey, A. C. (1986). *Psychosocial components of occupational therapy.* New York: Raven.

Rogers, C. (1980). *A way of being.* Boston: Houghton Mifflin.

Schultz, D. (1976). *Theories of personality.* Monterrey, CA: Brooks/Cole.

Sheehy, G. (1976). *Passages: Predictable crises of adult life.* New York: E. P. Dutton.

Sheehy, G. (1981). *Pathfinders: Overcoming the crises of adult life.* New York: E. P. Dutton.

Wilcox, M. (1979). *Developmental journey.* Nashville: Abbington Press.

Zemke, R., & Gratz, R. R. (1982). The role of theory: Erikson and occupational therapy. *Occupational Therapy in Mental Health, II*(3), 45-63.

Developmental
Activity Example 8-1
Ideal Man/Ideal Woman

This activity addresses Levinson's early adult transition, specifically, the tasks of finding a special woman or man and finding a mentor.

Materials: 12- x 18-inch sheets of white drawing paper, pastels, pencils, erasers, and tissues.

Directions: First look into your fantasy, and envision a person of the opposite sex whom you consider to be ideal, having all the qualities you would wish for in a mate, companion, and friend. What does that person look like? Notice hair, eyes, facial expression, stature, clothing, style of movement. What is that person doing? Perhaps he or she is sitting across from you at dinner, participating with you in an active sport, sitting by the fireside planning a new project with you, having lively interactions with others at a party, seriously engaging in a business venture, or walking alone on a deserted beach. When an image has come to mind, try to capture its essential qualities by drawing them.

Fold the paper in half and draw your first picture on the left half of the page. Never mind if your drawing does not look exactly like your mental image—just do the best that you can. You have 15 minutes for the drawing. After 10 minutes, next to your drawing make note of any particular personality traits, habits, attitudes, values, and other internal attributes possessed by the person you drew. Is this person sensitive, strong, energetic, intellectual, responsible, gentle? What talents and abilities does the person possess?

Now imagine a person of the same sex, whom you consider to be ideal. Maybe the person is someone whose accomplishments you admire or whose lifestyle seems appealing. Perhaps the person holds a position in life you aspire to or has talents you desire to develop in yourself. Do not think too much about this, but allow images to enter your mind, remembering that this will be a person you create, not necessarily someone you know. You may combine attributes of several people or just make up new ones. Keep in mind the images you consider most ideal, and when the image crystallizes, begin to draw it on the second side of your paper. Do the same as you did for the first part, considering physical appearance, activity or situation, and both external and internal traits. Write down those elements that cannot be defined by drawing (15 minutes).

Developmental
Activity Example 8-2
Times of Your Life Collage

This activity addresses Levinson's mid-life transition in providing an opportunity to review past accomplishments as well as unrealized expectations. It will assist clients in re-evaluating the past and present life structures in preparation for making changes in middle adulthood (Figure 8-1).

Materials: Variety of magazines suitable to patients, large posterboard, glue, scissors, and marker for each patient. If patients in the group are of similar or known ages, the posterboard may be set up ahead of time to provide a space for every 5 years of their lives up to their present ages.

0 to 5	5 to 10	10 to 15	15 to 20
20 to 25	25 to 30	30 to 35	35 to 40

Figure 8-1. Times of your life collage. Draw format on larger posterboard. Adapt ages for each member.

Directions: The object of this exercise is to get a temporal perspective on our lives and to see how the parts fit into the whole to make us the people we are today. The posterboard will represent the whole. Our life will begin on the upper left and proceed to the lower right, divided into time intervals of 5 years. Leave one space for the present. (Show example.) Now think about the events that occurred in each segment of your life, what you were like then, people who were in your life, places where you lived or traveled, accomplishments you achieved, and decisions you made. Then, look through the magazines and find pictures, words, and phrases that best describe the major event or aspect of each segment of your life up to and including the present.

This activity can take up to 2 hours. Depending on patient group, the project can be done on one day and discussed the next, or it can carry over several group sessions. Discussion should center around evaluation of events and account for spaces left blank. High and low points may be identified. Emotional responses to events or patterns may be identified. Are there patterns? Were there changes? How were the changes made? Markers may be used to identify highs, lows, and emotions surrounding events.

Change options should then be explored. What accounts for the decisions in your life? Were they made impulsively? Influenced by others? Done with careful planning? If you could go back and change parts of your life, what would you change? What do you wish you could add or delete? What was missing in your life development that you wish had been there?

A follow-up drawing can be added to this exercise, entitled "The Future." Planning the next 5 or 10 years can be done using the same collage techniques.

From Cole, M. B. *Group dynamics in occupational therapy: The theoretical basis and practice application of group intervention* (3rd ed.). Thorofare, NJ: SLACK Incorporated. © 2005 SLACK Incorporated.

Developmental
Activity Example 8-3
Fabric of Life

This simple weaving activity addresses the life review task of Levinson's late adult transition. It is in keeping with the views of Erikson and Jung as well. The use of colors, patterns, and materials encourage the incorporation of emotional and substantive memories or essences, as well as marker events (Figure 8-2). This exercise requires two or three 1-hour sessions for most groups.

Materials: Pencils, paper, and a medium paper bag for each group member to plan his or her project. A heavy wire circle (loom) 12 to 18 inches in diameter (warped with strong yarn dividing the circle into 16 equal parts, tied together in the center) and one pair of sharp scissors should be provided for each person. A large variety of fabric remnants (can be scraps from a seamstress or cut from old, donated clothes, curtains, sheets, tablecloths, etc.), trimmings, ribbons, and several colored balls of yarn. Fabrics should be cut into long 1-inch strips.

Directions: Fabrics are, for most of us, associated with clothing, home furnishings, draperies, bedsheets, and the like. They are adorning and surrounding us constantly, and although often not the focus of our attention, they influence our sensory experiences and our mood and color our lives in ways of which we may be unaware.

In this exercise, we will associate key events, places, and persons in our lives with a sensory awareness of the fabrics that may symbolize them. We will choose fabrics, trimmings, or ribbons to represent both events and significant others in our lives. In addition, each of us will choose one special yarn or fabric to represent ourselves. Begin by writing down any of the following that apply most to you. As you choose fabrics, trimmings, and ribbons for each memory, cut an arm's length of it and place it in your paper bag.

1. Birth and young childhood—Envision your room or most memorable environment as a child. What do you see? What can you feel? Is there a favorite blanket or stuffed toy? What color is there? How does the texture of the fabric feel to your touch? Choose a fabric or material from the collection to represent this association as closely as possible.
2. Parents—Envision each of your parents, either separately or together, doing whatever they ordinarily were doing when you were a child. How were they dressed? What was their favorite color? Style? Summon an image of each of your parents as you would like to remember them from childhood. Then choose a fabric to represent that image.

   Take a few minutes to re-experience visual, tactile, auditory, or olfactory memories (sights, sounds, textures, and smells) associated with each of the items to follow, and continue to select fabrics and place them in your bag.
3. Friends from childhood
4. Relatives and siblings
5. A childhood home (imagine your room)
6. First day of school (what did you wear?)
7. Communion, bar mitzvah, or joining a church
8. First date
9. First school dance
10. First boyfriend or girlfriend
11. Graduation
12. First job (or significant ones)
13. Marriage
14. First house or apartment
15. Death of loved one(s)
16. Important travels
17. Awards or promotions at work

Fabric of Life (continued)

Figure 8-2. Fabric of life.

18. Adult friends
19. Birth of children and their significant others
20. Marriage, graduation, or jobs of children
21. Birth of grandchildren
22. Organizations or committees
23 Adult hobbies or leisure activities
24. Other important events or milestones

Planning takes at least a 1-hour session and should be discussed before the session ends. Memories can be verbalized and elaborated. If desired, a small scrap of fabric can be taped to the paper and labeled after each item planned, so the group member will not forget what was chosen for which at the next session. Be sure to put names on paper bags. Planning paper can be folded and placed inside.

Developmental
Activity Example 8-3
Fabric of Life (continued)

Procedure for Weaving: Begin with the ball of yarn that represents you. Tie the end to the center and weave it under and over each warp thread, clockwise around the circle for five or six rows. This yarn will touch and become a part of all the other materials you have chosen. How much of each other material you use depends on how large a part its associated element played in your life. Begin with childhood and work chronologically, adding chosen materials and weaving them over and under with the yarn, around and around the circle. From time to time, rake the yarn toward the center with your fingers to push it together. End when you have used up all the materials selected. Wind the yarn (or add ribbon or trim) around and around the wire circle to cover it, and tie in a loop knot at the end to hang it on the wall. (See Figure 8-2 for example.)

Discussion should be encouraged during the weaving process, and the therapist will help patients as needed. Feelings about the project at the end are especially important. The doing process often evokes many hidden feelings that need to be expressed and explored. Is the review of life positive or negative? Which parts are positive or negative? What is missing? Patients should be encouraged to keep their own projects and to reflect on the significance of them, and not to use them as gifts, at least for a while. Remember, a life review is only the beginning of the task of evaluation and integration which Jung and Erikson have suggested is necessary for contentment in old age.

From Cole, M. B. *Group dynamics in occupational therapy: The theoretical basis and practice application of group intervention* (3rd ed.). Thorofare, NJ: SLACK Incorporated. © 2005 SLACK Incorporated.

Developmental
Activity Example 8-4
The Doctor's Dilemma

This activity refers to Kohlberg's fourth and fifth stages of moral development. The group's discussion is intended to cast doubt upon a strict "law and order" kind of reasoning about morality and to encourage empathy with more than one participant in a given situation.

Directions: First I will read you a story that has several characters who do not agree with one another. Listen carefully to the story, and then, as a group, decide who is right, who is wrong, and what should be done about the situation.

Story: Jenny was a healthy 24-year-old woman who went into the hospital unexpectedly to have her appendix removed. It was 8:00 p.m. and Dr. Strothers had just completed a long, tiring day of surgery. Jenny's sister Carol brought her to the hospital in terrible pain; it was evident that she needed to be operated on at once. The emergency room nurse, Eva, interviewed Jenny and prepared her for surgery. Eva wrote down on her report that Jenny had her last meal 1 hour ago, which put her at considerable risk of choking when given general anesthesia. However, the doctor did not read the report carefully. He operated anyway, and the patient choked to death on the table.

Carol was in shock; she suspected negligence and sued the doctor for $1 million. Although Jenny was not married and had no children, Carol missed her sister and felt that those who mistreated her sister should pay. But mostly, she could really use the money. She and her husband had just bought a house and had defaulted on the past few payments. $500,000 would just about pay off their mortgage, and prevent them from losing their home.

Eva, the nurse who prepared the report, was secretly in love with the doctor. Out of love, she offered to alter the report, changing the "1" hour since last meal to a "9." This would clear Dr. Strothers of any blame for Jenny's death. Eva saw that Dr. Strothers was a caring and brilliant young doctor, capable of saving many more lives if allowed to continue his practice. Of course, a verdict of guilty in the lawsuit would prevent him from ever practicing again. Eva was willing to give up nursing and take the blame for the man she loved. She hoped perhaps he would marry her if she did this, and after a brief jail sentence, they could live happily ever after.

Dr. Strothers was faced with a dilemma. Should he take the blame, plead guilty in the lawsuit, and give up his life's work? Should he accept Eva's offer to take the blame? Should he meet with Carol and offer to pay her $500,000 to withdraw the lawsuit? How should the story end? It is up to you.

From Cole, M. B. *Group dynamics in occupational therapy: The theoretical basis and practice application of group intervention* (3rd ed.). Thorofare, NJ: SLACK Incorporated. © 2005 SLACK Incorporated.

Developmental
Activity Example 8-5
Families of Clay

Margo Gross, MS, OTR/L, is acknowledged as the creator of this activity, which relates to Levinson's individuation in both the early adult and middle adult transitions.

Materials: A ball of soft clay, approximately 4 inches in diameter, a piece of cardboard or posterboard 18- x 24-inches for each member, clay modeling tools, water and paper towels for clean-up, markers, and small post-it notepads.

Directions: Divide your clay into sections for each member of your family, including yourself. Sculpt an abstract figure that represents how you feel about each person. Try to use nonconcrete representations. Arrange the people on the board in such a way as to describe the relationships in your family. Label each member.

Discussion: Discuss how you saw your family system at ages 5, 15, 25, 35, etc. How would you like to see the relationships in your family placed, ideally? What happened to the structure when new members were introduced? Geographical moves? Marriage or divorce? Death?

Individuals beginning to separate from their family of origin can look at the structure and their place in it from a distance. Assessing the aspects of learning derived from each parent, hidden messages, and alliances and conflicts between members is an important step in the individuation process. At mid-life, individuation takes on a qualitatively different process, as the role of parent to offspring ends and becoming caretaker for one's own aging parents is more of a reality. Whether or not family ties remain close, individuation continues psychologically as one ages. One's perception of each family member is altered as the individual becomes more fully integrated.

From Cole, M. B. *Group dynamics in occupational therapy: The theoretical basis and practice application of group intervention* (3rd ed.). Thorofare, NJ: SLACK Incorporated. © 2005 SLACK Incorporated.

Developmental
Activity Example 8-6
Eulogy for Yourself

Margo Gross, MS, OTR/L, is acknowledged as the creator of this activity, which addresses Levinson's middle and late life transitions.

Materials: Pencil and paper for each member.

Directions: This exercise will help you see your life more clearly from the perspective of your imagined death. Write the eulogy that your best friend might read at your funeral. Include any major accomplishments, special family relationships, contributions to the community, and values or morals that you strongly uphold. What has been the significance of your life, and how might you be leaving the world a better place?

Within the group format, pass your eulogy to the person at your right, and take turns reading them out loud. Record your response as you hear about your life in retrospect.

Discussion: What periods of your life were the most/least fulfilling in terms of career, family relationships, involvement in community life? Where were the major turning points? What values did you act on consistently? How can you plan to complete any unfinished business in the time left before your death?

This exercise has direct implications for those individuals approaching mid-life, where the sense of aging becomes more acute due to the beginning of the physical and cognitive decline. Their sense of mortality is accentuated by the change in generational status, by the aging of parental figures, and by the death or illness of friends or contemporaries.

Assessing the climb up the ladder of success and deciding whether earlier goals were attained or new goals need to be defined are aspects of this developmental period. The activity will reinforce the fact that each individual still has a period of life ahead to restructure a change to reach different or new goals.

For individuals in the late adult transition, the activity serves to assist in life review. It is a concrete way of seeing and hearing how the major themes and events in a life come together to unify the self.

From Cole, M. B. *Group dynamics in occupational therapy: The theoretical basis and practice application of group intervention* (3rd ed.). Thorofare, NJ: SLACK Incorporated. © 2005 SLACK Incorporated.

Developmental
Activity Example 8-7
Major Accomplishments

Margo Gross, MS, OTR/L, is acknowledged as the creator of this activity, which addresses Levinson's middle and late life transitions. Two 1-hour sessions are needed for this exercise.

Materials: 12- x 12-inch plywood boards for each member, sandpaper square, scissors, magazines, personal photographs if available, decoupage glue, water-based wood stain, rags, brushes, water and paper towels for clean-up, and permanent color markers.

Directions: Prepare the wood board by sanding the edges and corners and also both surfaces of the wood until smooth to the touch. Wipe away the sawdust. Brush the stain onto all sides of the wood in the color of your choice. Use a small rag to wipe off excess stain and set aside to dry. From the magazines, choose pictures and words that describe your major accomplishments up to the present time. Arrange them in front of you as you process the first session. Write your name on the back of your board with a marker, and place your clippings in a plain envelope with your name.

Bring any photographs, actual newspaper clippings, or mementos you have found at home to the second session. Arrange the clippings and photos on the board in a pleasing manner. You may wish to overlap the pictures, which means applying several coats of decoupage glue to adhere each layer of the design. Be sure to smooth the pictures well to eliminate air bubbles underneath, which can cause wrinkling of the pictures as the glue dries. Apply a final coat of glue to finish the plaque and give the project a glossy shine. Be sure to apply decoupage glue to the edges to seal and protect the plaque. When dry, a tooth hook may be applied to the center of the back for hanging.

Discussion: Depending on the transitional period in which members of the activity group are involved, the pictures chosen will represent feelings about their accomplishments to date. Individuals in the middle adult transition will use this activity to re-evaluate the past and take stock of their progress. For late adult transitions, the plaque serves as a life review. Persons facing retirement, changes in financial status, or widowhood may find the decoupage a concrete daily reminder of their self-worth, which may be shaky during such periods of adaptation. Categories of successes may be separated into family, career, or personal accomplishments. A discussion of how a future plaque might look will assist those in the process of designing a new life structure.

From Cole, M. B. *Group dynamics in occupational therapy: The theoretical basis and practice application of group intervention* (3rd ed.). Thorofare, NJ: SLACK Incorporated. © 2005 SLACK Incorporated.

Developmental
Activity Example 8-8
Exploring Sex Roles

Margo Gross, MS, OTR/L, is acknowledged as the creator of this activity, which addresses Levinson's early adult transition.

Materials: Worksheets and pens for each member, large newsprint pad with easel, and magic marker.

Directions: This activity is designed to explore and clarify sex roles in our lives. Using the headings provided, fill in the incomplete sentences, trying not to censor any ideas that come to mind, even if the statements seem to be contradictory. After 10 to 15 minutes, ask the group to stop writing and look over their answers. On the newsprint pad, write down the men's and women's responses as they are shared.

Discussion: Which items on your list seem the most powerful or important to you? Which items are self-imposed? Which show family influences? Which items are similar for the men? For the women? Which items from the opposite sex surprised you the most? How might your roles be the same or different from roles of your parents? Which did you neglect, which did you emphasize? Which items are age specific for you right now?

Exploring Sex Roles (continued)

Exploring Sex Roles Worksheet (Male)

If I were a woman, I could...
1.
2.
3.
4.
5.
Because I am a man, I must....
1.
2.
3.
4.
5.

Exploring Sex Roles Worksheet (Female)

If I were a man, I could...
1.
2.
3.
4.
5.
Because I am a woman, I must....
1.
2.
3.
4.
5.

Developmental
Activity Example 8-9
Childhood Games and Occupational Choice

Margo Gross, MS, OTR/L, is acknowledged as the creator of this activity, which addresses one of the life tasks of Levinson's early and middle adult transitions.

Materials: Worksheets and pencils.

Directions: Children from a young age, until they are well into adolescence, spend much of their free time in some form of play. Make a list of 10 childhood games that you remember playing. Think about games you played alone and ones you played informally with peers. Include both indoor and outdoor games, fantasy and make-believe, as well as group games and sports.

After you complete the list, analyze each game by placing the symbols next to it that best apply. Then apply these same symbols to your current occupation.

Discussion: What are the similarities and differences between your childhood play and current occupation? Consider whether your present occupation involves the characteristics of play that you enjoyed the most. Have you accepted or rejected aspects of yourself that you value and want to be a part of your life today?

From Cole, M. B. *Group dynamics in occupational therapy: The theoretical basis and practice application of group intervention* (3rd ed.). Thorofare, NJ: SLACK Incorporated. © 2005 SLACK Incorporated.

Developmental
Activity Example 8-9
Childhood Games and Occupational Choice (continued)

Childhood Games and Current Occupation Worksheet

Name:

Job title of current or most recent occupation:

List 10 childhood games you remember playing (before the age of 15):

1.

2.

3.

4.

5.

6.

7.

8.

9.

10.

After you complete the list, analyze each game by placing the symbols next to it that best apply:
M—Male oriented
F—Female oriented
U—Unstructured
S—Structured
A—Played alone
G—Played with others/groups
Ab—Abstract, fantasy oriented
C—Concrete, reality oriented
O—Objects or props necessary
M—Imagined or mentally created

Now apply these same symbols to your current occupation.

From Cole, M. B. *Group dynamics in occupational therapy: The theoretical basis and practice application of group intervention* (3rd ed.). Thorofare, NJ: SLACK Incorporated. © 2005 SLACK Incorporated.

Developmental
Activity Example 8-10
Reminiscence

Life review has a place in almost every developmental theory addressing the older adult. Erikson, Jung, and Levinson all define some form of re-evaluation of the meaning of one's life as its end draws nearer. Reminiscence is a review of past experiences, with a goal of establishing a sense of integrity and satisfaction with one's self through the process of remembering. Drawing, writing, and storytelling are creative ways to assist members in recalling their specific experiences. Once written or drawn, members should share through discussion. Some suggested themes are:

- Specific years or events: The Great Depression, World War II, The 50s, The 60s.
- What were you doing when... Pearl Harbor was bombed? Franklin D. Roosevelt died?
- What was the most difficult period in your life?
- When did you get your first car? First house?
- Describe your first date. First job. First child.
- Describe your first encounter with death (relative, close friend).
- What was your proudest moment?
- Whom do you admire most in your family?
- What values would you choose to leave to your children? To society?
- Bring in favorite music/songs from the past and discuss their significance.

It should be noted that reminiscence does not restore memory for persons who have cognitive deficits. However, persons with mild or moderate dementia often retain remote memories, and discussing these in groups can help them re-establish a sense of normal social functioning.

From Cole, M. B. *Group dynamics in occupational therapy: The theoretical basis and practice application of group intervention* (3rd ed.). Thorofare, NJ: SLACK Incorporated. © 2005 SLACK Incorporated.

Chapter 9

Sensorimotor Approaches

The sensorimotor approaches include a range of frames of reference that address motor, sensorimotor, perceptual, and cognitive problems due to developmental or acquired conditions affecting the brain. The motor control approaches in particular have undergone some major theoretical changes in recent years (Trombly & Radomski, 2002). This chapter will briefly review Trombly's Occupational Functioning Model (OFM), the task-oriented approach, motor learning theory, dynamical systems theory, and Carr and Shepherd's Motor Relearning (Sabari, 2002), as well as the more traditional approaches to motor control. The sensory integration (SI) theory of Ayres will also be briefly reviewed. This theory, which paved the way for group approaches, was devised by King and Ross. Extensive literature exists by and about all of these theorists, and the reader is referred to other books and articles for a more in-depth understanding of each specific theory.

Framework Focus

Traditionally, this approach has been used to facilitate learning or relearning of "motor skills" by applying controlled sensory input to specific "body structures" as defined in the *Occupational Therapy Practice Framework* (American Occupational Therapy Association [AOTA], 2002). "Body functions" such as learning, memory, and motor planning interact with body structures and environmental "contexts" to produce optimal occupational performance. SI moves beyond motor responses and addresses "processes skills," such as attending and listening, emotion modulation, eye-hand coordination, and academic learning ability. Current

evidence suggests that using motor facilitation techniques is most effective when practiced within specific "contexts" and "activity demands."

For occupational therapy, the primary use of this approach has been with developmental disabilities affecting the central nervous system (CNS) and those who have suffered trauma or disease to the CNS. However, recent studies of the brain have linked neurophysiological and CNS dysfunction to mental disorders as well. Applying SI principles of intervention with the geriatric population is increasing and shows promising results. Occupational therapy groups using this frame of reference should use activities that stimulate the senses, produce purposeful movement, promote cognition and affect, and use real-life tasks to approach the CNS in a systematic way.

Basic Assumptions

This frame of reference encompasses many theorists (and techniques), among them Trombly, Carr and Shepherd, Rood, the Bobaths (neurodevelopmental treatment [NDT]), Brunnstrom, and Ayres. These approaches are not necessarily intended to be used with groups, however, the principles of intervention can be applied when planning group activities. Examples of occupational therapy group intervention approaches using these theories are reviewed, including the writings of King and Ross. Some of these approaches make the assumption that brain function is hierarchical and rehabilitation follows a developmental sequence, while others view brain function as parallel and simultaneous and organize interventions around specific tasks. All of the theorists agree on

Table 9-1	Trombly's Occupational Functioning Model Hierarchy

- Sense of self-efficacy and self-esteem
- Satisfaction with life roles
- Competence in tasks of life roles
- Activities and habits
- Abilities and skills
- Developed capacities
- First level capacities
- Organic substrate

the importance of sensation in this process and the importance of practice and feedback in motor learning.

Trombly

In 1995, Catherine Trombly introduced her OFM in her Eleanor Clarke Slagle Lecture. She pointed out that when a client "got to choose an activity... the chosen activity was meaningful and kept the person interested and working" (Trombly, 1995, p. 960). Her model incorporates this idea in a "descending hierarchy of roles, tasks, activities, abilities, and capacities." The goal of her model is to "develop a sense of competency and self-esteem" (p. 961). She acknowledges that environment plays a much larger role in physical rehabilitation than was previously thought. In the OFM, "context and environment surround and permeate all levels of the occupational functioning hierarchy, but have a greater influence at the higher levels than the lower" (Trombly & Radomski, 2002, p. 9). This suggests that clients who have mastered the foundational capacities, abilities, and skills may be more appropriately treated in groups. For example, occupational therapists can compose groups of clients to work on valued roles in self-maintenance, self-advancement, or self-enhancement using a task-oriented approach. The group provides a social and cultural context within which each member is motivated to meet the task demand. Trombly calls this method of using tasks as intervention "occupation-as-end" (p. 6). See Table 9-1 for an overview of the OFM.

Task-Oriented Approach

This approach is based on the theories of motor learning and dynamical systems theory (described later). Functional tasks, chosen collaboratively by

client and occupational therapist, are believed to help organize motor behavior. Principles from learning theory are applied to the doing of meaningful tasks, which are graded and sequenced according to each client's needs and abilities. The client's occupational performance results from the interaction of multiple systems, both internal and external. From the *Occupational Therapy Practice Framework* perspective, "client factors," such as anatomy, physiology, and physical and mental functioning, are influenced by multiple "contexts" and "activity demands" in producing occupational performance. After CNS damage, a client's behavior may seem purposeless, but in this approach, all behavior is interpreted as a client's attempt to achieve functional goals. Each task requires practice and experimentation with a variety of strategies in multiple contexts in order for motor skills to be learned.

Bass-Haugen, Mathiowetz, and Flinn (2002) list the following five principles of the task-oriented approach:
1. Client-centered focus
2. Occupation-based focus
3. Person and environment
4. Practice and feedback
5. General treatment goals

Each will be reviewed briefly here.

Client-Centered Focus

Research shows that "clients who are actively engaged in their treatment show achievement in self-identified goals, increased functional independence at discharge, and (are) discharged to less restrictive environments (Gibson & Schkade, 1997)" (Trombly & Radomski, 2002, p. 484). Client priorities can be very task focused, and clients are often motivated by the wish to perform valued life roles. Occupational therapists form therapeutic relationships with clients during evaluation that involve a discussion of personal interests, values, and preferences; identification of meaningful life roles; and collaboration on goals and priorities. Choices of intervention tasks and decisions about group membership are a natural consequence of this continued collaboration. Clients with common goals can benefit from engaging in group tasks in which members participate in planning, implementation, group problem solving, outcome evaluation, and mutual feedback. The occupational therapist who facilitates a task-oriented group will contribute professional expertise and resources as needed or requested by client members. Some such groups will require more direction than others.

Occupation-Based Focus

This approach uses actual functional tasks as opposed to exercise to achieve movement goals. Tasks that are selected should be both meaningful and important to the client's life roles. "Life satisfaction is not determined by successful completion of a random set of functional tasks (changing a diaper...). Satisfaction or reward comes from the feeling that roles are fulfilled (parent...)" (Trombly & Radomski, 2002, p. 485). Selecting tasks collaboratively with clients and reinforcing their relevance to life roles is likely to enhance client motivation. However, clients need our assistance to avoid early failure with tasks that are initially too difficult. The occupational therapist must also carefully analyze the selected tasks and adapt or grade the task demand to match client abilities and learning needs.

Person and Environment

It is important for the occupational therapist to observe the performance of tasks that are difficult for the client. Many systems interact to influence occupational performance. Part of the occupational therapy intervention will be to identify both personal and environmental factors that facilitate or inhibit task performance so that adaptation of these factors can be explored. Client and occupational therapist can collaborate to develop strategies to prevent interfering variables and to adapt the task and environment to promote optimal functioning.

Practice and Feedback

Skill practice in a variety of settings is necessary for learning to occur. This reflects an important principle of motor learning, the principle of encoding specificity. According to this principle, events stored in memory are embedded in specific contexts, which limits the transfer or generalization of learning in a different context. Flinn and Radomski (2002) suggest using contextual interference by varying the context and the task for which a skill is practiced. This encourages more complex processing strategies, which include problem solving and adapting the skill in different situations. Motor learning theory also stresses the importance of feedback, both intrinsic and extrinsic. Intrinsic feedback is usually somatosensory or visual, experiencing the sensation of the movement. Extrinsic feedback comes from others. The occupational therapist may give feedback concurrently, coaching the client during task performance. This type of feedback is called knowledge of performance (KP). The outcome of task performance is called knowledge of result (KR). Research shows giving feedback on performance is more productive at the beginning stages of rehabilitation, and giving feedback on outcome or result is better if given intermittently. A decision needs to be made about whether to practice one part of a task (part learning) or the whole task (whole learning). A whole task is more readily stored in long-term memory than parts of a task. Storage and retrieval are both necessary for motor learning to occur.

General Goals

The overall goals of the client learning process are to discover the optimal movement patterns for task performance. Flexibility, efficiency, and effectiveness are important for any task, and these may develop as clients continue to practice skills in varying natural environments. Ultimately, clients need to develop problem-solving skills so that they can continue to identify their own solutions in both home and community environments.

Motor Learning Theory

Motor learning has been defined as a "set of processes associated with practice or experience leading to relatively permanent changes in the capacity for producing skilled action" (Shumway-Cook & Woollacott, 2001, p. 27). Central to this theory is the growing body of knowledge on neural plasticity. Organisms demonstrate an inherent capacity to self-organize throughout life. Neural plasticity is the ability of the nervous system to become more efficient at the cellular level and to change the way the whole system works by modifying neural connections. Short-term learning depends on short-term, or working, memory, which allows us to attend to a phone number long enough to dial it. This may be equated with the random access memory on a computer. Only when we "save" information to a hard drive on a computer can we then retrieve the information and use it later. Long-term memory acts in much the same way, as a necessary step in making permanent and lasting change. Occupational therapists are most interested in long-term modulation of synapses that results from experience. Using these principles, therapeutic activities can be devised by occupational therapists to effect lasting changes in motor functioning for clients.

Schmidt (1988) identified four basic concepts for motor learning.

1. Learning is a process of acquiring the capability for skilled action.
2. Learning results from experience or practice.
3. Learning cannot be measured directly, rather it is inferred from behavior.
4. Learning produces relatively permanent changes in behavior.

Motor learning during rehabilitation occurs in three stages, according to Fitts and Posner (1967). At first, the client attempts to understand the nature of the task. The occupational therapist discusses various strategies for doing the task and evaluating performance. This is the cognitive stage. The second, associative stage, involves refining and perfecting the skill through practice. The third stage occurs when the skill becomes habitual, and a low degree of attention is required for optimal performance. This is called the autonomous stage.

Dynamical Systems Theory

Applied to physical disabilities, this theory defines motor control as a blend of reflexes and voluntary control that is dependent on the demands of both task and environment. The CNS interprets cues from the environment and involves multiple subsystems when planning to reach desired goals. In contrast to hierarchical models, this is seen as "parallel distributed processing" in which many signals may be processed simultaneously among many brain structures. Movement is then generated by an open-loop feed-forward system with emphasis on anticipatory postural adjustments made as part of the total movement pattern. Behavior, therefore, is a product of the interaction between the individual, the task, and multiple environmental factors (Bowler, 1999).

Carr and Shepherd

Carr and Shepherd (1987, 1998) developed a Motor Relearning Program (MRP), which focuses on teaching clients how to use feedback to modify their performance. These theorists use dynamical systems theory, which views changes in neural connections as initiated by environmental opportunities. In other words, they assume that voluntary movements are initiated by functional task goals instead of exercise. An important principle of dynamical systems theory is attraction states, or preferred patterns of movement. A deeply entrenched movement pattern can become a barrier to lasting change. For example, if a person develops a faulty golf swing and uses it many times, it is very difficult to unlearn. It is the same with maladaptive movement patterns following brain damage. If the pattern is new and unpracticed (shallow), it is much easier to change. Control parameters are those factors that influence preferred patterns of movement. For example, a wet floor or an icy sidewalk will alter one's movement patterns while walking. Some control parameters are external, while others are internal. For example, fatigue might be an internal factor that alters one's pattern of walking.

Carr and Shepherd use four principles of intervention to shape long-term learning:

1. Oral instruction: The most important aspects of movement are used to create an objective goal (e.g., "touch the spoon handle").
2. Visual demonstration: The therapist models the movement for the client. Photographs and drawings can also be used. The demonstration focuses on the most essential task components.
3. Manual guidance: The occupational therapist moves the client through a sequence, attending to inhibition of constraining components.
4. Accurate and timely feedback: Feedback is offered to reinforce actual improvements in performance. While effort can be acknowledged, it should not be treated in the same way as actual improvement.

In dealing with motor abnormalities, four general categories of motor performance are addressed:

1. Standing up and sitting down
2. Walking
3. Reaching and manipulation
4. Balance

Carr and Shepherd (1998) have devised an assessment tool, the Motor Assessment Scale

Table 9-2	Carr and Shepherd's Motor Assessment Scale Categories

- Supine to side lying on intact side
- Supine to sitting on edge of bed
- Balanced sitting
- Sitting to standing
- Upper arm functions
- Hand movements
- Advanced hand activities

(MAS), using a seven-point scale to evaluate seven specific movements related to the above categories. These movements are listed in Table 9-2. For the full assessment scale, see Carr and Shepherd (1987).

An important aspect of the Carr and Shepherd intervention technique is grading the activity demand. The following are guidelines for grading an activity to elicit specific motor response patterns:

- Change the position of the person, the seating, the support, or the alignment.
- Change object placement, position relative to body, or distance.
- Change the object characteristics, weight, size, one- vs. two-handed lifting.
- Change temporal demands, such as using stationary vs. moving objects.

Carr and Shepherd (1998) go on to define the essential features of each movement category addressed by their theory. Potentially, the most interesting category to be addressed by group intervention is the fourth: reach and manipulation. This category is said to have the greatest number of degrees of freedom, or potential variations in complexity of movement. This is addressed by combining several movements into synergistic combinations. Relearning of reach and grasp requires initial passive stretch of the shoulder muscles to maintain range of motion. This passive stretching using the unaffected arm might be one example of an activity that can be learned in a group format, perhaps while moving to music or incorporating visualization. Client members might learn to observe one another and offer feedback using guidelines modeled by the occupational therapist facilitator.

Traditional Neurophysiological Approaches

The following group of theories have come to be known as the reflex-hierarchical models of motor control. The reflexive basis of human movement has been challenged in recent years by research that suggests that motor behavior is not primarily controlled by the CNS in a top-down hierarchy. The dynamical systems theory and the motor learning theory have cast doubt as to the legitimacy of some of these earlier theories, which discouraged the use of functional tasks for fear of developing "splinter skills" or skills learned by rote, which skipped ahead of the normal developmental sequence. Thus, doubt is cast upon approaches that emphasize adherence to a developmental sequence at the expense of functional performance (Trombly & Radomski, 2002, p. 142). However, these theorists continue to influence practice, and some, such as NDT, are being researched and updated.

Rood

Margaret Rood's work preceded most of the other theorists covered in this chapter, and her ideas seem to have inspired many of the concepts of SI developed later. Rood was the first to focus on the importance of reflexes. Rood (1954) states:

...motor patterns are developed from fundamental reflex patterns present at birth which are utilized and gradually modified through sensory stimuli until the highest control is gained on the conscious cortical level. It seemed to me then, that if it were possible to apply the proper sensory stimuli to the appropriate sensory receptor as it is utilized in normal sequential development, it might be possible to elicit motor responses reflexively and by following neurophysiological principles, and establish proper motor engrams.

Table 9-3	Rood's Eight Ontogenetic Motor Patterns

1. Supine withdrawal
2. Segmental rolling
3. Pivot prone (prone extension)
4. Neck cocontraction
5. Supporting self on elbows
6. All-fours movement patterns
7. Standing
8. Walking

Rood's (1954) theory has four basic components:

1. Sensory input is required for normalization of tone and evocation of desired muscular responses.
2. Sensorimotor control is developmentally based.
3. Movement is purposeful.
4. Repetition of movement is necessary for learning.

Most occupational therapists recognize Rood's techniques of facilitation and inhibition. Light stroking, brushing, icing, and joint compression are used to facilitate movement. Joint approximation (light compression), neutral warmth, pressure on tendon insertion, and slow rhythmical movement are used to inhibit unwanted movement. Rood recommended the facilitation of normal movement in a developmental sequence. First, phasic reciprocal contraction, such as flexion to extension and back, is practiced repeatedly until learned. Next, stabilization through cocontraction of major muscle groups is facilitated. A third phase combines these, practicing movement imposed on stabilization, and a final phase incorporates the development of skilled movement. Table 9-3 states Rood's eight ontogenetic motor patterns.

This sequence gives occupational therapists some very specific guidelines for planning movement activities for clients with neurodevelopmental disorders. When planning group intervention, each client's unique developmental level with respect to movement needs to be carefully considered. Movement groups can be set up at many levels but should progress from earlier to later stages in the ontogenetic sequence. Clients should not be asked to perform movements at higher levels than they are capable. Positioning is a primary concern, especially at the lower levels. It may involve the extensive use of mats, bolsters, beach balls, or other specialized equipment.

Many games can be devised that involve pushing and pulling, throwing and catching, and rolling and creeping to move the body from one place to another. These activities should be set up to incorporate the correct therapeutic movement sequences for each client, while the clients are participating in goal-directed activities.

The Bobaths

Dr. and Mrs. Bobath are a neurologist and a physiotherapist from England who originated the therapeutic technique best known as "neurodevelopmental therapy," or NDT (Bobath, 1972). One of their most important contributions to theory is their focus on sensorimotor learning. It is not movement itself but the sensation of movement that is learned and remembered. Much of the Bobaths' work was done on children with cerebral palsy and adult stroke clients. The techniques are widely known and used but little researched prior to 1990, according to Levit (2002). Since the Bobaths' deaths in 1990, the Neurodevelopmental Treatment Association in the United States, as well as similar groups in other countries, have been working to update the theoretical basis and practice techniques for NDT. Although it addresses mainly the motor and sensory components of performance, NDT intervention is individualized to meet specific client goals and represents an "interactive process among the individual, caregivers, and members of the interdisciplinary team" (Levit, 2002, p. 523). The approach works best when all helpers, including family members, use the same approach.

Following the Bobaths' focus on sensation, their handling of children with cerebral palsy, and subsequently of adults with hemiplegia, concentrated on repetition of correct motor responses. The

Table 9-4	Brunnstrom's Six Stages of Recovery

1. Flaccidity, no voluntary movement
2. Synergies or minimal voluntary movement
3. Synergies performed voluntarily
4. Some deviation from synergy
5. Independent or isolated movement
6. Individual joint movement nearly normal with minimal spasticity

assumption is that when clients experience normal movement, this results in correct sensory feedback to the CNS. NDT involves teaching the client how correct movement feels (Trombly & Radomski, 2002). To this end, great effort is made to inhibit primitive reflexes through "reflex inhibiting patterns" (RIPs) (Trombly & Radomski, 2002, p. 525) and to elicit righting and equilibrium responses.

In NDT, sensory stimulation is regulated with great care. Weight bearing, placing and holding, tapping, and joint compression are used to activate normal movement and posture. However, these stimuli are withdrawn as soon as an abnormal response occurs. In hemiplegia, sensory deficits are interpreted as an indication of poor prognosis for regaining normal control of movement. Stress is avoided, since it is thought to promote abnormal tone and movement.

After stroke or head trauma, the sequence of relearning movement approximates normal development. While compensatory movement that uses one-handed techniques is discouraged, tasks that are client priorities may be practiced using bilateral movements and key points of control. Some researchers have demonstrated that an approach that combines traditional NDT with instruction in home exercise showed greater improvement in functional control than NDT alone (Sunderlund et al., 1992). Therapist assistance is needed initially to inhibit abnormal movement patterns during task performance. Recovery from stroke and trauma generally involves a flaccid stage followed by a spastic stage. Many specific exercises and handling are suggested in each of these stages following the developmental process. These involve positioning, weight bearing, holding and placing, balance reactions, and protective extension, among others. Trombly and Radomski (2002) suggest a good source of both individual and group activities based on the Bobath NDT approach is Eggers' *Occupational Therapy in the Treatment of Adult Hemiplegia* (1983).

Brunnstrom

Unlike the other theorists so far, Signe Brunnstrom took an opposite view of the use of reflexes. Her basic assumption was that as normal development progresses, spinal cord and brain stem reflexes become modified and their components rearranged into purposeful movement through the CNS. Therefore, reflexes can and should be used to elicit movement where none exists as part of a normal sequence (Trombly & Radomski, 2002). Both proprioceptive (resistive) and exteroceptive (tactile) stimuli are used to elicit reflexes, and the client is encouraged to think about the movement that results and try to gain control of that movement.

The Brunnstrom approach seeks to elicit associated reactions and synergies. For example, resistive stimuli are believed to achieve both reflexive movement on the noninvolved side and similar synergistic movement on the involved side. A synergy is defined as the total flexion or extension movement of a joint or limb. Six stages of recovery are defined by Brunnstrom for the upper and lower extremity as listed in Table 9-4.

These are specifically defined, and interested students are encouraged to read about specific assessment and treatment techniques in Brunnstrom's *Movement Therapy in Hemiplegia* (1970).

Groups using the principles of NDT, as well as other neurodevelopmental theories, may be designed with clients who have achieved a fair degree of voluntary movement. Exercise groups, movement to music, and simple games are best suited to these clients, many of whom are likely to have language and cognitive problems as well.

Ayres

A. Jean Ayres is credited with the founding of the theory of sensory integration, or SI, in the

1960s. Her researched focused on sensory processing in an attempt to explain the underlying causes of behavioral and motor difficulties and learning problems in children. SI is a process approach that assumes that remediating underlying neurological processes will improve a child's motor coordination and ability to attend and learn in the classroom. In the 1970s, efficacy studies failed to validate this assumption; thus, educators concluded that process-oriented interventions with children's learning and behavior problems were generally ineffective (Hammill, 1993; Mulligan, 2002). The current paradigm in education generally rejects all process approaches in favor of direct instruction and training, such as teaching handwriting. Although SI techniques are frequently used by school-based occupational therapists, the approach is still questioned by educators.

Two basic assumptions currently dominate SI theory: neuroplasticity and a hierarchical view of the CNS. Neuroplasticity of the brain refers to its ability to adapt and change. According to Mulligan (2002), an abundance of evidence exists to support the concept of neuroplasticity. The concept of CNS hierarchy has been challenged in recent years. However, as it is still a central concept in SI theory, we will review Ayres' original ideas here. SI largely focuses on the remediation of brain stem functions as a way to improve functional skills. Ayres refers to the normal developmental sequence in her study of the use of sensory input. She suggests four levels of the sensory integrative process. Her concept of foundation skills implies that lower level (brain stem) functions precede higher levels in Stages 1 through 4.

Primary Level

At this level, Ayres (1974) identifies the three basic sensory systems as vestibular, proprioceptive, and tactile. Visual and auditory are acknowledged but not thought to play a major integrative role in this early stage. Touch is cited as the basis for the infant's first emotional bond with mother. The processing of these initial touch sensations is seen to be responsible for establishing a basic sense of security.

The proprioceptive and vestibular senses offer another kind of basic security--gravitational security. These help the child develop balance for standing and walking and prevents the fear of falling. This level includes the eye movements, posture, balance, muscle tone, and gravitational security all resulting from the vestibular and proprioceptive integration. Sucking, eating, the moth-er-child bond, and tactile comfort are seen as the result of integration of tactile sensations.

Second Level

At this level, the three basic senses are integrated into a body precept, coordination of the two sides of the body, motor planning, attention span, activity level, and emotional stability. Sensory information from vestibular, proprioceptive, and tactile receptors are used to form precepts, or maps, of the body that are stored in the brain. With this mechanism, one is constantly aware of where his or her body is and what it is doing. This precept has information about right and left sides of the body, which allow the two sides to work bilaterally to accomplish tasks. The precept also allows a person to plan motor actions (e.g., catching a ball or feeding him- or herself). The organization of sensory input by the brain is also reflected in the ability to focus attention and adjust the level or pace of activity. Hyperactivity, hypoactivity, and the inability to attend are thus explained by poor integration at the secondary level of SI.

Third Level

Speech and language, eye-hand coordination, visual perception, and purposeful activity are possible at this level due to the impact of auditory and visual sensations. According to Ayres (1974), the vestibular and auditory systems are intimately related. The vestibular system, as stated above, is responsible for the ability to attend to what is heard. Language comprehension likewise begins with the child's touching, moving, lifting, and otherwise interacting with the objects in his or her environment. Only through this experience can he or she begin to appreciate the unique properties of an object and know its name. Visual perception is also seen as an end product of earlier SI; how big something is, how far away it is, and what its relationship is to other parts of the environment are all experienced first by reaching and touching. The visual experience is thus intimately related to the tactile and vestibular systems as well. With an understanding of what he or she hears and what he or she sees, the child's actions with respect to the environment can be purposeful. Visual sensation directs the child's hand to reach out to pet the kitten. He or she alters his or her posture to keep his or her balance as the kitten moves under his or her touch. The child hears the kitten purr and repeats the action. Visual, auditory, tactile, and vestibular systems all work together to help the

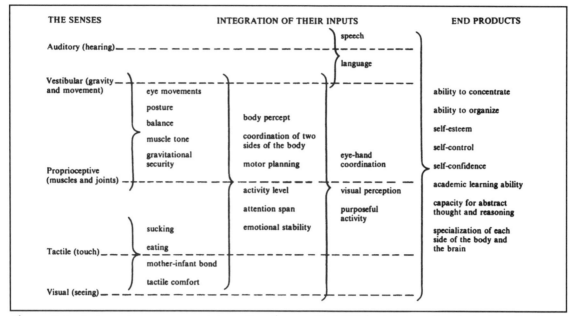

THE SENSES | INTEGRATION OF THEIR INPUTS | END PRODUCTS

Figure 9-1. A. Jean Ayres sensory integration theory. (© 1979 by Western Psychological Services. Reprinted from *Sensory Integration and the Child* by permission of the publisher, Western Psychological Services, 12031 Wilshire Blvd., Los Angeles, CA 90025.)

child explore and learn about his or her environment.

Fourth Level

The fourth and final level of SI includes the following end products: the ability to organize and concentrate, self-esteem, control and confidence, academic learning ability, capacity for abstract thought and reasoning, and development of dominance and hemispheric specialization. From Ayres' (1974) point of view, it does little good for occupational therapists to attempt to directly teach these skills when the earlier stages of integration are not adequately developed. This point of view has been challenged in recent years.

Skilled voluntary fine motor hand movement, for example, cannot be taught to the disabled child by giving practice exercises. Ayres describes the development of hand movement as a sequence of many steps:

- Control of neck and eye movements
- Trunk stability and balance
- Scapular and shoulder stability and movement
- Elbow motion
- Gross grasp
- Wrist positioning and movement
- Release of grasp
- Forearm supination and pronation
- Individual finger manipulation

Overlapping this sequence is the coordination of visual and sensorimotor mechanisms. Movements begin as spinal reflexes and are modified and refined to achieve a behavioral goal. In this way, reflex movement becomes voluntary. Regarding the role of sensation in this process, Ayres states two basic assumptions: (1) "reflex movements (which) are the precursor to and the foundation of voluntary movement... are elicited by sensory stimuli" and (2) "ongoing motor learning and behavior are strongly influenced by if not dependent on incoming sensation" (Ayres, 1979). She further reflects that although reflex movement can be elicited by direct stimulation, voluntary movement must be purposeful. A great deal has been written about sensory integrative function, and the reader is referred to Ayres' *The Development of Sensory Integrative Theory and Practice* (1974) *and Sensory Integration and the Child* (1979) for a more in-depth discussion (Figure 9-1).

Theoretical Updates

A systems view of brain function has largely replaced the hierarchical view. According to systems theory, the brain works as an integrated, holistic system. Fisher and Murray (1991) describe an updated view, that SI dysfunction results from a number of interrelated systems that are not functioning optimally. Recent practice tends to combine SI techniques with other approaches that incorporate research evidence from multiple sources.

The spiral of development, a newly developed addition, combines Ayres' original theory with studies of normal development, systems theory, and humanistic psychology. As children spiral upward toward maturity, their development includes the adaptive use of sensory information in the context of sensorimotor activities to further develop the sensory integrative capacity of the brain. Children's natural tendencies to explore and master their environment move them ever closer to self-actualization (Bundy, Lane, & Murray, 2002).

Group Approaches

King

While most of the research of Ayres and her associates applies to children, several occupational therapists have written about the treatment of mentally ill adults using neurodevelopmental and sensory integrative techniques. The best known of these is Lorna Jean King, who pioneered the use of SI approaches with chronic schizophrenic adults.

Lorna Jean King has noted the lack of SI in both schizophrenic and autistic clients by observing the kinds of sensory stimulation they seek from the environment. For example, she evaluates a retarded and autistic adolescent by observing his or her preference for vibratory input (plays with a hand-held vibrator), proprioceptive input (constant self-hugging), and calming vestibular input (distractible and disruptive behavior is reduced by slow swinging and rocking) (Larrington, 1987).

Paul Schilder noted as early as the 1930s that schizophrenic clients are markedly underreactive to vestibular stimulation as measured by postrotary nystagmus (rapid eye movements) (King, 1974). King linked the vestibular system abnormalities with the postural and movement limitations (pacing, adduction, and internal rotation) observed in the chronic process schizophrenic client, more currently called the negative symptom schizophrenic (Figure 9-2). Process schizophrenia is a subtype of schizophrenia, a mental disorder that develops insidiously from childhood and is not the result of a severe or recognizable stress. Process schizophrenics do not respond readily to medical or behavioral intervention and so tend to be chronically institutionalized.

Figure 9-2. Postural abnormalities due to faulty proprioceptive feedback in the person with process schizophrenia (flexion, adduction, internal rotation).

King refers to numerous studies of the neurological deficits in schizophrenia (and also autism) that link faulty vestibular and proprioceptive processing to schizophrenic symptoms. Some of these symptoms include perceptual deficits, feelings of fatigue and slow movement, postural insecurity (fear of falling), concrete thinking, and lack of emotional response. King's hypothesis is that some schizophrenic clients have "defective proprioceptive feedback mechanisms, the vestibular component in particular being underreactive in its role in the sensorimotor integration" (King, 1974, p. 534).

Considering today's emphasis on the biochemical etiology of all mental illness (including schizophrenia), King's theory of the central role of movement in altering biochemical states, as well as biochemistry affecting movement, remains timely. Movement and sensation are known to produce chemical changes just as taking medication produces changes in brain chemistry. Furthermore, King (1974) states:

...this model... applies not only to etiology but also to treatment. Although we cannot be sure which chemicals to alter, or in what direction, we can intervene in the motor behavior of the individual with the knowledge that there will be effects upon the thought processes and upon biochemistry. (p. 534)

In later publications, King notes the role of activities in coping with stress. A strenuous action, or "fight or flight" response to stress (citing Gal & Lazarus, 1975), was found to be responsible for the rapid metabolism of stress hormones, thus preventing secondary damage to the system. This suggests that strenuous or heavy work activity can serve to normalize the neurotransmitter balance that has been deranged by stress (King, 1978, 1988).

The intervention techniques King utilizes in treating groups of chronic schizophrenic clients are adaptations of the techniques Ayres used with children. They are gross motor movement activities aimed at normalizing patterns of excessive flexion, adduction, and internal rotation and increasing range of motion. Vestibular and tactile stimulation are provided through the use of the standard props—hammocks, scooter boards, balls, and blankets. Heavy work patterns suggested by Rood in King (1974) resisted use of tonic muscle groups, and cocontraction patterns are also incorporated. Other equipment King has added are parachutes, balloons, and beanbag chairs.

King suggests two criteria for the selection of activities: (1) attention must not be centered upon the motor process but rather on the object or outcome and (2) the activity must be pleasurable and evoke smiles, laughter, and feelings of fun. Clients should not have to think about what they are doing or how they move; the goal is to elicit spontaneous movement and affect. Vestibular and proprioceptive processing occur at the brainstem level and produce automatic responses, not cortical (voluntary) responses. Therefore, if a ball is thrown to a client and his or her hands extend spontaneously to catch it, we can assume that this automatic action reflects adaptive vestibular processing at the brainstem level. The goal of group activities using this frame of reference is to stimulate the sensory processing systems so that they will function more adaptively. As occupational therapists, we see spontaneous and purposeful motor responses as evidence that we are reaching that goal.

Ross

Mildred Ross further developed the use of sensory integrative theory and techniques with the chronic population. She extended the use of the SI approach to the elderly, the neurologically impaired, the Alzheimer's client, the mentally retarded, and the long-term chronic client of any age with disabilities that prevent adequate functioning in the community (Ross, 1997; Ross & Bachner, 2004). Ross developed her group techniques over more than 20 years of clinical experience. Her group sessions occur in five stages, which move developmentally from alerting activities involving tactile, kinesthetic, and proprioceptive input to graded opportunities for organized cognitive thought and behavior (Table 9-5). The following is a summary of Ross's five-stage groups.

Stage I

Stage I acknowledges the presence of each member to each other member of the group. Introductions or saying names can easily accomplish this. The purpose of the session is established by the therapist or group members in Stage I, and this orients members to the session. Explanations should be kept brief and on a level the members can understand. The attention of members should be captured in Stage I.

Stage II

Stage II provides maximum exertion in movement. A variety of gross motor movement is suggested here, incorporating all three planes—horizontal, vertical, and sagittal. Exercise, dance patterns, or games may be adapted for this stage. Pleasure, communication, and interaction or "cohesiveness" are possible goals. The effect of this stage is to stimulate or excite.

Stage III

Stage III emphasizes perceptual-motor skills. Activities may be chosen that require less vigorous movement and more judgment and focus action to accomplish a purposeful task. Making a fruit salad or drawing a picture are examples. The activities should be short-term and able to be finished in 30 minutes or less. This stage should have the effect of calming and focusing.

Table 9-5	Adapting Ross' Five-Stage Groups: Alerting vs. Calming Sensory Stimuli	
	Alerting	*Calming*
Environment	Bright light, bright colors, high contrasts, loud sounds, rapid rhythms, uneven sounds	Low light, pastel colors, similar hues, soft melodic sounds, slow even rhythms, closing one's eyes
Smell/Taste	Pungent odors, cold/hot foods/ liquids, crunchy, strong flavors	Sweet or herbal smells, smooth textures, mild flavor, temperate foods
Touch/Movement	Light touch, sudden touch, rapid movement, rotation or changing direction, jumping/hitting/ clapping	Steady moderate pressure, slow rhythmic movement, vibration, slowly rotating movement, holding on, hugging

Stage IV

Stage IV is the time for cognitive stimulation. A discussion of the previous stages, memory games, or poetry reading are suggested by Ross. "This is the opportunity for cortical controls to be demonstrated through organized behavior such as impulse control or creative expression. It is the highest point for display of attentiveness and group cohesiveness" (Ross, 1997, p. 9). The length of this stage may be changed depending on the activity chosen and the level and interest of the group. Music or current events discussion may take a major portion of the time, while a short inspiring poem may take less than 5 minutes. Preparation for closure should be kept in mind in selecting activities for this stage.

Stage V

Stage V provides resolution and termination. A way to say goodbye, when to meet next, or suggestions of what to do next time might serve as endings. When the therapist feels that the group was good, it may be appropriate to verbalize this in summarizing. Statements of satisfaction with the group by the therapist and clients can achieve a sense of peacefulness at its end.

Role of the Therapist

Using Ross's stages, the therapist plans and leads the activity, guided by knowledge of the principles of sensorimotor integration and activity

analysis but taking his or her cues from the group as well. The occupational therapist must be quite skilled to lead this kind of group effectively, keeping control while gently encouraging members to get involved. The stages provide a clear structure around which to plan appropriate activities. Ross, in *Integrative Group Therapy: Mobilizing Coping Abilities With the Five Stage Group*, offers excellent guidelines for considering when an activity should be introduced and how it should be presented (1997). Application for adults with developmental disabilities are extensively outlined in Ross and Bachner (2004).

Function and Dysfunction

In the sensorimotor frames of reference, functioning may be viewed as adequate when a person is able to learn and use all of the adaptive skills characteristic of his or her age. Since there is assumed to be a sequence of neurological and physiological development, dysfunction can be defined as a lag in development causing the client to function below his or her age level. An adult is dysfunctional when neurological or physiological malfunctioning interferes with normal daily activity and participation in life. This view of dysfunction in any illness encourages the identification of a physical cause. Even mental illness, as King has discussed, can respond to a neurodevelopmental intervention approach that follows the guidelines of early development. In using movement and games, the client's active participation is encouraged to produce an adaptive response in activities that are both functional and meaningful.

Change and Motivation

Change in neurophysiological functioning is thought to be brought about through several methods. Physical activity can produce change through its effect on muscle tone, muscle strength, and range of motion. Physical activity has also been shown to produce chemical changes; this is how the "runner's high" has been explained. During occupational therapy activities, changes in brain and body function can be brought about through sensory stimulation and repetition of movement. Using the traditional theories, change occurs in a specific sequence and progresses stage by stage up the hierarchy toward maturity. In an illness that has left clients without normal movement patterns and sensory processing skills, a baseline level must be established through careful sensorimotor assessment. Then, through a repetition of the developmental sequence, sensory and motor components of activity can be utilized by the occupational therapist in such a way as to facilitate subcortical learning. Automatic movement and postural responses will precede more advanced cognitive responses. The changes we look for in the sensorimotor frames can often be seen as spontaneous self-corrections, such as an increased state of alertness or a more functional body posture. These normalized neurological states can then serve as building blocks for working on more skilled purposeful movements and the use of language in interactions within groups.

As Ross points out, activities we offer clients can have powerful effects on the CNS. These effects can be both positive and negative. Activities should be carefully planned to approach the CNS in a way that it can accept and handle and to do so in a way that facilitates positive change. The occupational therapist does this through control and limitation of sensory input (Ross, 1997).

Change from the motor learning perspective comes about through repetition of a sequence of actions in performing functional tasks. This repetition in varied contexts and environments encourages the formation of new or alternate neural pathways that circumvent damaged areas. When linked with self-directed goals, repetition of adaptive strategies, and environmental adaptation, practice, and feedback, pave the way for habituation of

adapted motor and process skills (Bass-Haugen et al., 2002).

Motivation comes in the form of accepting the challenge to be a more active participant in life. Clients, after illness or injury, may be motivated to go back to work and to do things the way they used to. The lack of motivation comes when they expect too much change too fast, and therefore, they feel they have failed. With long-term physical dysfunction, clients may be unable to modify their goals or accept new methods for meeting their needs. Chronic illness may leave clients without hope. When cognitive impairment accompanies the physical or emotional dysfunction, long-term goals may no longer be understood. The spontaneous urge to advance one's development must often be rekindled after illness. Interventions such as sensory stimulation and movement play can encourage the client with chronic illness to pursue more active participation with others and the environment. Once success or pleasure is experienced, clients may be more motivated.

Group Intervention

King and Ross have given some helpful guidelines on how to structure groups. Gross motor activities are the common element. While movement activities are used extensively with pediatrics and physical dysfunction populations, movement is too often overlooked as an effective media for psychosocial dysfunction and geriatrics. As occupational therapists, we need to expand our repertoire of tools to include more activities involving movement. Much of our training in physiology, neuroanatomy, and sensorimotor integration prepares us well for doing so. Perhaps our level of comfort in using movement with our clients is not as high as it could be. Often occupational therapists need to be comfortable with their own ability to move and play before they are able to share this with clients.

Role of the Occupational Therapist

In the sensorimotor frames, the occupational therapist is a directive leader. The therapist needs a fairly thorough knowledge of neurodevelopment, neurophysiology, and SI in order to lead these groups competently. In most cases, clients with which we are working are at low levels of functioning. Often verbal communication is at a minimum, and it is through imitation and role modeling that our clients perform activities therapeutically. The occupational therapist plans movement, sensory, or cognitive activities that match their level and are relatively sure to succeed. The concept of the "just-right challenge" applies here. Activities should interest and challenge the clients but should not be so complex as to overwhelm them. In movement groups as described by King, Ross, and Levy, the occupational therapist is the undeniable leader. He or she comes prepared with equipment and ideas and guides the group from start to finish, taking cues from clients as needed along the way.

Neurodevelopmentally-based movement groups can be effective with some higher cognitive level populations as well. When this is done, care should be taken to explain the purpose thoroughly so that clients understand how the exercises and movements will help them.

Goals

Some of the goals mentioned by the various theorists may be summarized as follows:

- Provide sensory stimulation and opportunities for adaptive response. The client will develop skill in sensorimotor performance and strengthen normal sensorimotor integration.
- Improve and maintain muscle tone, posture, and motor planning. The client will demonstrate these successfully during participation in activities.
- Motivate the client to participate. The client will respond to stimulation by imitating or initiating activity.
- Facilitate the development of higher level cognitive skills through the integration and assimilation of lower level skills. The client will demonstrate higher level skills through participation in activity.
- Provide multiple opportunities for practice of functional and meaningful tasks. Group members can support one another, provide valuable feedback, and benefit from group problem solving.
- Achieve a sense of mastery and well-being. The client will demonstrate positive affective responses during participation in activity.

Specific goals for individual clients may be easily set and measured. All of the goals may be worked on appropriately through the use of group activities.

Examples of Activities

Movement activities of all types may be adapted in this frame of reference, from simple calisthenics to dance and sports, to laying bricks and digging in the garden. When working with adult populations, the therapist must be careful not to make the activities seem too childish.

New Games

One particularly rich source of activities that are adaptable is the handbook of the New Games Foundation (Fluegelman, 1976). The New Games Foundation is an organization that originated at San Francisco State College in 1966 as a resistance to the Vietnam War. The group was against any type of competition, even in sports, so they designed games that provided opportunities for individuals to express aggressiveness without anyone winning or losing. The games were designed for all ages and levels of activity, and since 1974, every few years they publish another book of newly invented games; see Activity Examples 9-1 and 9-2.

The New Games followers suggest what occupational therapists already know: that all the games can be adapted by changing the rules or that new games can be invented to meet the special needs and goals of our clients.

Parachute Games

King suggests parachute play as effective for spontaneous range of motion and postural correction as well as vestibular-proprioceptive stimulation (Figure 9-3). A real parachute (with no strings) works best and can be obtained in surplus stores or sports equipment supply catalogs.

Parachute games (Activity Example 9-3) are rich in sensorimotor integration potential. The basic movement involved requires reaching high above the head, an extension of the shoulders, elbows, and wrists to the full range of motion. The head tends to roll back as the client looks at the effect of his or her movement, the parachute rising high in the air. Lowering the parachute to below the knee requires the client to flex the spine forward at the waist and to extend the head forward, again following the movement of the parachute. The motion of the head and joints provides both proprioceptive and vestibular stimulation. Other movements may also be analyzed in this manner to aid in intervention planning to meet specific goals.

Figure 9-3. Parachute play.

Bioenergetics Groups

These are groups aimed at the expression of feelings through movement. The major spokesman for this approach to movement is Alexander Lowen. Lowen's bioenergetics exercises were developed from his bioenergetics theory of personality, which is understood in terms of the body and its energetic processes (Lowen & Lowen, 1977). More recently, Lowen's workshops have been offered as an extension of the myofascial release therapy workshops given by John Barnes, a physical therapist. Bioenergetic exercises can offer occupational therapists guidelines in the use of breathing and movement exercises to heighten emotional awareness and expression. Some of the bioenergetics exercises can release very powerful feelings and should not be done without training. However, the basic concept is useful in planning expressive exercises in moderation. For further information about this approach, the reader is referred to Lowen and Lowen's book, *The Way to Vibrant Health* (1977).

The activity groups discussed in Activity Examples 9-4 and 9-5 are based on this concept and have been used with adult clients with mental illness who are inhibited in the expression of feelings. In doing these activities, the occupational therapist should be careful not to overstimulate potentially volatile clients. The exercises should not be done with clients who are excitable or at risk for violent behavior. These neurophysiological techniques are especially well-suited to intervention with depression.

Exercise Groups

Exercise to music or dance activities has good potential as a therapeutic tool. Circle or group dancing is usually best suited to our purpose in occupational therapy. In physical disability areas where goals involve maintaining and increasing strength and range of motion, group activities that accomplish these goals are more enjoyable and motivating than individual exercise programs. A good example of this type of group is the "Range of Motion Dance," an exercise program for clients with rheumatoid arthritis developed by Diane Harlowe and Patricia Yu at St. Mary's Hospital Medical Center in Madison, Wisconsin (Van Deusen & Harlowe, 1987). This is a guided fantasy done with groups of clients with arthritis seated in chairs. The exercises, while following the story, go systematically through the range of motion for nearly every joint in the body. Once the sequence of motions is learned, it can be repeated by the clients at home by listening to the story on an audiotape. Greenfield and Godinez have introduced a similar group for clients with stroke, called "Self Range of Motion Exercises" (Greenfield & Godinez, 1989). They have defined eight skill levels for these exercises, ranging from complete dependence on the therapist leader to independence in performing the exercises.

In doing such groups, it is important to use the potential of the group to provide mutual support, encouragement, and feedback. Do not let the activity speak for itself; combine it with verbal reinforcement, progress checks, and education about how and why it is helping. It is generally the social and emotional aspects of a group that keep members coming back.

Ross' Five-Stage Groups

Mildred Ross gives us a sequence of specific guidelines for the selection of activities. Since the five-stage group is designed for severely impaired and chronic populations, movement and sensory stimulation are key elements of activity. "A routine of organized sequences enhances the likelihood of an automatic habitual response" (Ross, 1997, p. 2). The purpose of the five separate organized sequences is to motivate interaction with the environment. Sensory stimulation produces the heightened arousal and alertness to one's surroundings that maximizes the potential for adaptive responses. The outcome must be calm alertness that makes adults ready to move on in an organized way to the next activity of the day.

Table 9-5 may be useful in creating and modifying activities to help accommodate and manage the behaviors that emerge during the five-stage group.

Activity Examples 9-6 and 9-7 suggest specific organized sequences. In Ross' book *Integrative Group Therapy*, many other activity sequences are suggested. Because different populations have differences in their abilities to integrate sensory information, the examples given cover medium (Activity Example 9-6) and low (Activity Example 9-7) levels of processing skill.

Movement Therapy Groups With Handicapped Children

Sophie Levitt (1982) suggests therapeutic group work using a neurodevelopmental approach for children with cerebral palsy and motor delay. Both play groups and structured groups are seen as more effective than individual intervention for several reasons. The group often curtails rebellion and encourages cooperation. Children imitate other children and often instruct each other in doing what is required. Children seem to be able to concentrate more than twice as long with the stimulation of the group setting (1 to 1.5 hours as opposed to 20 minutes individually, Levitt reports). Levitt emphasizes the interdisciplinary nature of these groups. Occupational and physical therapists, nurses, speech therapists, and teachers all contribute to planning and implementing the activity.

In groups with handicapped children, it is not useful to group by diagnosis. Children should be selected for the groups according to their functional problems. The basis of selection may be motor problems such as poor grasp and release, poor balance, or recurring abnormal movement patterns or postures. The developmental or cognitive level of group members should be similar. Some children who are too severely involved to be aware of the group may not be appropriate. The selected group should be capable of working together and establishing a degree of group spirit. The specific activities should be selected according to the deficits of the members (Levitt, 1982).

It is evident that adults as well as children should be treated in groups of similar developmental level and that the same principles for selection and planning apply. It would be encouraging to see more groups of physically disabled adults treated in a manner that encourages interaction and takes advantage of general group dynamics principles. Some more current resources for groups with children are Mannix's self-esteem activities for secondary students with special needs (1996) and Mannix's social skills activities for special children (1993).

Task-Oriented Groups for Physical Disabilities

Client-centered interviews will determine which goals and tasks have priority for clients with acquired brain damage. Clients who have reached a level of voluntary control may benefit from groups that address similar goals. Activity Example 9-8 uses the materials for a cooking task as the basis for practice of reach and grasp. It uses the principle of variation of strategies by presenting objects of different shapes, sizes, and weights, which are placed at different shelf levels, to achieve optimal learning.

Music in Movement Groups

The use of music in therapy groups has been mentioned briefly. Music has qualities that can both relax and invigorate; it can energize a group, distract it, or put it to sleep. The choice of music should be made with care; instrumental rather than vocal may be less distracting. The clients' level of stimulation should be closely monitored, as Ross suggests. Music can change the mood of the group, but the key is to do it gradually; the music should match the mood of the clients to begin with, and then change little by little, accompanied by appropriate movement activities. It can arouse emotion easily because it has an effect on the body and the mind. Selection of music may depend to a great extent on what you want to accomplish with the client. With clients with depression, the therapist may want to energize them by playing music with a lively beat. Clients susceptible to anxiety might benefit more from slow, mellow rhythms and ballads that soothe the nerves. In any case, occupational therapists usually use music in combination with movement activities, and it is the activity that should remain the focus with the music providing an appropriate background.

Group Leadership

Introduction

In neurodevelopmental groups, the explanation of purpose should match the clients' ability to understand it. The level of cognition is the most important factor, and this varies widely in groups using the neurodevelopmental approach.

The warm-up is essential and takes on a somewhat different emphasis here. The warm-up should prepare the members for the activity not only psychologically, but physiologically as well. As Ross has stressed, there is a systematic way to approach the CNS (1997). If members are unable to screen out nonessential sensory stimulation, they may be overloaded very quickly. With client populations that are at risk for this, such as those with stroke, head trauma, autism, developmental delay, or chronic mental illness, the warm-up can offer limited and gradually increasing stimuli to test the group for an acceptable level of sensory stimulation.

Likewise, with the physically ill, the warm-up may be used as a testing experience to determine what level of physical exercise can be tolerated. Naturally, the occupational therapist has evaluated the client members prior to the group planning, so he or she should already be aware of the limits of safety. However, clients' conditions will vary on a daily (or hourly) basis and changes need to be taken into account. Based on the warm-up, the time frame or the activity itself may have to be modified.

Activity

The activities used will vary widely depending on the client population. Sensorimotor or cognitive-perceptual tasks are most common. Activities will generally address some aspect of neurological or physical functioning and will facilitate some kind of adaptive response. Unlike previously described frames of reference, there may be several short-term activities planned during each session. The activities are organized and sequenced according to neurophysiological theory, so that simpler sensorimotor activities can build up to advanced, more complex activities. Likewise, high stimulation activities are followed by slower, more calming ones, so that the CNS does not get overstimulated. Materials that facilitate movement, like mats, balls, props, and pillows, are often used. Craft activities or work activities that incorporate gross motor actions are useful. Materials and environments may be set up to provide cues for functional tasks so that activity demand matches or challenges the performance capacities of clients. Timing depends on the endurance and attention span of members, and sessions can be relatively short, 30 to 50 minutes.

Sharing and Processing

Sharing in movement groups occurs within the bounds of the activity. Clients can observe each other's movements; the cognitive or symbolic meaning of the movement is really not the point and therefore, not necessary to share. Processing involves expressing feelings about the group, and when possible, should be done verbally. Verbal processing can reveal hidden resistances and bring out other notable problems clients have while participating in the activity.

Generalizing and Application

The principles learned are associated with the effects of activity or movement of various kinds on the body and the emotions. The knowledge of the therapist may be shared with the group, when appropriate, to facilitate this learning. For example, a group of clients with depression may notice that after the physical expression of anger and hostility, they feel more energy. The lesson in this is that expression of feeling is natural and healthy. The application is to find ways to express feeling without hurting others or otherwise getting into trouble.

Application, even with clients at a lower cognitive level, may involve learning to repeat a desired adaptive response. When movement activities result in spontaneous laughter, for example, the pleasure of this response may motivate the client to repeat the movement that produced it. The neurodevelopmental response to movement activities tends to be spontaneous and not planned. As clients integrate new movement patterns into their repertoire, they will use them spontaneously at times outside of the group. The goal is to stimulate the development of higher level skills and more adaptive functioning in the client's everyday life.

Neither generalization nor application need to be separate phases of the sensorimotor group. The verbal summary is sufficient to reinforce this learning. However, discussion of learning and applications in life activities can be useful for those clients who are capable of such verbalization and insight.

Bibliography

American Occupational Therapy Association. (2002). *Occupational therapy practice framework: Domain and process.* Bethesda, MD: Author.

Ayres, A. J. (1974). *The development of sensory integrative theory and practice.* Dubuque, IA: Kendall Hunt.

Ayres, A. J. (1979). *Sensory integration and the child.* Los Angeles: Western Psychological Services.

Bass-Haugen, J., Mathiowetz, V., & Flinn, N. (2002) Optimizing motor behavior using the occupational therapy task oriented approach. In C. Trombly & M. V. Radomski (Eds.), *Occupational therapy for physical dysfunction* (5th ed.). Philadelphia: Lippincott, Williams and Wilkins.

Bobath, B. (1972). The neurodevelopmental approach to treatment. In P. Pearson (Ed.), *Physical therapy services in developmental disabilities.* Springfield, IL: Charles Thomas.

Bowler, D. (1999). Functional improvement through motor learning. Presentation handout given in White Plains, NY sponsored by Preventionworks, Nov. 14th, 1999.

Brunnstrom, S. (1970). *Movement therapy in hemiplegia.* New York: Harper & Row.

Bundy, A. C., Lane, S. J., & Murray, E. A. (2002). *Sensory integration: Theory and practice* (2nd ed.). Philadelphia: F. A. Davis.

Carr, J. H., & Shepherd, R. B. (1987). *A motor learning program for stroke* (2nd ed.). Rockville, MD: Aspen.

Carr, J. H., & Shepherd, R. B. (1998). *Neurological rehabilitation: Optomizing motor performance.* Oxford: Butter worth-Heinemann.

Eggers, O. (1983). *Occupational therapy in the treatment of adult hemiplegia.* London: William Heinemann Medical Books.

Fisher, A., & Murray, E. A. (1991). Introduction to sensory integration theory. In M. Fisher, E. A. Murray, & A. Bundy (Eds.), *Sensory integration: Theory and practice.* Philadelphia: F. A. Davis.

Fitts, P., & Posner, M. (1967). *Human performance.* Belmont, CA: Brooks/Cole.

Flinn, N., & Radomski, M. (2002). Learning. In C. Trombly & M. Radomski (Eds.), *Occupational therapy for physical dysfunction* (5th ed.). Philadelphia: Lippincott, Williams & Wilkins.

Fluegelman, A. (1976). *The new games book.* Garden City, NY: Doubleday.

Gal, R., & Lazarus, R. S. (1975). The role of activity in anticipating and confronting stressful situations. *Journal of Human Stress, 4,* 4-20.

Greenfield, J. M., & Godinez, M. (1989). Clients with stroke learn independence by leading their own therapy group. *OT Week,* April 20.

Hammill, D. (1993). A brief look at the learning disabilities movement in the United States. *Journal of Learning Disabilities, 26,* 295-310.

King, L. J. (1974). A sensory integrative approach to schizophrenia. *American Journal of Occupational Therapy, 28,* 529-536.

King, L. J. (1978). Toward a science of adaptive responses. Slagle lecture. *American Journal of Occupational Therapy, 32,* 429-437.

King, L. J. (1988). *Occupational therapy and neuropsychiatry in mental health focus.* Rockville, MD: American Occupational Therapy Association.

Larrington, G. (1987). Sensory integration based program with a severely retarded autistic teenager: An occupational therapy case report. In Z. Mailloux (Ed.), *Sensory integrative approaches in occupational therapy.* New York: Haworth Press.

Levit, K. (2002). Optimizing motor behavior using the Bobath approach. In C. Trombly & M. V. Radomski (Eds.), *Occupational therapy for physical dysfunction* (5th ed.). Philadelphia: Lippincott, Williams and Wilkins.

Levitt, S. (1982). *Treatment of cerebral palsy and motor delay.* Boston: Blackwell Scientific Publications.

Lowen, A., & Lowen, L. (1977). *The way to vibrant health.* New York: Harper and Row.

Mannix, D. (1993). *Social skills activities for special children.* New York: Prentice Hall.

Mannix, D. (1996). *Self-esteem activities for secondary students with special needs.* New York: Simon & Schuster.

Mulligan, S. (2002). Advances in sensory integration research. In A. C. Bundy, S. J. Lane, & E. A. Murray (Eds.), *Sensory integration: Theory and practice* (2nd ed.). Philadelphia: F. A. Davis.

Rood, M. S. (1954). Neurophysiological reactions as a basis for physical therapy. *Phys Therapy Rev, 34,* 444-449.

Ross, M. (1997). *Integrative group therapy: Mobilizing coping abilities with the five stage group.* Bethesda, MD: American Occupational Therapy Association.

Ross, M., & Bachner, S. (Eds.). (2004). *Adults with developmental disabilities: Current approaches in occupational therapy.* Bethesda, MD: American Occupational Therapy Association.

Sabari, J. S. (2002). Optimizing motor control using the Carr and Shepherd approach. In C. Trombly & M. V. Radomski (Eds.), *Occupational therapy for physical dysfunction* (5th ed.). Philadelphia: Lippincott, Williams & Wilkins.

Schmidt. (1988). *Motor control and learning: A behavioral emphasis* (2nd ed.). Champaign, IL: Human Kinetics.

Shumway-Cook, A., & Woollacott, M. (Eds.). (2001). *Motor control: Theory & practical application* (2nd ed.). Philadelphia: Lippincott, Williams & Wilkins.

Sunderland, A., Tinson, D., Bradley, E., Fletcher, D., Langton Hewer, R., & Wade, D. (1992). Enhanced physical therapy improves recovery of arm function after stroke. *Journal of Neurology, Neurosurgery, & Psychiatry, 55,* 530-535.

Trombly, C. (1995). Occupation: Purposefulness and meaningfulness as therapeutic mechanisms. *American Journal of Occupational Therapy, 49,* 960-972.

Trombly, C., & Radomski, M. V. (Eds.). (2002). *Occupational therapy for physical dysfunction* (5th ed.). Baltimore: Williams and Wilkins.

Van Deusen, J., & Harlowe, D. (1987). The efficacy of the ROM dance program for adults with rheumatoid arthritis. *American Journal of Occupational Therapy, 41,* 90-95.

Sensorimotor

Activity Example 9-1

Blob

The Blob begins as a game of tag. When the person who is "it" catches someone, that person joins hands and becomes part of the Blob. Only the outside hand on either end of the Blob can snatch runaway players. Thus, the insidious Blob keeps growing, cornering stray runners and forcing them to join up. In large groups, the Blob may split itself into parts and organize raiding parties to round up the last few strays. Boundaries must be set for this game, so eventually everyone is caught. "The thrilling climax occurs when there's only one player left to put up a heroic last ditch stand on behalf of humanity" (Fluegelman, 1976, p. 107). The last survivor can start the next Blob as the game continues.

This game is obviously for people who are ambulatory, have good balance and coordination, and have enough cognitive understanding to be able to follow simple rules. Blob is a simple concept that can be fun even for those who do not grasp its deeper implications. Done inside a room with the elderly, a therapist can talk the group through any difficulties, or he or she can begin by being the Blob. It may be done slowly or quickly to adapt to patient ability, and it provides light exercise with an element of fun and challenge.

Sensorimotor

Activity Example 9-2

People to People

Here is a new game that is made for occupational therapy. It is especially good for integrating movement, motor planning, and cognition. Everyone chooses a partner and the game begins with a rhythmic clapping and snapping in unison (clap-clap-right hand, snap-snap-left hand). The caller names two body parts, one on the right snap, the other on the left snap (e.g., "elbow to ear"). On the next snap-snap the whole group repeats "elbow to ear" while simultaneously one partner places his elbow on the other partner's ear. The caller continues to name body parts, trying to challenge the group by naming obscure anatomical structures (esophagus to gastrocnemius) or forcing them to take awkward positions. When the caller gets tired of this, he may call out "people to people." Then everyone must change partners, and in the confusion, the caller grabs a partner, leaving another member to become the new caller.

Adaptations for this game are endless. At the very least, it is a great socialization ice breaker, sure to get everyone laughing. It is also an excellent way for occupational therapy students to study their anatomy. Patients can practice bilateral coordination (clapping and snapping), motor planning (touching parts with partner), body awareness (identifying parts), and cognition (naming and recognizing body parts). A fair amount of balance, coordination, and visual-motor integration are required to perform this activity successfully. Care should be taken with this and other games requiring touch that patients are not threatened by the close proximity to others.

The New Games followers suggest what occupational therapists already know—all the games can be adapted by changing the rules, or that new games can be invented to meet the special needs and goals of our patients.

From Cole, M. B. *Group dynamics in occupational therapy: The theoretical basis and practice application of group intervention* (3rd ed.). Thorofare, NJ: SLACK Incorporated. © 2005 SLACK Incorporated.

Sensorimotor

Activity Example 9-3

Parachute Games

All the games begin with group members holding an edge of the parachute at even intervals. It will take a few tries to move the parachute up over heads and down to the knees in unison to "catch the air." When the group has accomplished this, members can take turns running under the chute and exchanging places with one another across the circle. Other variations of parachute play are as follows:

- Popcorn—When the parachute is down, a few tennis balls can be tossed in the center. The group makes the balls "pop" into the air and catches them with the parachute.

- Round the World—One ball is placed in the center of the parachute. The group is instructed to work together to make the ball roll around the edge of the parachute by moving it in unison.

- Down the Drain—Two colored balls are placed in the parachute. One side (blue ball) tries to get the other side's ball (red ball) to drop through the hole in the middle of the parachute.

- Secret Club—Billow the parachute by the unified above the head, below the knees motion of the group. Then on the count of three, group members bring the parachute edge down behind their backs and proceed to sit on the edge of the parachute. The air in the middle produces a "tent" in which the "secret club" can meet (but not for long or the air can get very stale!).

- Shark—The members gather up the edge of the chute at just about waist level until a "calm sea" is produced. Then the "shark" ducks under and stalks the group with one finger pointing up touching the parachute from below, so that his or her movements may be observed from the top of the parachute. At an unexpected moment, the shark grabs the legs of an unsuspecting group member. The "victim" screams loudly as he or she is pulled under to become the next "shark." Two or three sharks at a time may be used in larger groups.

From Cole, M. B. *Group dynamics in occupational therapy: The theoretical basis and practice application of group intervention* (3rd ed.). Thorofare, NJ: SLACK Incorporated. © 2005 SLACK Incorporated.

Sensorimotor

Activity Example 9-4

Expressing Anger With Movement

Materials: Exercise mats or thick carpeting and pillows.

Directions: Give directions for each step of the sequence and allow members to take the time they need for each step.

1. Lie down on your back on the mat and extend both legs. Kick your legs rhythmically and allow your energy to flow into this motion. Take a few minutes to do this, setting your own pace.

2. Stand up and form a circle. Kick alternately with the right, then the left leg into the center of the circle.

3. Clench your fists and as you kick into the center of the circle, say "No!" Louder!

4. What other words can we say? As members make suggestions, have the whole group try them. Try punching into the center of the circle and saying words or making sounds.

5. Rest a few minutes and concentrate on breathing. Walk slowly around the circle, then turn and walk the other way. The slow walking has a calming effect after the excitement of kicking and punching.

6. Lie down on stomach with pillow in front of you. Punch pillow with right and left fists in a rhythmic motion. Do this for a few minutes and set your own pace.

7. As you punch the pillow, say "No!" If you feel like kicking also, allow yourself to do this.

8. If you would like, give the pillow a name. (Therapists should do this with caution, so as not to arouse too much anger.)

9. After a few minutes, wind down and just breathe slowly, resting head on pillow.

10. Stand up again when rested. Shrug shoulders in a backward roll and loosen tension in the neck area.

11. As patients shrug, say "Get off my back!" Louder!

12. Sit in a circle and massage muscles in back of neck. Each person massages the back of the person in front of him or her.

This exercise must be processed so that clients are not left with unresolved angry feelings. One goal is awareness of anger so that its appropriate expression can be discussed. Another goal is eliciting normal movement patterns subcortically. The careful planning and adaptation of this type of activity can utilize the concepts of Rood, NDT, PNF, Brunnstrom, or sensory integration.

Sensorimotor

Activity Example 9-5

Acting Out Feelings

Materials: Twenty index cards with feeling words, paper, pencils, and stopwatch. Words for cards are lonely, disgusted, excited, pleased, annoyed, infuriated, friendly, jealous, miserable, crabby, ecstatic, impatient, giddy, silly, moody, spacy, frightened, terrified, hopeless, hurt. Other feeling words may be added or substituted.

Directions: Each member draws a card and takes 30 seconds to act out the feeling on the card. Someone should be designated as timekeeper. Players may make sounds, but no words are allowed. Players can walk back and forth in front of the group, sit, stand, lie down, and make gestures and facial expressions. The entire 30 seconds should be used. Nonverbal interaction with other members may be allowed as long as no one is hurt.

Members do not shout out their guesses; this is not charades. When time is up, group members write down what they think the feeling is. As each "mini-drama" ends, members read out their feeling words and discuss why they thought so. After a brief discussion, the player shows the group the card. Members continue to draw cards and act out feelings until they are all used.

Sensorimotor

Activity Example 9-6

Ross Five-Stage Group for Medium/Verbal Members

Materials: Six to eight clients, blackboard and chalk (or newsprint pad and large marker), and a basketball. Arrange chairs in a circle.

Directions: Stage I (5 minutes)—The therapist introduces self and states, "We are all going to exercise our muscles and our brains so we can share ideas and learn from each other. To begin, I'd like each of you to take a turn coming up to the board and writing your name." The chalk is handed to the first volunteer, who sits back done when finished. The group will read each name aloud as it is written. Note that everyone is needed to complete the circle; gather any late or distracted members.

Stage II (10 to 15 minutes)—An agitated group is organized by asking members to pass the basketball from one to another with both hands while sitting. Members may then stand and bounce the ball to each other across the circle. Members take turns walking around the outside of the circle bouncing the basketball; then the members stand in a circle, facing right, an arm's length apart from each other. They must pass the basketball between their legs to the person behind them. The whole group jogs around the outside of the circle of chairs for maximum exertion. Members face left, arm's length apart, and pass the basketball backwards over their heads to the person behind them. The group can create its own movement sequences by requiring the ball to be passed without hands, or from member to member in a predetermined pattern.

Stage III (15 minutes)—Members move chairs back a few feet before sitting down, thus expanding the circle. A large, empty wastebasket is placed in the center. Members take turns bouncing the basketball once and trying to get it in the "basket." The group can be split into "teams," keeping score on the board. If teams are uneven, reshuffling should occur. Blocking may be done if skill permits for "offensive and defensive play." Members of teams sit alternately and attempt to block winning plays with arm movements. Different colored bandannas may be tied around the members' necks or heads to signify the different teams.

End group with a series of stretches (e.g., pantomime throwing a free point, reaching for the hoop, and blocking). Finally, pantomime congratulating each other on a winning game. Check level of excitement; use a calming strategy from Table 9-1 if needed.

Stage IV (15 minutes)—Discussion of favorite sports can follow. Each member takes a turn remembering an experience involving a sport. What athletics do members know? Admire? Dislike? What do they remember about Winter or Summer Olympics? What about leisure or solitary sports, such as swimming, fishing, or bicycling? The goal of the discussion is to learn about each other and from each other about different sports. Encourage members to ask each other questions or respond to one another's comments.

If discussion is somewhat beyond the group, substitute taking turns with the chalk and drawing a piece of sports equipment on the board. Have the group guess what it is or what sport uses the equipment. Examples include fishing line with hook, swimming pool, boxing glove, golf club, baseball bat, tennis racquet, pair of skis. Congratulate the group for sharing their knowledge and experience with each other.

Stage V—To summarize, the therapist asks members to remember parts of the session. "What things did we do today? Which did you like best? What did you learn about each other?" End with a firm handshake and say goodbye by name as each member leaves.

From Cole, M. B. *Group dynamics in occupational therapy: The theoretical basis and practice application of group intervention* (3rd ed.). Thorofare, NJ: SLACK Incorporated. © 2005 SLACK Incorporated.

Sensorimotor

Activity Example 9-7

Ross Five-Stage Group for Low/Nonverbal Members

Materials: Hand lotion, candle, balloons, party favor blowers, card table, cards with different colors, 10 to 12 pairs of matching objects, tray, and bag.

Directions: Stage I—Clients sit in a circle. The therapist greets each member by name and asks everyone to hold out their hands. A dot of herbal-smelling hand lotion is squeezed into their palms; the therapist demonstrates rubbing it into the hands. Ask members to notice how it smells. A vanilla or spice-scented candle is then passed from member to member, and sniffing is encouraged.

Stage II—Every member chooses a colored, blown-up, 6-inch diameter balloon to hold between their hands. "Don't let go… don't drop it… hold onto it." The therapist then asks members to imitate holding it out in front, above the head, swinging to the left and the right (shoulder height), gently throwing and catching it, and touching the balloon to knees, ankles, floor, lap, chin, and each shoulder.

Put on music, such as a waltz tempo (e.g., Strauss) or a song that suits the members' age group. Ask the group to stand and imitate movements to the music: swinging the balloon back and forth, up and down, and around in a circle.

Batting balloons in the air begins as another song is played. Members try to keep all the balloons in the air until the music ends. Observe behavior and modify as needed.

Stage III—All balloons are collected except one. The therapist passes this balloon with his or her elbows and asks a member to begin passing it around the circle with no hands. This can be done sitting or standing. If it is someone's birthday, ask the members to sing "Happy Birthday" (many persons who no longer speak can still sing). Party blowers are passed out and everyone practices blowing by imitating the therapist. A small table is set up and balloons are placed on the table. Members attempt to knock all the balloons off the table using the party blowers (again, no hands). Pick them all up and do it again. Passing a single balloon from one side of the table to the other can follow.

Stage IV—Cards with different colors are passed to each member. Colored cards matching these are placed down on the table. Members take turns choosing a card from the table until they find one that matches.

The therapist makes a board or tray with 10 or 12 common objects. Matching objects are placed in a bag. Members draw an object, guessing what it is by touch if they can, and pointing to the matching object on the tray. The they look at the object to see if they guessed correctly.

Stage V—Play a short waltz tape and ask members to stand and join hands for a group sway.

From Cole, M. B. *Group dynamics in occupational therapy: The theoretical basis and practice application of group intervention* (3rd ed.). Thorofare, NJ: SLACK Incorporated. © 2005 SLACK Incorporated.

Activity Example 9-8

Grocery Game

Goal: Upper extremity strengthening, grasp and release practice, and improvement in efficiency of movement using a variety of shapes, sizes, and weights.

Position: Six members, seated in wheelchairs in a circle, no table.

Timing: Warm up: 5 to 10 minutes

Activity: 10 to 15 minutes

Discussion: 20 to 30 minutes

Summary: 5 minutes

Materials: Six each of the following: 8 oz. can of beans, 16 oz. can of tomato sauce, 1 lb. box of pasta, large yellow onions, 5 lb. bag of flour, individually wrapped roll of paper towels, cloves of garlic, 1 liter bottles of soda, brown paper grocery bags. (Any eight items may be used, vary number and weight according to client needs. Avoid glass containers.) One of each item will be in a brown paper grocery bag. The remaining five of each item is stored in a visible location in the room, using varying levels of reaching difficulty. (Activity should be graded to match member skills and abilities.)

Description

Introduction: All of you have discussed with me your difficulties with reaching and handling objects since your illness or injury. The only way to get better at lifting and handling objects is by practicing. Today we are going to use these grocery items to play a game. This will make exercise and practice more fun.

Warm-Up: Therapist allows each member to choose one item from a grocery bag. Members hold the item with one or both of their hands, and briefly discuss the best way to reach for and grasp this item. Taking turns, each member will pass one item to the person on the right, and continue passing the item around the circle. To add a challenge, members may pass more than one item at a time. Continue several times, ask members to keep track of how many times they reached for and grasped each item. Each member will end up holding only one item. Discuss any difficulties members had with this activity.

Activity: For the next part of the game, I'm going to ask each of you to "go shopping" right here in this room. The first part of the game is for each of you to look around the room and locate where I have stored five more of the item you are now holding. Some of them are high up, and you'll have to reach up to get them. Some are eye level, and some are low down. (Members take turns locating and pointing to the stored items. Members may help each other do this.)

Why do you think I put the items where they are? (May process member comments. Pass out grocery bags, encourage/help members to "open" the bags and balance them on their laps.) The goal of this activity is to collect one of each item and place them in your shopping bag. You have 10 minutes to complete this activity. Does everyone understand the directions? Who will volunteer to repeat the directions for the group? (Repeat directions as needed, answer member questions.) I will give you a 1-minute warning. You may begin.

When time is up, return to original circle with grocery bags. Members write names on the grocery bags, and count how many items they retrieved, and which ones (if any) are missing.

Sharing: Please take turns telling the group how many items you retrieved, what is still missing, and what problems you had in doing this activity. (Encourage members to respond to each other and share some of their problem-solving strategies.)

Processing:

- How did you feel about playing the grocery game? (Elicit both positive and negative feelings without judgment.)
- What did you like about the activity? What did you dislike? Why?
- What conflicts occurred when more than one of you went for the same item at the same time?
- What help did you receive from or give to other members? How did you feel about that?

From Cole, M. B. *Group dynamics in occupational therapy: The theoretical basis and practice application of group intervention* (3rd ed.). Thorofare, NJ: SLACK Incorporated. © 2005 SLACK Incorporated.

Activity Example 9-8
Grocery Game (continued)

Generalizing:
- What physical skills did we need to do this activity?
- What mental skills did we need?
- What was hardest to do? What was easiest?
- What mental and physical strategies did we use to deal with the difficult parts?
- How can we help each other with activities like this?
- What did you learn about yourself from doing this? What did you learn about others?

Application (everyone answers these questions for him- or herself):
- What tasks do you do at home that require these same skills?
- What places in the community require us to do something like this?
- What jobs have you held that require this kind of activity?
- How does where we store different items affect our ability to function at home?
- How could you change where you keep the things you need to do projects at home?
- Who can help you to reach or lift things when you cannot do it yourself?
- Why is it important for you to have the skill and ability to gather items for a project?
- What can you do to practice these skills at home?

Summary (ask a member to summarize):
- What did we do in group today?
- What skills did we learn or practice?
- Please remember the ways you plan to practice these skills at home.
- I really appreciated how hard everyone worked in group today.
- I especially noticed... (give individual feedback to each member)
- We'll meet again at... See you then.

From Cole, M. B. *Group dynamics in occupational therapy: The theoretical basis and practice application of group intervention* (3rd ed.). Thorofare, NJ: SLACK Incorporated. © 2005 SLACK Incorporated.

Chapter 10

A Model of Human Occupation Approach

The Model of Human Occupation (MOHO) emerged around 1980 as a further definition of the theory of occupational behavior developed by Mary Reilly (1962). The central idea of occupational behavior theory is that engagement in activity or occupation in itself will produce and maintain health. Human achievement and daily occupation are identified as the focal point for the development of the model of human occupation (Kielhofner, 2002). White (1959) is credited with introducing the concept of the human need for competence and achievement. Kielhofner, Burke, and Igi (1980) expanded on these concepts and combined them with general systems theory. They describe the human being as an open system, define the various parts of the system (volitional, habituation, and performance subsystems), and describe how it interacts with other systems (culture, tasks, social norms, human and nonhuman environment). The MOHO can be viewed as a superstructure that organizes concepts and expresses them in terms that can be readily applied to evaluation and intervention.

and culture" (2002, p. 2). As a therapeutic approach, it is holistic and universally applicable across ages, cultures, and disabilities. MOHO views the person as an open system, which has the capacity to reorganize itself or be reorganized. Injury or illness can bring about unwelcome change that disrupts both daily occupations and life occupations. The function of occupational therapy is to evaluate all aspects of the system and to facilitate an adaptive reorganization so that order can be restored. The subsystems within the client include volitional, which incorporates occupational choices of performance areas of occupation; habituation, which incorporates occupational performance patterns; and performance, which incorporates both performance skills and client factors. External parts of the system include all of the contexts defined by the *Occupational Therapy Practice Framework* (AOTA, 2002). Perhaps because of its broadness, MOHO "will not address all the problems faced by a client, requiring the therapist to actively use other models along with it" (Kielhofner, 2002, p. 3).

Framework Focus

MOHO is sometimes identified as an "overarching" theory because it is so broad. As such, MOHO touches upon just about every domain of the *Occupational Therapy Practice Framework* (American Occupational Therapy Association [AOTA], 2002). According to Kielhofner, human "occupation is complex and multifaceted. Occupation encompasses a wide range of doing that occurs in the context of time, space, society,

Basic Assumptions

The Human Open System

The basic assumption in applying systems theory to human functioning is that man is an open system that can change and develop through interaction with the environment (Kielhofner, 1978). The human open system is described as a cyclical process involving output, feedback, input, and

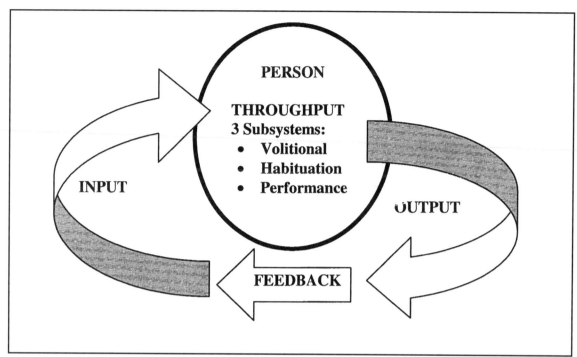

Figure 10-1. The human open system. (Adapted from Kielhofner, G. [Ed.]. [2002]. *A model of human occupation: Theory and application* [3rd ed.]. Baltimore: Williams & Wilkins.)

throughput (Kielhofner & Burke, 1985). The human being gives output to the environment, receives feedback in the form of input from the environment, and experiences throughput, a process of change and adaptation of the person resulting from the feedback given (Figure 10-1). The system is divided into parts for the purpose of examining (evaluation) and influencing (intervention) its processes.

The Three Internal Subsystems

Following systems theory, throughput occurs within the three internal subsystems: volitional, habituation, and performance capacity, which comprise the internal organization of the human system. These subsystems are consolidated and heterarchical (i.e., they are interdependent with one another, contributing equally to the human system as a whole). The volitional subsystem maintains a belief in one's self and one's values, and exerts influence in choosing one's occupations and initiating occupational behavior. The habituation subsystem organizes and maintains occupational behavior in routines and role patterns (habit maps and role scripts). The performance subsystem has been separated into intrinsic and extrinsic components (Kielhofner, Forsyth, & Barrett,

2003). Performance capacity refers to the status of mental and physical skills and abilities within the individual, while extrinsic performance describes actual engagement in occupational behavior during participation in life. The three subsystems work together in an integrated fashion to maintain the balance of work, play, and self-care activities (see Figure 10-1).

The Volitional Subsystem

The volitional process involves anticipating, experiencing, choosing, and interpreting occupational behavior (Kielhofner, 2002, p. 44). This system serves to direct and energize the other subsystems toward desired goals. However, this motivating force is highly influenced by the other subsystems (state of fatigue, habitual patterns) as well as external circumstances. Cultural common sense defines one's perceptions of one's self and one's environment and creates the context for occupational choices. Choices for occupation can be immediate (activities for today) or long-term (career choices, committed relationships). The three main components of this subsystem are: personal causation, values, and interests. Personal causation refers to a belief in one's self and is related to feelings of competence. A healthy individual is thought to possess needed skills (sense of personal capacity) and to believe him- or herself to be capable of using these skills to have a desired effect on the environment (self-efficacy). A person who believes in him- or herself expects to succeed through the use of his or her own abilities. A person who lacks a sense of personal causation may feel that what happens is controlled by fate or external circumstance. Such a person feels helpless to cope with the functional problems resulting from illness and disability.

Values in the MOHO refer to the meaningfulness of activities. Individuals are thought to spend time doing activities that have meaning and are thought to be good or morally right. For example, if a student thinks that having a college degree is good, he or she may work very hard at reading, writing, and studying, activities that will help him or her achieve that goal. Clients often find themselves unable to perform activities that they consider to be important or meaningful, such as going back to work. A reprioritizing of values might be an intervention goal. Using this model, clients can find alternate ways to perform a work role that are within their capabilities.

Interests in this model are defined as tendencies to find certain occupations attractive and pleasurable. If a person enjoys a particular activity, he or she may be inclined to participate in it frequently or for longer periods of time. Interests related to work, play, and self-care activities and are not limited to recreational endeavors. Occupational choices are highly influenced by the activities one finds attractive. A healthy individual uses his or her interests to guide present action and to plan the use of time. A person lacking in interests may need help in exploring his or her environment and in finding pleasure in activities.

In summary, the volitional subsystem guides the occupational behavior of the individual in ways that are meaningful and pleasurable and are likely to have a desired effect on the environment.

The Habituation Subsystem

The concept of "habit training" dates back to the practice of Eleanor Clarke Slagle, reflected by the writings of Adolph Meyer. He describes the "systematic engagement of interest and concern about the actual use of time and work (as) an obligation and a necessity" in the treatment of chronic illness (Meyer, 1982, p. 81). The organization of activities throughout the day is the concern of the habituation subsystem, as conceptualized by the MOHO. Roles and habits are its components.

Habits are routine or typical ways in which a person performs tasks. Their familiarity provides a sense of stability and well-being that comes with predictability. For example, a morning routine may involve getting up at 7 a.m., bathing, dressing, and eating breakfast. Habits can decrease the effort required to perform tasks by making them so routine that they are almost automatic. Consider the effort needed to find one's way to a new place of work. After driving the same route for several days, one recognizes familiar landmarks and the trip requires much less conscious thought. This routine allows the individual to save his or her energy for the more challenging activities of the day.

However, research has shown that habits are not just mindless repetitions of behavior. Rather, they operate as habit maps, or guidelines, which must be improvised to accommodate each new circumstance. Habit maps include thoughts and perceptions as well as action sequences. Young (1988) views habits as internalized intuitive knowledge, which gives us our bearings (orients us) and allows us to anticipate the next step in familiar temporal, physical, and social surroundings. According to Young, habits that are shared by a social group are called "customs" and are the carriers of culture. They are the rules for living that keep us in harmony with our social environment (Young, 1988).

Illness often results in a breakdown of normal routines. Occupational therapy may be needed to relearn and reorganize one's habits after illness. Being in a familiar surrounding may provide a way for persons to maintain order in the face of illness or disability. MOHO stresses the importance of a familiar and safe habitat and the necessity of assessing one's habitual ways of doing things. Often the initial intervention in occupational therapy is to reinforce familiar routines and existing skills.

A role is a position or status within a social group, along with its accompanying obligations and expectations and related cluster of attitudes and actions. Some typical roles are worker, parent, family member, student, and volunteer. Functional individuals generally internalize and enact a variety of life roles and find it necessary to achieve a balance of these if they are to maintain order in their lives. The roles we play have an organizing effect on how we use time. The worker role and the family member role, for example, each require the performance of defined tasks that must be balanced and planned for if the day is to flow smoothly.

According to Kielhofner (2002), every role has a role script. Role scripts guide comprehension of social expectations and construction of performance actions (p. 73). Similar to habits, roles guide our improvisation of behavior, which changes and adapts continually. The role of a parent in the family, for example, suggests various tasks concerned with providing food and shelter; maintaining the household; and providing instruction, authority, and guidance for the children. The parent role also constrains behavior because parents are expected to set an example for their children, and to refrain from activities (gambling, alcohol abuse) that would be detrimental to the family unit. Some role scripts are more flexible than others. As circumstances change, role expectations may require rethinking and their script adaptation.

Our clients may lack social roles or may find it difficult to meet the obligations and expectations of their roles. The focus of therapeutic intervention may be the development of new roles and/or the planning and modification of activities required within chosen roles. For evaluation and intervention purposes, grouping clients who wish to continue in similar roles, such as returning to work or maintaining a home, allows persons with disabilities to share ideas and provide mutual support for adapting their role scripts to accommodate physical, emotional, or cognitive limitations.

In addition to role modification or loss, Hammel (1999) points out the necessity for persons with acquired disability to learn a new self-manager role, which involves the management of medical, functional, economic, and social aspects of a disability. The degree to which this role is internalized can influence the person's independence in the community and the successful performance of other life roles. An occupational therapist might establish a group for clients with newly acquired disabilities and provide a structure for clients to help one another in learning this new role.

The Performance Capacity Subsystem

Performance capacity is the ability for doing things. This subsystem includes both objective and subjective client factors required to perform purposeful activities. Components, or foundation abilities, include musculoskeletal, neurological, cardiopulmonary, and cognitive images. Three types of skills are identified as part of subjective experience: perceptual-motor, process, and communication/interaction skills. The intrinsic part of performance has been relabeled "performance capacity," and the extrinsic part is called "occupational performance." A person's performance, as linked to the output of the human open system, is called "participation." These updates, adapted from Kielhofner, Forsyth, and Barrett (2003), are diagrammed in Figure 10-2.

The volitional and habituation subsystems can only perform to the extent that existing capacities and skills will allow. Therefore, a lack of skills can prevent the needed organization of roles and habits, the pursuit of interests, and the accomplishment of valued goals. In this area, occupational therapy may treat deficit areas using other frames of reference, such as biomechanical or sensory integration, in a fragmented fashion. Authors of the updated MOHO theory caution against this "reductionistic" practice. The application of physiological, psychological, or biomechanical theory should always be in service to the more basic human need to engage in meaningful occupations.

Interaction With the Environment

The three subsystems discussed above are part of the throughput process of the human open system. Output, feedback, and input define the system's interaction with the environment. Since the health and adaptation of the individual is dependent on this interaction, the environment represents a vital part of the MOHO. The MOHO first defines the influences of the environment on occupational behavior as opportunities, resources, demands, and/or constraints. Secondly, environments themselves are defined as physical or social and occupation-specific settings.

Every environment offers the opportunity for a prescribed range of behaviors. The behavior that is selected depends upon the interaction of the person (intentions, habits, and skills) and the objects and circumstances of the context. Each environment affords opportunities and resources within a range of possibilities. For example, a university environment offers multiple opportunities for academic and technical learning. Classrooms, laboratories, libraries or study areas, and office hours for dialogue with professors all suggest different modes of learning. Environmental press is the expectation of performance or behavior placed on an individual by a given environment (Barris, 1985). For example, a health club environment requires the individual to dress in a defined manner and to demonstrate a certain level of physical skill. Individuals generally seek out environments that fit their interests and their level of skill. Individuals who are disabled may find themselves

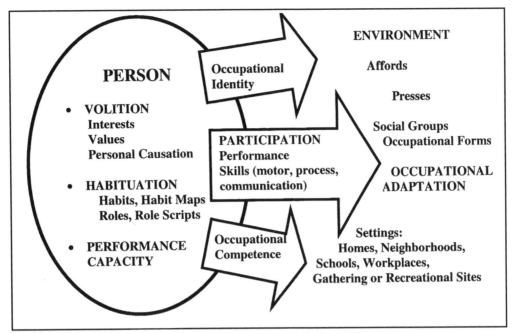

Figure 10-2. Expanded MOHO. (Adapted from Kielhofner, G., Forsyth, K., & Barrett, L. [2003]. The model of human occupation. In E. Crepeau, E. Cohn, & B. Boyt Schell [Eds.], *Willard & Spackman's occupational therapy.* Philadelphia: Lippincott, Williams & Wilkins.)

in environments that do not match their competence level and may need the services of an occupational therapist to help them change either their skill level or their environment.

Environments are described in both physical and social contexts. Physical environments operate according to the laws of science. They may be natural (untouched by humans) or fabricated (buildings, automobiles, roads, airports). Objects within these environments may also be man-made (clothes, dishes) or may occur naturally (trees, seashells). These environments are organized according to various purposes, and their contents and arrangement greatly influence human occupational behavior.

Social environments consist of social groups and occupational forms. Social groups, which assemble and meet regularly, define and assign occupational roles to individuals within them (a family, a corporation). An occupational form, according to Nelson (1988), is "the preexisting structure that elicits, guides, or structures subsequent human performance" (p. 633). For example, dinner is an occupational form that is accepted across cultures. Each culture has its unique ways of obtaining and preparing food, as well as acceptable ways of consuming it. Kielhofner defines occupational forms as "rule-bound sequences of

action which are at once coherent, oriented to a purpose, sustained in collective knowledge, culturally recognizable, and named" (2002). Many rules apply to the term dinner. It implies a certain time of day, usually the early evening in American culture, and a time sequence (beverage, appetizer, salad, main course, bread and butter, dessert). It consists of foods from different groups (proteins, fruits and vegetables, breads and grains, dairy), cooked, chopped, diced, or otherwise combined in culturally prescribed ways. It is coherent in that a number of separate tasks are involved, such as shopping (gathering ingredients), cooking according to certain recipes, using certain tools (plates, glasses, utensils), and interacting in socially acceptable ways (blessing the food before eating, polite dinner conversation). The obvious purpose of dinner is to sustain life by supplying food to the body, but its purpose is also social, such as a time for a man and woman to get to know one another (dinner date) or for the family to communicate and be together (family dinner). This example demonstrates both the immediate/physical and the symbolic/cultural nature of occupational forms.

Occupational behavior settings combine the physical and social environments in ways recognizable to most people. These include: homes, neighborhoods, schools, workplaces, and gathering or recreational sites. These are settings that should be evaluated by occupational therapists when planning and facilitating patient adaptation. Habituation refers to features within these settings that are familiar and that suggest, guide, and sustain purposeful occupational behavior.

Occupational Adaptation

Occupational adaptation develops from repeated interactions with the environment and consists of two elements: occupational identity and occupational competence. Occupational identity is defined by Kielhofner et al. (2003) as "the cumulative sense of who people are and wish to become as occupational beings" (p. 216). Sustained patterns of occupational performance lead to a person's occupational competence, which also results from experience. Occupational identity and occupational competence both develop as a result of feedback from the environment.

A general outline for organizing data about the human open system is found in Table 10-1.

For definitions and elaboration of all these terms, the reader is referred to Kielhofner's *A Model of Human Occupation* (2002). Additionally, current updates on MOHO may be found at the following Web site: www.moho.uic.edu.

Function and Dysfunction

When the human open system is functioning optimally, order exists within the system. This means that the individual competently performs everyday tasks of daily life in a routine and satisfying way (Rogers, 1982). This "order" produces and maintains a state of health in the individual. If a person can describe a typical day at work or home, identify a number of social roles he or she performs, and express satisfaction with these, then he or she is seen to be healthy.

Kielhofner (2002) defines occupational dysfunction as "difficulty performing, organizing, or choosing occupations." The causes of occupational dysfunction are "multifaceted" and can include both intrinsic and extrinsic contributors. A lack of order in one's life can be recognized in disordered daily routines, a lack of social roles, and/or dissatisfaction with any aspect of the person's life structure. When disorder exists, the occupational therapist evaluates the client to determine what parts of the system are not operating properly. Kielhofner suggests specific kinds of disorder within each subsystem, including ineffective or unrealistic

views of personal causation, disruption in intrinsic motivation, poor decision-making capacity, role dysfunction, disruption of habits, temporal dysfunction, disorder of environmental interactions, and disorder of performance components.

MOHO has specified three levels of occupational functioning:

1. Exploration
2. Competence
3. Achievement (Reilly, 1974)

These have also been called levels of arousal and accomplishment (Kaplan, 1986; Kielhofner, 1988). Exploration is the lowest level and involves curious investigation of one's self and one's potential for action in conjunction with the properties of the environment. Competence involves striving to meet the demands of a situation through the development of skills and their organization. Achievement includes striving for excellence and the successful performance of roles.

Concurrent levels of occupational dysfunction are also described as inefficacy, incompetence, and helplessness. Inefficacy, the least dysfunctional level, implies a reduction of motivation, satisfaction, or control (Bruce & Borg, 2002).

There are dozens of assessment tools originating from this frame of reference, which can help occupational therapists to specify which parts of the system are disordered or malfunctioning. The state of order or disorder is easily observed in the client's occupational behavior.

Change and Motivation

Change in the MOHO involves the restoration of order in the person's internal and external life structure. In recovering from illness, this often means restructuring a person's daily routines and re-establishing role performance. For example, Angie's roles were office administrator, wife, and mother of a 5-year-old son. When, at age 35, she was hospitalized for depression following a bitter divorce, all of her roles became inactive. The occupational therapist collaborated with Angie in restructuring her life so that she could resume her roles as worker and mother. Angie was able to volunteer while in the hospital to help maintain her administrative skills. She arranged to have dinner with her son each evening and to take him on an outing one day on the weekend. In restoring these roles, Angie was able to organize her already existing skills into a normal daily routine. She showered and dressed each morning, went to her

Table 10-1	Components of the Model of Human Occupation

INTERNAL	(Components/ Examples)	EXTERNAL	(Components/ Examples)
Volitional Subsystem		**Natural Environment**	Mountains, beach
Personal Causation	Knowledge of capacity (I can ski)	**Fabricated Environment**	House, airport, car, factory, supermarket
	Sense of efficacy (I can learn in college)	**Objects**	Clothes, dishes, machines, tools
Choices for Occupation	Activity choice (I need to buy milk)	**Social Environment**	
	Occupational choice (I want to be a doctor)	**Social Groups**	Family, corporation
Values	Personal convictions (be kind to others)	**Occupational Forms**	Driving a car, skiing, shopping, working
	Sense of obligation (always return what you borrow)	**Occupational Behavior**	
Interests	Attraction (loves reading, conversing)	**Settings:**	Homes
	Preference (enjoys the outdoors)		Neighborhoods
Habituation Subsystem			Schools
Habits	Routines (getting dressed for work)		Workplaces
	Habit maps (operate a computer, adapt for different uses)		Gathering or recreational sites
Roles	Internalized roles (teacher, spouse, parent, friend)		
	Role scripts (teaching = papers, preparing/giving lectures, etc.)		
Performance Capacity (mind, brain, body)	Musculoskeletal, neurological, cardiopulmonary, cognitive images	**Occupational adaptation:** motor, process, communication, interaction skills	Occupational identity, occupational competence

volunteer job each day, and met her son at a relative's house for dinner each evening. At night, she returned to the hospital.

The preceding therapy program addressed the habituation and performance subsystems. Grieving over the loss of her role as spouse was dealt with in counseling and resulted in the addition of several activities to allow Angie to make new social contacts, like joining a tennis club and attending weekly meetings of a church social club.

The therapeutic work is not in what activity is chosen but in getting Angie moving toward the regular performance of desired occupational behaviors. Normal, everyday activities are the media used, and the client herself makes the choices of activity, with the help and guidance of the occupational therapist.

Motivation in this frame of reference is attributed to an innate urge to explore and master the environment. Many writers have been credited with the elaboration of this concept, which is said to have a biological basis (Kielhofner, 1988). The best known of these is R. H. White (1960) who contributed the ideas of competence, adaptation, and motivation. Motivation speaks to the meaningfulness of activities. The meaning in occupation is derived not only from the individual, but from the context of his or her social and cultural environment. Part of the occupational therapist's job is not only to restore individual task performance but also to identify and restore meaningful roles in society.

A major value of the MOHO lies in its holistic view of the individual and its helpfulness in organizing data about patients' specific dysfunctions. Many examples exist in the literature of the application of the MOHO in identifying patterns of occupational dysfunction.

Group Intervention

Most of the literature on the MOHO does not address group treatment specifically. However, several aspects of its superstructure are helpful in program planning. For example, a balanced occupational therapy program is ensured when one incorporates group activities addressing the areas of self-care, work, and leisure. Another concept was to organize a program by using the three levels of occupational functioning. Kathy Kaplan (1986, 1988) writes about a group program for short-term psychiatry using group activities at the levels of exploration, competence, and achievement.

Exploration level groups incorporate simple activities to help the most severely disorganized clients to develop basic process skills (planning and problem solving), perceptual motor skills, and communication/interaction skills. The occupational therapist selects the activities and organizes the environment. The group is structured in four stages:
1. Orientation and introductions
2. Warm-up activities
3. Selected activities
4. Wrap-up

Kaplan calls this type of group a "directive group." An exercise group is another example of an explorative level group.

At the competence level, it is assumed that the clients have basic skills but may need to integrate them into habit patterns: "These groups are designed to help patients identify goals, interests, and needs for meaning and action" (Kaplan, 1986, p. 476). Some examples of groups at this level are task groups and activity planning groups.

Groups at the achievement level are designed to help clients integrate skills into daily life roles (Kaplan, 1986). Examples of achievement level groups are assertiveness training and leisure awareness. For more information on the directive group, the reader is also referred to Kaplan's *Directive Group Therapy* (1988).

Group Structure and Limitations

Within the components of the three subsystems, the most useful concept for organizing groups is roles. Roles help define the goals for clients and will dictate the kinds of skills that will need to be restored or strengthened. Therefore, in MOHO, it is best to disregard diagnosis and focus on the social roles persons intend to return to or find. Grouping persons according to their need to maintain a home, care for children, socialize, participate in recreational activities, or engage in gainful employment allows them to learn from and support each other in adapting their routines, role scripts, and environments to accommodate physical or mental limitations.

It has been stated that the use of the MOHO is not limited by age or diagnosis. Functional levels are organized by levels of arousal and achievement and by the components of the three subsystems that are functioning within the human open system. The focus of occupational therapy in the MOHO is on activities and tasks and not on emotions or process.

Role of the Therapist

The therapist in MOHO plays the role of an adviser and collaborator. He/she counsels the patients in the various aspects of occupational functioning. Kaplan's "directive group" is so named because of the "active and supportive way in which the group leaders elicit adaptive behaviors and structure the environment to assure maximum participation of all the members" (Kaplan, 1986, p. 477). This role of leader as "director" is necessary for groups that have severely disorganized occupational behavior. However, even at this level, the occupational therapist encourages the active participation of the clients. The occupational therapist continues at higher levels to facilitate, not direct. Thus, the clients' sense of control and personal efficacy is reinforced by the occupational therapist as the client continues to acquire new skills and make personal choices.

Goals

Goals are not discussed as a separate issue in the MOHO. The goal is to restore order in daily functioning, both internal and external. Therefore, the goal of group treatment may be seen as finding and engaging in meaningful occupations and meaningful roles in society. Group intervention goals are concerned with performance of normal daily occupations: work, daily living tasks, and play. They may involve any or all of the three subsystems. In the volitional subsystem, exploration of values and rekindling the urge to explore and master the environment may be goals. Habit formation or the acquisition of new roles may be goals in the habituation subsystem. Learning and practicing the skills necessary to perform the tasks of one's chosen or valued roles can be goals in the performance subsystem.

Examples of Activities

An updated criterion for placing clients in groups, according to Janice Burke, co-founder of MOHO, is to group them according to their anticipated social roles (1997, personal communication). Common roles, such as homemaker, caregiver, worker, or student, all suggest clusters of skills and tasks that may be selected for group activities. MOHO stresses the use of the client's normal daily activities as the modalities of choice. Groups designed around common roles, as Burke has suggested, can incorporate specific tasks or skills that need to be practiced or adapted. The more common

media used in therapeutic groups include cooking, money management, home maintenance skills, parenting skills, leisure planning, and work skills. The client's own interests guide activity selection, and the focus is on the real problems of everyday living. Some kinds of activities necessitate longer sessions. The environment is important in providing feedback to the patient and challenging him or her to further exploration.

Part of the activity planning should address the intended roles and social environments the members will seek out or return to after recovery. Skills and tasks will seem meaningless unless they are connected to meaningful roles that reconnect them with their social groups and help them fulfill a useful purpose. This connection with society and with culture is what sets MOHO groups apart from groups in other frames of reference.

Some occupational therapy group activities used in a program based on the MOHO are described in Activity Examples 10-1 through 10-4.

Group Leadership

In this frame of reference, the activity or occupation itself is considered health producing, and the need to take great pains to share it or understand its process is de-emphasized. In keeping with the greater emphasis on activities, two steps in the seven-step process have been eliminated: sharing and processing. There are longer and more frequent group meetings, and activities tend to be longer or ongoing, so that discussions of general principles and application are not necessary during every session. However, the introduction and summary should be done without fail and should serve the purposes outlined in Chapter 1.

Introduction

Greetings and description of the purpose are done thoroughly at the outset of each activity. A warm-up is optional and can be used to set the mood or energize patients if appropriate. The expectations may be general and somewhat tentative as the members will have input and make choices as the group progresses. The time frame often varies according to the activity and therefore should be started at the beginning of each session.

Activity

The thrust of all MOHO group activities should be moving patients toward meaningful roles in their own social environments. Persons with similar roles or intended roles are grouped together so that their task choices are likely to be similar also. At the exploratory level, the activities selected for groups are generally designed to help patients develop specific skills. Patients who need to work on these skills are grouped together. For example, those who need to develop routines for self-care might do a series of skill building sessions such as maintaining fingernails and toenails; doing laundry; selecting appropriate clothing; applying make-up; shaving; and caring for teeth, hair, and skin.

At the competence level, choices are encouraged so that patients can apply their skills and organize them into habit patterns (Kaplan, 1986). Patients may be encouraged to set their own goals within the group context. For example, the title of the group may be "time management," and within that theme, patients may plan their own individual time schedules with tasks that are meaningful for them in their own social/cultural contexts.

Achievement level groups focus on life roles such as work support, leisure planning, and values clarification.

Generalizing and Application

The meaning of the activity is discussed with the group as outlined in Chapter 1. This is done after the activity is completed and focuses on how the activity relates to the life roles of the members. Similarities and differences among group members are de-emphasized. For example, in the vocational readiness group described earlier, the skills learned in doing a leather craft project may be generalized to a patient's actual job. Concentration, efficient use of tools, work neatness, and finishing on time are skills necessary for both. This kind of discussion leads directly into application. A group discussion in the vocational readiness group will necessarily focus on individual application of skills, as patients' vocational plans differ widely. Feedback from the occupational therapist on results of the vocational rating scale should also be presented in the group. The group focus is useful to confirm the therapist's observations and give a stronger message to patients. For example, a member may have done very careful work and showed considerable manual skills, but he or she may have taken excessive time to do so. The reality of the workplace is not only to do quality work, but also to meet deadlines. The group discussion may help the patient see the necessity to compromise and perhaps curb his or her perfectionistic tendencies.

Summary

The summary should review the purpose and goals of the group and determine what the group accomplished. Focus on individual achievements and strengths should be confirmed. The skills learned may be general or different for each member, and their application should be reinforced in the summary. Future plans, goal achievement, and life roles to which occupational therapy activities apply may be discussed by each member as part of the summary.

Bibliography

American Occupational Therapy Association. (2002). Occupational therapy practice framework: Domain and process. *American Journal of Occupational Therapy, 56,* 609-629.

Barris, R. (1985). Occupation as interaction with the environment. In G. Kielhofner (Ed.), *A model of human occupation: Theory and application.* Baltimore: Williams & Wilkins.

Bruce, M. A., & Borg, B. (2002). *Frames of reference in psychosocial occupational therapy.* Thorofare, NJ: SLACK Incorporated.

Hammel, J. (1999). The life rope: A transactional approach to exploring worker and life role development. *Work: A Journal of Prevention, Assessment and Rehabilitation, 12,* 47-60.

Kaplan, K. (1986). The directive group: Short-term treatment for psychiatric patients with a minimal level of functioning. *American Journal of Occupational Therapy, 40,* 474-481.

Kaplan, K. (1988). *Directive group therapy.* Thorofare, NJ: SLACK Incorporated.

Katz, N. (1988). Interest checklist: A factor analytical study. *Occupational Therapy in Mental Health, 1,* 45-55.

Kielhofner, G. (1978).General systems theory: Implications for theory and action in occupational therapy. *American Journal of Occupational Therapy, 32,* 637-645.

Kielhofner, G. (1988). Model of human occupation. In S. Robinson (Ed.), *Mental health focus.* Rockville, MD: American Occupational Therapy Association.

Kielhofner, G. (Ed.). (2002). *A model of human occupation: Theory and application* (3rd ed.). Baltimore: Williams & Wilkins.

Kielhofner, G., & Burke, J. (1985). Components and determinants of occupation. In G. Kielhofner (Ed.), *A model of human occupation: Theory and Application.* Baltimore: Williams & Wilkins.

Kielhofner, G., Burke, J., & Igi, C. (1980). A model of human occupation, part 4. *American Journal of Occupational Therapy, 34,* 572-581.

Kielhofner, G., Forsyth, K., & Barrett, L. (2003). The model of human occupation. In E. Crepeau, E. Cohn, & B. Boyt Schell (Eds.), *Willard & Spackman's occupational therapy*. Philadelphia: Lippincott, Williams & Wilkins.

Lindquist, J., Mack, W., & Parham, L. D. (1982). A synthesis of occupational behavior and sensory integration concepts in theory and practice, part 2: Clinical applications. *American Journal of Occupational Therapy, 36*, 433-437.

Mack, W., Lindquist, J., & Parham, L. D. (1982). A synthesis of occupational behavior and sensory integration concepts in theory and practice, part 1: Theoretical foundations. *American Journal of Occupational Therapy, 36*, 365-374.

Meyer, A. (1982). The philosophy of occupational therapy. Reprinted from the Archives of Occupational Therapy (Vol 1, pp. 1-10) in *Occupational Therapy in Mental Health, 2*, 79-89.

Nelson, D. (1988). Occupation: Form and performance. *American Journal of Occupational Therapy, 42*, 633-641.

Reilly, M. (1962). Occupational therapy can be one of the great ideas of 20th century medicine. *American Journal of Occupational Therapy, 16*, 1-9.

Reilly, M. (1974). An explanation of play. In M. Reilly (Ed.), *Play as exploratory learning: Studies of curiosity behavior* (pp. 117-155). Beverly Hills, CA: Sage Publications.

Rogers, J. (1982). Order and disorder in medicine and occupational therapy. *American Journal of Occupational Therapy, 36*, 29-35.

White, R. H. (1959). Motivation reconsidered: The concept of competence. *Psychological Review, 66*, 126-134.

White, R. H. (1960). *Competence and the psychosexual stages of development. Nebraska Symposium on Motivation*. Lincoln: University of Nebraska.

Young, M. (1988). *The metronomic society: Natural rhythms and human timetables*. Cambridge, MA: Harvard University Press.

MOHO

Activity Example 10-1

The Special Events Group

This group is designed for exploratory level clients (chronic mentally ill) whose social relations and daily routines are severely disordered. The purpose is to increase orientation, to expand their level of awareness to the world outside themselves, and to work on time planning and social skills. The focus is on events in people's lives, such as holidays, birthdays, welcomes, and goodbyes, and how to celebrate them. The group is organized by the month, and begins with a planning session at the beginning of each month. The group meets for 2-hour sessions.

Materials: Posterboard with lines drawn up like a monthly calendar. Other materials are colored markers, colored paper, scissors, glue, blank cards and envelopes, cake mixes and frosting ingredients, large sheet cake pan, cake decorating kit, two large punch bowls, ingredients for punch, cake knife, serving ladle, paper supplies for parties, birthday candles, coffee maker, cream and sugar, and access to a kitchen for baking.

Directions: For a typical month, October.
Week 1—Organize monthly calendar (Figure 10-3).
Write name of month and numbers. Therapist begins by writing "1" on the day the month begins. Identify season and decorate calendar with designs appropriate for the season: pumpkins, cornstalks, leaves. Identify holidays for that month and write on calendar or decorate with appropriate symbols. Survey all patients and staff on ward to find out whose birthday is in October and write on calendar. Identify one day for the whole ward to celebrate October birthdays and Halloween and write on calendar.

Post the calendar in a prominent place on the ward. Other events, such as discharge dates and arrival or departure of staff, may also be added.

Plan what tasks need to be done for the celebration (e.g., make cards, bake cake, shop for supplies, think about masks or costumes for Halloween theme) and decide when to do each.

Week 2—Make cards. Identify birthday people and write names on index cards. Each member makes one card. If there are not enough birthdays, make some for Halloween, too. Each patient designs the card and writes the name and message inside. Stencils and markers, colored paper shapes, scissors, and glue should be available for the less "artistic."

Clients then circulate around the ward gathering signatures for the cards. A shopping list is made for needed refreshment items, eggs and milk for cake, ingredients for punch, etc. (The therapist does the actual shopping.)

Week 3—Bake cake and decorate. Group meets in kitchen. Needed items should be set out on table ahead of time (e.g., bowls, mixing spoons, measuring cups and spoons, eggs, confectioner's sugar, cake decorating supplies, etc.). The large sheet cake pan holds two complete cake mixes, so the recipe should be doubled (assuming a ward size of 20 or more).

The group divides into work teams and roles to accomplish this.
- Cake bakers—Recipe reader, measurer, mixer, timer
- Frosting makers—Recipe reader, measurer, mixer
- Designers—Choose motif or theme, border design, colors, and message

Activity Example 10-1
The Special Events Group (continued)

			October			
S	M	T	W	Th	F	S

Figure 10-3. Special events group monthly calendar.

Supply frosting makers with desired food coloring. Trace motif design on paper (jack o'lantern) and cut out. Write out message on paper and check spelling of "Happy Birthday" and "Happy Halloween."

Members learn to use decorating kit to decorate cake, frost in white, do border, trace motif, and write message. All may help with this "fun" part, and all help clean up (Figure 10-4).

When finished, the entire cake is frozen to be used the next week. The ward is informed of the date and the exact time and place are decided at a ward community meeting. Permission of staff is necessary.

Week 4—Celebration. Preparation time is 1 hour. Take cake out of freezer 2 hours ahead. Cover a large table with a sheet in the party room. Set up chairs in a large circle. Set out punch bowls and make punch. Make coffee in coffee maker, set out cream and sugar. Set out plates, forks, cake knife, cake, cups, ladle, spoons, and napkins. Bring the cards. Put the birthday candles on the cake. Bring matches or a lighter. When everything is ready, gather clients and staff.

Party—Estimate time is 30 minutes. Give a toast. Members serve everyone punch, but do not drink it right away, save it for the toast. The whole group is asked to take turns proposing toasts or sharing wishes with honored members. Members lead group in singing "Happy Birthday." Candles are lit. Birthday people must come forward and blow out candles. Group members serve cake to all. Members serve themselves last. Informal socializing occurs while cake is being served. People help themselves to more punch or coffee.

Activity Example 10-1
The Special Events Group (continued)

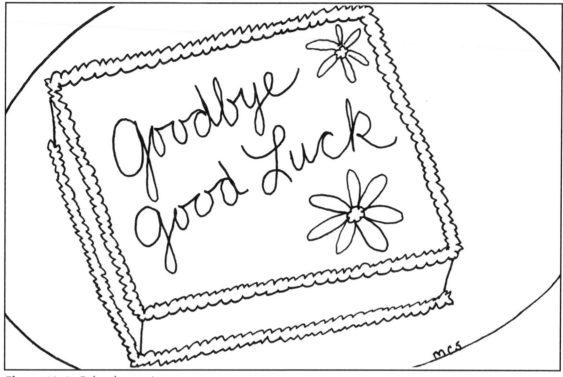

Figure 10-4. Cake decoration.

Clean up and discussion—Estimated time is 30 minutes. All members help clean up. When finished, group gathers in a meeting room to discuss and evaluate what roles members played, give feedback, verbalize what skills were learned, and discuss how to apply skills.

MOHO

Activity Example 10-2

Vocational Readiness Group

This group uses craft or office activities to explore interests and practice work-related skills. The group runs for 4 weeks and has been used with clients with acute mental health conditions or substance abuse. Appropriate members are those whose goal is to take on a work role after discharge. Group meets in 2-hour sessions. The goals of the group involve all three MOHO subsystems.

1. Volitional—Clients identify and explore their interests by selecting to do craft or office tasks.
2. Habituation—Clients gain and/or maintain good work habits, such as punctuality and following directions, in anticipation of regaining the worker role.
3. Performance—Clients practice basic work skills such as concentration, organization of time and materials, quality of workmanship, and task follow-through. Specific skills like typing and woodworking may also be learned and practiced.

Materials: Two typewriters, access to a copy machine, file cabinet with files and labels, typing tutorial manual, typing paper, workbench with vise, electric drill, band saw, pine boards, plywood, wood patterns, sandpaper, painting supplies, leather work supplies, belt blanks and key fob blanks, buckles, rivets, stamping tools, punch, mallets, bowls of water, sponges, and written directions for making several projects at several different levels of complexity.

Directions: Week 1—Evaluation and project choice. Members begin by doing a Work Activity Checklist. The basis for this is Noomi Katz's adaptation of Matsutsuyu's Interest Checklist (Katz, 1988.) For this group, the checklist has been modified to include work-related activities. The scale has been designed to include five work categories as follows.

MOHO
Activity Example 10-2
Vocational Readiness Group (continued)

1. **Office Work**
   Typing
   Using computers
   Filing
   Answering phones
   Using calculator
   Accounting and math
   Writing letters
   Opening mail
   Making appointments
   Supervising employees

2. **Building and Construction**
   Electrical wiring
   Pipe fitting
   Assembling parts
   Working on cars
   Woodworking
   Refinishing furniture
   Installing carpeting
   Landscaping
   Gardening
   House painting

3. **Communications/Teaching**
   Writing articles
   Making posters
   Painting signs
   Broadcasting news
   Introducing people
   Reading books

   Giving lectures
   Giving exams
   Taking notes
   Teaching children

4. **Sales/Service**
   Showing houses
   Selling clothing
   Doing make-up
   Serving food
   Styling hair
   Giving sales pitches
   Giving fashion shows
   Travel planning
   Dining with clients
   Planning conferences

5. **Home Maintenance**
   Washing dishes
   Mopping floors
   Cooking
   Wallpapering
   Arranging furniture
   Grocery shopping
   Menu planning
   Doing laundry
   Mixing drinks
   Washing windows

From Cole, M. B. *Group dynamics in occupational therapy: The theoretical basis and practice application of group intervention* (3rd ed.). Thorofare, NJ: SLACK Incorporated. © 2005 SLACK Incorporated.

Vocational Readiness Group (continued)

Work Activity Checklist

Activity	INTEREST			PAST PERFORMANCE			FUTURE	
	Some	Casual	None	Usual	Some	Never	Yes	No
Typing	❑	❑	❑	❑	❑	❑	❑	❑
Electrical wiring	❑	❑	❑	❑	❑	❑	❑	❑
Writing articles	❑	❑	❑	❑	❑	❑	❑	❑
Showing houses	❑	❑	❑	❑	❑	❑	❑	❑
Washing dishes	❑	❑	❑	❑	❑	❑	❑	❑
Using computers	❑	❑	❑	❑	❑	❑	❑	❑
Pipe fitting	❑	❑	❑	❑	❑	❑	❑	❑
Making posters	❑	❑	❑	❑	❑	❑	❑	❑
Selling clothing	❑	❑	❑	❑	❑	❑	❑	❑
Mopping floors	❑	❑	❑	❑	❑	❑	❑	❑
Filing	❑	❑	❑	❑	❑	❑	❑	❑
Assembling parts	❑	❑	❑	❑	❑	❑	❑	❑
Painting signs	❑	❑	❑	❑	❑	❑	❑	❑
Doing make-up	❑	❑	❑	❑	❑	❑	❑	❑
Cooking	❑	❑	❑	❑	❑	❑	❑	❑
Answering phones	❑	❑	❑	❑	❑	❑	❑	❑
Working on cars	❑	❑	❑	❑	❑	❑	❑	❑
Broadcasting news	❑	❑	❑	❑	❑	❑	❑	❑
Serving food	❑	❑	❑	❑	❑	❑	❑	❑
Wallpapering	❑	❑	❑	❑	❑	❑	❑	❑
Using calculator	❑	❑	❑	❑	❑	❑	❑	❑
Woodworking	❑	❑	❑	❑	❑	❑	❑	❑
Introducing people	❑	❑	❑	❑	❑	❑	❑	❑
Styling hair	❑	❑	❑	❑	❑	❑	❑	❑
Arranging furniture	❑	❑	❑	❑	❑	❑	❑	❑
Accounting and math	❑	❑	❑	❑	❑	❑	❑	❑
Refinishing furniture	❑	❑	❑	❑	❑	❑	❑	❑
Reading books	❑	❑	❑	❑	❑	❑	❑	❑
Giving sales pitches	❑	❑	❑	❑	❑	❑	❑	❑
Grocery shopping	❑	❑	❑	❑	❑	❑	❑	❑
Writing letters	❑	❑	❑	❑	❑	❑	❑	❑
Installing carpeting	❑	❑	❑	❑	❑	❑	❑	❑
Giving lectures	❑	❑	❑	❑	❑	❑	❑	❑
Giving fashion shows	❑	❑	❑	❑	❑	❑	❑	❑
Menu planning	❑	❑	❑	❑	❑	❑	❑	❑
Opening mail	❑	❑	❑	❑	❑	❑	❑	❑
Landscaping	❑	❑	❑	❑	❑	❑	❑	❑
Giving exams	❑	❑	❑	❑	❑	❑	❑	❑
Travel planning	❑	❑	❑	❑	❑	❑	❑	❑
Doing laundry	❑	❑	❑	❑	❑	❑	❑	❑
Making appointments	❑	❑	❑	❑	❑	❑	❑	❑
Gardening	❑	❑	❑	❑	❑	❑	❑	❑
Taking notes	❑	❑	❑	❑	❑	❑	❑	❑
Dining with clients	❑	❑	❑	❑	❑	❑	❑	❑
Mixing drinks	❑	❑	❑	❑	❑	❑	❑	❑
Supervising employees	❑	❑	❑	❑	❑	❑	❑	❑
House painting	❑	❑	❑	❑	❑	❑	❑	❑
Teaching children	❑	❑	❑	❑	❑	❑	❑	❑
Planning conferences	❑	❑	❑	❑	❑	❑	❑	❑
Washing windows	❑	❑	❑	❑	❑	❑	❑	❑

MOHO
Activity Example 10-2
Vocational Readiness Group (continued)

The checklist is discussed with regard to interests, past work history, and satisfaction with current work skills. The expectations for the group are then shared. Members are expected to:

- Arrive on time or give prior notification of absence
- Appear well-groomed and dressed in clean work clothes
- Follow directions for project/task
- Respond positively to supervision
- Effectively deal with frustration
- Ask for help when needed
- Work independently
- Learn necessary skills
- Follow through on task (meet deadlines); strive for quality of workmanship

Several starter projects should be ready with written directions for each client. Members may choose projects based on their interests and skills, and get started for the remaining time. Examples of starter craft projects are leather key fobs with stamped initials and border, wood wall plaque made from precut 6- x 8-inch pine board with picture to decoupage, or a wood trivet made from a kit. Examples of starter work projects are typing a short letter or sorting tiles by color. Starter projects are intended to teach basic skills and allow the therapist to evaluate client's manual and cognitive abilities.

Weeks 2 through 4—Clients complete projects as assigned by the therapist. Each client works independently on a different project. At the end of each session, members are evaluated with the Work Behavior Rating Scale and results are discussed with the clients.

From Cole, M. B. *Group dynamics in occupational therapy: The theoretical basis and practice application of group intervention* (3rd ed.). Thorofare, NJ: SLACK Incorporated. © 2005 SLACK Incorporated.

Work Behavior Rating Scale					
Name			*Dates*		
Arrives on time (gives prior notice of valid absence)					
Appropriate appearance (well-groomed, clean work clothing)					
Follows directions					
Responds positively to supervision					
Effectively deals with frustration					
Asks for help when needed					
Works independently					
Learns necessary skills					
Follows through on tasks (meets deadlines)					

Scale: 1 = Independent and correct
2 = Requires some assistance
3 = Requires much assistance
4 = Is dependent or unmotivated

MOHO
Activity Example 10-3
The Perfect Parent

This activity is designed for parents who have arthritis or other physical illness involving chronic pain or limitation, who wish to continue being good parents to their young children.

Materials: Worksheets and pencils.

Directions: Have members begin by giving their names and then the names and ages of children living with them. "The purpose of today's activity is to identify some specific concerns involving your ability to care for your children as you deal with the chronic pain and limitations of arthritis." Hand out worksheets and pencils, and give 15 minutes to complete. Areas to consider for parental tasks are meal preparation, dressing, shopping, family events, school-related activities, sports, cultural and social activities, developing special talents or interests, and nurturing/emotional support.

Discussion: The group shares areas of concern from their individual worksheets. Priorities may be discussed, and ideas for coping with conflicts may be shared.

MOHO
Activity Example 10-3
The Perfect Parent (continued)

The Perfect Parent Worksheet

Write name and age of each child:

List and describe five tasks you must perform for your children before 9:00 a.m. on a typical school day.
1.

2.

3.

4.

5.

List five tasks your children would appreciate your doing for them before they return home from school.
1.

2.

3.

4.

5.

List five tasks you must do for your children after 5:00 p.m. on a typical school day.
1.

2.

3.

4.

5.

Go back over the above lists and place a * next to those tasks that present potential problems for you in terms of physical exertion or endurance, time constraints, or conflicting obligations.

From Cole, M. B. *Group dynamics in occupational therapy: The theoretical basis and practice application of group intervention* (3rd ed.). Thorofare, NJ: SLACK Incorporated. © 2005 SLACK Incorporated.

MOHO

Activity Example 10-3

The Perfect Parent (continued)

The Perfect Parent Schedule Worksheet

Directions: Write the tasks listed on the preceding page in the column "Things I Want to Do for My Children" at the appropriate times. Then, in the next column, schedule in your own needs for rest, exercise, socialization, and other obligations. Put a * next to possible conflicts between these.

Typical School Day	*Things I Want to Do for My Children*	*Things I Need to Do for Myself*
6:00 a.m.		
7:00 a.m.		
8:00 a.m.		
9:00 a.m.		
10:00 a.m.		
11:00 a.m.		
12:00 p.m.		
1:00 p.m.		
2:00 p.m.		
3:00 p.m.		
4:00 p.m.		
5:00 p.m.		
6:00 p.m.		
7:00 p.m.		
8:00 p.m.		
9:00 p.m.		
10:00 p.m.		
11:00 p.m. or later		

Conflict areas:

Coping strategies:

From Cole, M. B. *Group dynamics in occupational therapy: The theoretical basis and practice application of group intervention* (3rd ed.). Thorofare, NJ: SLACK Incorporated. © 2005 SLACK Incorporated.

MOHO
Activity Example 10-4
Forming Good Habits

This activity is designed for persons whose daily structure have been disrupted by illness or injury. It starts at the beginning again, with self-care, and assists with building a supportive environment. This activity may require two or three sessions to complete, depending on attention span of members. Contact with family member or caregiver is needed for follow-up.

Materials: 3- x 5-inch cards with pictures of toothbrush, toothpaste, glass, shower or bathtub, bathmat, soap, wash-cloth, towel, razor, shaving cream, cosmetics, nail file, nail clippers, hand lotion, hairbrush, comb, shampoo, conditioner, and a variety of clothing items appropriate to season and age of members. A second set of cards contains pictures of dishes, utensils, breakfast items, kitchen sink/dishwasher, sponge, broom, dustpan, and trashcan. Duplicate cards should be made for each member. Pictures may be cut out of magazines as needed for this activity. Posterboards, glue or tape, and broad black markers are needed for the second part of this activity.

Directions: Members introduce themselves and discuss familiar morning routines they can remember having in the past. Cards for bathing, dental care, shaving, hair care, and make-up are distributed, and members are asked to select those items used in the morning and place them in sequence in front of them on the table. Items may be sorted into categories and each given separately, depending on the skill level of group members. Dressing and breakfast cards are given in a likewise manner.

Discussion: How can members learn good morning habits? What is the best sequence of tasks for each individual? What is your home environment like? Where can you keep the items pictured on the cards so that you can find them easily each day?

Follow-Up: Posterboards are distributed with labels at the top of each: Grooming and Bathing, Dressing, Eating Breakfast, and Cleaning Up. Each member selects appropriate cards and pastes or tapes them to the posterboard in the desired sequence. Members take the posterboards home with them and obtain assistance in gathering the items and finding appropriate storage for the items. The posters serve as reminders until sequences are repeated often enough to form good daily habits of self-care.

From Cole, M. B. *Group dynamics in occupational therapy: The theoretical basis and practice application of group intervention* (3rd ed.). Thorofare, NJ: SLACK Incorporated. © 2005 SLACK Incorporated.

Section Three

Planning an Occupational Therapy Group

Introduction

This section returns the student to experiential learning. Chapter 11 provides a stepwise structure for the application of theory with client populations, while Chapters 12 and 13 take the form of guided learning experiences.

With the advent of client-centered practice, it is no longer acceptable to simply match theory and technique to a diagnosis. Occupational therapists must take into account client priorities and preferences, activity patterns, and contexts when planning groups for evaluation and intervention. Accordingly, the first step in planning group is to assess client needs. Selecting members for groups was discussed in Chapter 3 as part of the client-centered evaluation. In this section, we will consider designing groups both as intervention and as a part of the process of evaluation.

In Chapter 11, the first learning exercise requires the student to identify a context for occupational therapy intervention. Since occupational therapists work in community as well as institutional settings, a broad range of potential client groups may be considered. For students with limited experience, visits to local community settings are highly recommended. Occupational therapists cannot design effective groups without first gaining a firsthand understanding of the people for whom their groups are designed.

The next step in group planning is selecting a frame of reference that best fits the client needs identified. This sequence reflects both the Occupational Performance Process Model outlined by Fearing, Law, and Clark (1997), and the *Occupational Therapy Practice Framework* (American Occupational Therapy Association [AOTA], 2002). Guidelines are offered for the application of theories discussed in Section Two. This step allows students to review the evidence within the various theoretical perspectives and to consider alternate approaches to client occupational concerns. When an approach is selected, its principles will then guide the process of setting goals, adapting environments, and designing therapeutic group activities.

Concurrently with theory application, the occupational therapist reviews the profession's practice domain to provide a focus for the group design. When client group members have identified specific occupational concerns and priorities, these will guide the selection of group goals, activities, and structure. Groups may be designed to meet multiple goals and to facilitate client involvement in the intervention process. When clients need assistance with sorting out their concerns and priorities, groups may be designed to facilitate self-awareness through learning experiences and group feedback. Observing client occupational performance within the group structure provides valuable insights during the evaluation process as well as intervention.

The group protocol assignment requires the student to design and structure a sequence of six group sessions with a common theme. This gives the student an opportunity to synthesize and integrate the various aspects of clinical thinking that define occupational therapy: client evaluation, theory review and application, consideration of the various domains of occupation, and application of the therapeutic use of the self through the seven steps of group leadership.

Chapter 12, A Group Laboratory Experience, offers a group membership experience as a context for learning about group dynamics. This chapter follows the guidelines of the group protocol described in Chapter 11, and thus provides an example of a group intervention designed for students called "Developing Your Professional Self." As a laboratory experience, these sessions can be beneficial for students as they approach the clinical training phase of their education. In the 10 years we have been offering these groups for second semester juniors, the feedback from students has been excellent. In addition to learning and applying the principles of group dynamics, students have found the feedback for themselves invaluable for their own professional growth.

Respect for diversity is a professional priority, as well as a guiding principle of client-centered practice. To assist students with the application of this principle, Chapter 13, "Developing Cultural Competence," offers an additional laboratory experience for students

Law and Mills (1998) point out that in client-centered practice:

> ...clients of occupational therapy come from many different backgrounds, have encountered different life experiences, and have made choices regarding occupation that are unique to them and the situation in which they live. A fundamental concept of client-centered occupational therapy is that therapists show respect for the choices that clients have made, choices they will make, and their personal methods of coping. (p. 9)

This chapter applies Wells and Black's (2000) cultural competency model in a series of six group sessions, which can be directly applied in the classroom or as a continuing education series for practicing therapists.

These experiences facilitate the application of theory in practice. The process of this text has gone from concrete (the seven-step format), to abstract (the frames), and then back to concrete (the protocol). This is not unlike the clinical reasoning process itself, which swings back and forth between the empirical and the hypothetical as the therapy process progresses. A good group plan involves the empirical collection of data about clients' occupational functioning in disability and health, the formation of a hypothesis about what kind of group activity might be helpful, and a method for evaluation of treatment outcome after implementation (empirical again). The laboratory experiences for students demonstrate this process.

Finally, as part of the practical application of theory to group planning, the student is encouraged to think about how Cole's seven-step group leadership is changed and adapted with each frame of reference. As a learning guide, a chart comparing group leadership in the six frames of reference is presented in Appendix E.

Bibliography

American Occupational Therapy Association. (2002). Occupational therapy practice framework: Domain and process. *American Journal of Occupational Therapy, 56*, 609-639.

Fearing, V., Law, M., & Clark, J. (1997). An occupational performance process model: Fostering client and therapist alliances. *Canadian Journal of Occupational Therapy, 64*, 7-15.

Law, M., & Mills, J. (1998). Client-centered occupational therapy. In M. Law (Ed.), *Client-centered occupational therapy* (pp. 1-18). Thorofare, NJ: SLACK Incorporated.

Wells, S., & Black, R. (2000). *Cultural competency for health professionals.* Bethesda, MD: American Occupational Therapy Association.

Chapter 11

Writing a Group Protocol

The group protocol is an extensive and detailed outline of a group to be planned by the occupational therapist for a specific client population. Recent group theory suggests that careful planning greatly influences group outcome (see Gersick study in Chapter 2). This exercise is intended to prepare students and therapists to plan effective programs to meet the needs of clients with a wide variety of characteristics, using multiple frames of reference.

This method of group intervention planning fits well with the *Occupational Therapy Practice Framework's* concept of designing group interventions for populations (American Occupational Therapy Association [AOTA], 2002). The members selected for groups should have common population characteristics (e.g., young mothers with arthritis or unemployed workers with depression) so that their occupational needs and priorities can be evaluated as a group, and interventions can be designed that will have meaning for all members. Given the importance that the framework process places on collaboration, client profiles should be formed as a part of the group member selection process. Care should be taken to orient each member to the format and purpose of the group prior to its inception, leaving no doubt as to why he or she has been assigned to a particular group. The introduction to the group session can then serve as a reminder of the group's intended purpose, and the summary serves as an outcomes review as described in Chapter 1.

Several steps have been outlined to clarify our clinical thinking about groups. They are:
- Identifying your client population
- Selecting a frame of reference
- Selecting a focus for intervention
- Writing a group intervention outline
- Planning individual sessions

Identifying Your Client Population

For the purposes of learning, the student should choose one of the following intervention settings in which occupational therapists typically work with clients. This will be the client population around which you will plan your group.
- Adolescent intensive psychiatric rehabilitation treatment team
- Adult inpatient detoxification
- 28-day rehabilitation facility for drug and alcohol use disorders
- Stroke recovery unit
- Community Clubhouse for chronic mental health
- Day treatment program for adults with traumatic brain injury
- Group home for adults with developmental disabilities
- Community program for adults with physical disability (specify one type)
- Geriatrics, skilled nursing facility
- Cardiac recovery client community group
- Hand injury clinic
- Hospice terminal illness (specify one type) group
- Senior center prevention/education

- Injury prevention in the workplace: health insurance seminar for employees
- Dementia home care: client and family/caregiver sessions

Settings should be chosen on the basis of interest, prior experience, or curiosity. The planning will incorporate a process of familiarization with the chosen population. Since most students do not have much experience, it is advisable to contact a local intervention center and arrange a visit. Prior fieldwork and volunteer experience is also helpful. It is impossible to plan an effective group intervention without some knowledge of the population for which it is intended.

Another way to become more familiar with the population you choose is to do some reference reading. Many excellent books are available describing specific diagnostic categories, such as Alzheimer's disease, multiple sclerosis, drug abuse, eating disorders, and mental retardation. Reading case studies of people with these disorders is particularly helpful.

Probably the most motivating way to choose a client population is personal experience. Many students have friends or relatives who may have a disorder that fits one of the listed categories. Writing a group protocol for a specific individual and others with the same disorder gives the student the advantage of greater personal understanding. It may be easier to imagine the impact of certain group activities and the barriers that may need to be addressed.

For those students who are unfamiliar with some of the diagnoses mentioned or implied in the list of populations, a short research assignment may be appropriate prior to attempting Worksheet 11-1. Once the clients in a given setting are defined with respect to diagnosis, one or two of the most common illnesses can be researched in medical textbooks. In a real-life setting, a needs assessment is the preferred format for defining the population because it includes collaboration with potential clients.

How to Do a Needs Assessment

Some students may have the opportunity to work with organizations in the community or to work with nontraditional populations. For these settings, the student should perform a needs assessment in lieu of a population worksheet. Brownson (2001) outlines some helpful steps in performing a needs assessment at schools, work-

sites, community agencies, and assisted living or other health care environments for the proposed population for whom your group will be directed. The purpose of community interventions with well populations is to educate and strive to achieve pre-planned objectives such as changes in lifestyle; changes in knowledge, attitudes, skills, or behaviors; and maintenance of improvement in function or health.

A needs assessment is a systematic set of procedures to identify and describe specific areas of need for a given population, which leads to a clear set of goals and objectives for the program (group). The steps are as follows:

1. Gather background data: Do an Internet search or literature search on the organization for whom you are designing a group. Research various aspects of the population you already know, such as adolescents and discipline problems if you are working with a local high school. Choose at least three topics to summarize.

2. Identify participants for a survey: Involve the potential participants by collaborating with them concerning their perceptions of the needs, problems, or circumstances that you might potentially address. There are several methods for eliciting potential participant input. Students should choose one of the following:

   a. Written survey: Design a one-page survey containing both closed- (yes/no) and open-ended questions about the topics of concern. Give it to 20 people and make arrangements for returning it by having someone collect it or by mail. Since participation is voluntary, you can expect less than half the surveys to be returned.

   b. Face-to-face interviews: Arrange to meet with a limited number (five or six) of potential participants one at a time. Come prepared with specific questions that will serve as both a guideline and a reminder to gather all the information you intended.

   c. Telephone interviews: Although this is not the preferred method, it may be more time efficient. Be sure you have specific questions and a quick way to record the answers before calling. Interview 10 people and keep track of answers to consider for later analysis.

Worksheet 11-1
Client Population

1. Population choice (choose an intervention setting from those listed previously)

2. Population definition

    a. Identify two centers nearby that work with this population. Call or visit these centers to familiarize your-self with the context and clients. Choose one of the centers to answer the questions on the remainder of this sheet.

	First Resource	Second Resource
Center name:		
Telephone number:		
Address:		
Contact person or occupational therapist:		

    b. Describe client characteristics typical of the center.
    Criteria for admission to center/program:
    Age range; male/female/both:
    Health conditions and approximate percentages:
    Clients' education level and socioeconomic status (average or range):
    Clients' living situation:
    Range of cultural backgrounds of clients:
    Occupation/work status (a few typical examples):

    c. Predict rehabilitation potential.
    Approximate level of cognitive functioning (high, medium, low):
    Describe physical limitations (acute or chronic):
    Verbal ability/interaction potential:
    Desired outcomes for program as a whole:

3. Describe the social and cultural context where a group intervention would occur.
    Facility's mission:
    Criteria for admission:
    Funding source(s):
    Staff disciplines (members of the treatment team):
    Staff/client ratio:
    Types of interventions offered:
    Frame of reference (if known):

d. Key informants: Ask your contact person to identify people who would be most helpful in identifying needs of your potential population and limit your surveys or interviews to just a few people (three or four).

e. Focus group: Invite a small group (eight or less) of potential participants to meet for a brief discussion of their perceptions, problems, and needs relative to your group intervention idea. This is the preferred way to assess the needs of a group of participants because you can also observe their social skills and modes of interaction in a group.

3. Use secondary data, such as archives, prior surveys, and reports by related organizations or agencies. If other "volunteers" or "fieldwork students" have worked with this population before, consult their notes, reports, or summaries. Find out what has already been tried so that you do not repeat past errors. If you cannot find data interview your contact person (fieldwork supervisor) regarding what group strategies have been effective in the past.

4. Analyze the data: Look at answers to survey/interview questions and find a way to summarize this information for the purposes of group planning. It is not necessary to do a statistical analysis, but charts or graphs are an easy way to get a visual picture of the results. For example, if you would like to do a weight control group for overweight adolescents at a local school, your survey questions might address issues of self-image; facts of height, weight, and diet; and amount of and attitude toward physical activity. Part of your summary will confirm the extent of obesity in this specific group and compare that with information you have previously gathered from the Internet regarding adolescent obesity in the general population. Another issue to summarize is the strength of interest your responses indicate in attending a group that focuses on weight control. Self-esteem might be a factor that motivates adolescents to attend such a group, and that can be a part of your "marketing" strategy.

5. Write a profile of the "typical" participant. Include gender, age, educational and cultural factors, diversity factors, family background, and client factors such as verbal and problem-solving skills, functional capacities, and barriers to participation. In a real community setting, you will need to define the inclusionary and exclusionary criteria for membership in your proposed group and share this information with potential sources of member referral.

The needs assessment is included here as a possible alternative to the Population Worksheet. If opportunities exist for planning community groups, students have much to gain from designing a group protocol for a "real" population rather than an imagined one.

Students who choose this option should now move on to the next step, choosing a frame of reference.

Selecting a Frame of Reference

After you describe your client population, the next decision to make is what frame of reference to use. There are several factors to consider in this decision. The preceding six chapters can be consulted for a better understanding of the choices. While there are many frames of references in occupational therapy, for this assignment, try to stick with one of the seven included in this text. While personal beliefs usually have some influence over frame of reference selection, students should become competent in using all of them.

The major factor in the selection should be what is likely to work best for the client. Sometimes the intervention setting has an identified frame of reference, and if so, the occupational therapist should find an occupational therapy frame of reference that is compatible with it. Some helpful factors to consider are:

- View of function and dysfunction
- Client physical and cognitive level of function
- Change strategies
- View of motivation
- Intervention time frame
- Intervention options

View of Function and Dysfunction

Each frame of reference has its unique point of view of disability. Looking at your client population, compare their abilities and disabilities with the explanations of function and dysfunction given in each frame of reference. Which frame best explains the function and dysfunction you see in your clients? Why?

Client Physical and Cognitive Level of Functioning

Some frames of reference have a greater usefulness for higher functioning clients, while some relate better to lower levels of functioning. Which frame offers intervention guidelines that have been effective for your clients' level of functioning? Summarize guidelines given to your clients.

Change Strategies

Another way the frames of reference differ is in their view of the change process. Some depend on the therapeutic relationship or on group interaction to facilitate change, while others rely more heavily on the components of tasks and activities or on the environment. Think about what changes your clients need to make. Then look at the explanations given by the frames of reference on how change takes place. Which do you think might work the best for your clients? Why?

View of Motivation

How motivated are your clients? What forces do you think might motivate them to make positive changes? Each frame of reference explains motivation differently. The existential/humanistic view is freedom from anxiety and self-actualization. The ego adaptive, developmental, and neurophysiological frames of reference and Model of Human Occupation describe a drive toward mastery, but each defines something different to be mastered. The cognitive behavioral approach looks at various forms of reinforcement as the motivator. The goal of most of our occupational therapy groups is to help clients achieve a higher level of function or adaptation. However, it is not enough for the therapist to be motivated. We need to think about our clients' motivation as well. Which frame of reference best explains how our clients could be motivated? Why?

Intervention Time Frame

Some frames of reference work best for long-term intervention that encourages the development of relationships and insight, while others lend themselves to more immediate goals. For the purposes of this assignment, the intervention runs for six 1-hour sessions. But these could be spread out once a week for 6 weeks or condensed into two sessions a day for 3 days. If there is no center mentioned, what would be the most likely setting for the client population you have chosen? Acute settings can be assumed to average 10 days to 2 weeks. Substance abuse programs are generally 1 to 4 weeks of intensive intervention. Day treatment can go on for a year or more, and chronic conditions can be treated for a lifetime. How long are your clients likely to be in treatment? Which frame of reference best fits the time frame at your identified intervention center?

Intervention Options

Each frame of reference has different guidelines for activity selection. Some have specific suggestions, while others are more flexible and able to be adapted. Which frame of reference offers intervention options that would interest you? What are they? Which frame of reference offers intervention options that would interest your clients and/or best meet their needs? What are some options you might choose?

Selecting a Focus for Intervention

The *Occupational Therapy Practice Framework* (AOTA, 2002) outlines the domains of concern for occupational therapy and the process of evaluation, intervention, and outcomes that enables "engagement in occupation" and "supports participation in life."

The framework domain lists and defines six categories related to human occupation. The order in which the terms are presented has no bearing on their relative importance (see Appendix D).

1. Performance in areas of occupation includes activities of daily living, instrumental activities of daily living, education, work, play, leisure, and social participation.
2. Performance skills include motor skills, process skills, and communication/interaction skills.
3. Performance patterns include habits, routines, and roles.
4. Seven contexts are specified: cultural, physical, social, personal, spiritual, temporal, and virtual.
5. Activity demands are listed as follows: objects used and their properties, space demands, social demands, sequencing and timing, required actions, required body functions, and required body structures.

6. Finally, client factors are specified as body functions and body structures. This aspect includes both mental and physical functions or capacities.

The document goes on to define each of the terms. For definitions, please refer to the original publication. All of the above-mentioned areas can potentially shape group interventions.

The best strategy is to go over the document in Appendix D and decide what parts of the domain your clients most need to work on or improve. In practice, occupational therapists would collaborate with clients in choosing the most meaningful options. Most clients have more than one, and activities in occupational therapy can be designed to address several of these areas. After looking over the document, use Worksheet 11-2 to list 10 areas that your client population may need to work on.

The *Occupational Therapy Practice Framework* process lists five intervention approaches:

1. Create, promote (health promotion)
2. Establish, restore (remediation, restoration)
3. Maintain
4. Modify (compensation, adaptation)
5. Prevent (disability prevention)

Using these intervention approaches, write a statement about each domain area you have listed, incorporating one of these five approaches on the worksheet. For example, a group of home maintainers with arthritis might work on instrumental activities of daily living to establish energy conservation strategies. Statements may be either general or specific. These statements will help the therapist define the scope of the group. For example, sessions might include several instrumental activities of daily living, such as child rearing, home establishment and management, shopping, meal preparation and cleanup, and care of pets, or its focus may be modifying the activity demands for only one of these areas, such as meal preparation and cleanup for all six sessions. In the next section, these identified aspects of intervention can help us to formulate goals for our group.

Writing a Group Intervention Outline

Once the client population is chosen and the frame of reference and aspects of intervention have been identified, the next step is to write a general outline. The outline should include all the factors inherent in designing a group. The general outline includes the following headings:

- Group title
- Author
- Frame of reference
- Purpose
- Group membership and size
- Group goals and rationale
- Outcome criteria
- Method
- Time and place of meeting
- Supplies and cost
- References

This outline is intended to include not only the ingredients of an effective group intervention protocol but also factors that will be of interest to administrators. Often, occupational therapists are asked to present a group protocol to administrators prior to implementation. Administrators will need to consider factors such as group size, space, scheduling, and cost. The plan you present must not only be therapeutically sound, but also cost-effective.

Group Title

The name of a group is often the client's first impression of the role occupational therapy will play in treatment. Choose it with care. Not only should a title accurately reflect the goals and content of the group, but it should also attract the client's interest. Some examples of good titles are "Developing Self-Identity" (a group for substance abusing adolescents), "Art for Social Skills" (a group for persons with chronic mental illness), and "Re-Entering Your Kitchen" (a group for postoperative cardiac clients).

Author

This includes your name and professional title (e.g., Jane Doe, OTS).

Frame of Reference

State the frame of reference you have decided to use to guide your approach to clients, organization of intervention groups, and selection of activities. A single sentence on why this frame of reference is appropriate will suffice. For example: "The cognitive behavioral approach has been widely used

Worksheet 11-2
Selecting an Intervention Focus

List 10 areas of the occupational therapy domain that your clients may want or need to work on, using Appendix D as your guide.

1.

2.

3.

4.

5.

6.

7.

8.

9.

10.

Use the framework intervention approaches to define the most appropriate focus for each domain listed above, using one of these five approaches: create/promote, establish/restore, maintain, modify, or prevent.

Define the scope of your intervention and discuss reasons why this scope is appropriate for your client population.

with substance abuse clients, and it seems to help them change their own behavior by learning new ways of thinking about their lives."

Purpose

The purpose of the group is the group's general intent. Overall goals of the group should be stated, as well as the general nature of the activities to be used. This section should be short, preferably no longer than three sentences and should summarize the overall scope of the group plan. For example, "The purpose of a leisure planning group might be to assist clients whose disability requires a loss of the worker role in identifying and planning leisure activities to meet their social and emotional needs. Clients will complete written exercises, participate in group discussions, and plan and carry out individual leisure activities as part of group requirements."

Group Membership and Size

The client population for which your group is intended should be described in as much detail as possible. Not only general diagnostic factors but factors like age, functional level, gender, and role identity might be included. For purposes of referral, both inclusionary and exclusionary criteria should be described here. Inclusionary criteria describes characteristics that are appropriate for your group. Exclusionary describes characteristics that are not appropriate. Some activities are appropriate for specific groups only, while others encompass a wide variety of characteristics. A target population should always be identified to give the group a focus. Broader applicability of the protocol should be described in a separate paragraph.

For the purposes of this assignment, the size of groups will be limited to three to eight members. It is generally not cost-effective to treat groups of less than three and not effective intervention for more than eight. The size of a group will depend on many factors, such as the degree of impairment, the need for individual attention, and the complexity of the tasks, to name a few. Group membership may be open or closed. A closed group includes all the same clients at every session for the duration of the group. An open group allows members to be added or dropped from session to session. It is generally easier to plan for closed groups, since the membership is predictable and a sense of belonging is developed. Open groups are more practical for most intervention settings and are a necessity

in acute settings in which clients come and go rapidly. This assignment requires you to plan a closed group. This allows the student to plan specific sessions without having to adapt to unexpected changes in membership.

Group Goals and Rationale

The goals of a group are the specific intervention aims that are intended to be met by individuals participating in the group. No less than three and no more than eight goals should be stated. Less than three usually means that goals are too vague and therefore not useful in planning specific activities. More than eight gives the group too broad a focus. Ideally, there should be at least one specific goal for each individual session planned. However, since there is usually more than one goal met with any given activity, the exact number will vary.

Goals should be stated in measurable terms. They should state what the client will do (i.e., define, discuss, report, demonstrate). Vague terms like "learn," "understand," and "develop" should be avoided; "attend" and "participate" are generally not enough of a description to be meaningful. Well-written goals are the backbone of any well-designed group. They will make the rest of the group easier to plan and the outcome easier to measure. For example, the goals of a money management group might be:

- Recognize the need for a budget.
- List monthly income and expenses.
- Demonstrate ability to follow a budget for 1 week.
- Demonstrate specific banking skills.
- List anticipated needs and expenses.
- Practice comparative shopping techniques and skills to reduce impulse buying.

Once these goals are identified, the activities used to reach the goals will logically follow. Perhaps each group session can focus on a different goal, or several sessions can include more than one goal. For example, the fourth goal can be addressed by giving each client samples of a check register, check, deposit slip, and withdrawal slip. Simple addition and subtraction can be practiced and included when appropriate. Use of a banking machine or telephone banking can be taught and practiced. The outcome of this activity can be measured by examining the completed forms and watching the demonstrated procedures. Specific activities and measured outcomes should follow logically from each stated goal. Rationale for goal selection should relate goals to the chosen client population and its inherent problems. This section should explain why the goals you selected are appropriate. Limitations of the group should be mentioned—for which clients are these goals inappropriate? For example, clients who will be institutionalized may not need the skills. Precautions that may need to be taken should also be mentioned in the rationale. Adaptations that can be made to make the group useful to a wider variety of clients, perhaps in settings other than the target setting, should be mentioned here as well. For example, in the case of the money management group, the same goals can be applied to any group of clients with the goal of living independently.

Outcome Criteria

The desired results of the group should be stated in behavioral terms. By the end of the group, each client should be able to show how he or she has progressed. The therapist needs to develop a measurable way to demonstrate the effectiveness of the group to the client, the administrator, and to those responsible for payment of services. Specific procedures should be outlined, such as a pre/post questionnaire or a pre/post rating scale for each client. An appropriate assessment tool can be identified, if one exists, or evaluation can be specific for the group.

Outcome criteria have a direct relationship to the client goals. However, the outcomes also need to relate in some way to engagement in occupations and participation in life. This necessitates greater emphasis on the application part of group discussion during each session, where clients discuss how they will apply this particular group experience to their own lives. It would be appropriate for the therapist to take this opportunity to remind group members how their comments relate to outcome. The topic could be introduced as a discussion question, and feedback from the therapist and other members could occur spontaneously. However, if verbal feedback is used, the therapist should specify where and how this information is to be recorded. The easiest way to keep track of session by session progress is to create an observation check sheet or brief comment form ahead of time.

Therefore, for learning purposes, both pre/post test, assessment, or questionnaire (such as the Group Member Progress Rating outlined in the next chapter) and a weekly outcomes documentation worksheet must accompany your group outline as separate worksheets.

Method

An outline of the media to be used and the kind of leadership offered are key elements here. Media can be as simple as structured discussions and as complex as learning to build a small engine. Most activities are fair game. However, complex media that require special training, such as biofeedback, systematic desensitization, bioenergetics, and psychodrama, should not be used. Therapeutic interventions that are the traditional roles of other disciplines, such as family therapy, unstructured verbal psychotherapy, or dietary planning, should also be avoided.

The kind of leadership offered depends upon the therapist's frame of reference. If a psychoeducational format is used, the therapist may include short lectures on skills to be learned (see Chapter 13 for example). The therapist's frame of reference will determine the type of introduction and explanation given to clients during each session. The group protocol should reflect a consistent frame of reference. If a psychoanalytic, developmental, or cognitive behavioral approach is used, more emphasis may be placed on group interaction. Cognitive perceptual, cognitive disabilities, or sensorimotor groups for lower level clients require more structured environments with carefully planned therapist assistance.

Time and Place of Meeting

Several design elements should be described in this section. For the purposes of this assignment, the time will be limited to six 1-hour sessions. The scheduling of sessions will vary according to the intervention setting. Chronic settings will accommodate weekly sessions. Acute settings may require daily meetings. The length of sessions will vary with client attention span and type of activity chosen.

The place of meeting should be chosen with specific requirements in mind. In an actual intervention setting, a room can be identified. For the purposes of this assignment, only the characteristics of the setting should be described. The following environmental factors could be included:
- Size of room
- Contents (tables, chairs, cabinets, sink, etc.)
- Lighting, windows

- Visual factors (bare walls or more home-like)
- Door opened or closed
- Noise factors (not next to gym or bathroom)
- Accessibility of medical assistance (special telephone equipment needed, if any; kitchen for cooking activities)
- Availability of assistance from therapist
- Safety factors

This assignment will not limit any of these factors. A good room description will take into consideration the characteristics of the client population chosen, as well as the activities to be included.

Supplies and Cost

The sum total of all materials and supplies and their total cost is listed here. It is recognized that copies of forms and paper and pencils or pens are generally available in most settings at no cost. Items other than these should be listed. If specific items such as videotapes or assessment materials are to be used, the name and address of the source of these should also be listed. This section will probably have to be done after specific sessions are outlined.

References

List all references that were used to create the material for the group sessions, including short lectures, forms to be used as worksheets, and other copyrighted materials. References should use the format of the American Psychological Association (2001):

Books: Author, date, title, publisher, place of publication.

Articles: Author, date, title of article, journal name, volume, and pages.

Materials: Name of item (such as videotape, if used), name and address of source, company, center or hospital, telephone number, and approximate cost.

Planning Individual Sessions

A group session outline should be written for each of the six sessions of your group.

Headings are as follows:
- Session
- Group title
- Session title
- Format (time sequence)

- Supplies
- Description: Each of the seven steps numbered in order: 1) introduction, including warm-up, educational concepts, or purpose; 2) activity including instructions; 3) sharing including procedures used; and 4 through 7) discussion questions in processing, generalizing, application, and summary

Session

The session number (Session ___ of 6) out of total number of sessions planned indicates sequence. Your group sessions should be planned in logical order, from simple to complex, superficial to deep, general to specific, etc. In a closed group, the sessions should build on one another so that general group principles can be applied. It would make sense for the first session to be somewhat introductory, so that members begin to know not only the subject of the group, but each other as well. Subjects of a more personal nature should be saved for later in the sequence when members know one another better. The last session needs to deal with summary and termination of the group. The way you sequence the sessions will depend somewhat on your chosen population.

Group Title

This is the title of the group as a whole (e.g., "Money Management").

Session Title

Like the group title, each session should be labeled with a word or phrase describing either the content or the goal for that session.

Format

This is a short outline stating what will happen when. For example, a session in "Balancing Your Checkbook" might have the following format:

15 minutes—Review last week

15 minutes—Introductory short lecture

15 minutes—Complete sample checkbook worksheet

10 minutes—Check answers with calculator

20 minutes—Discuss specific problems and summarize importance of balancing checkbook

60 minutes—Total

You need not include this last total figure, but make sure your timing fits the total time allotted for the group.

Supplies

This category includes a complete list of what is needed to complete the group. Do not assume clients will be carrying pens and pencils with them or will be wearing a watch. The supply list should include the correct number of each item needed. For a "Balancing Your Checkbook" session, supplies for a group of five clients would include the following:

5 worksheets (attach copy)

5 pencils

5 pocket calculators

1 large pad and 1 marker (for therapist to illustrate process)

Description

This is a step-by-step description of what will be included:

1) The introduction should be fully described, including warm-up (if appropriate), explanation of purpose, expectations, and time frame. If there are educational concepts which illuminate the purpose, these must be outlined.

2) Activity: If worksheets are to be written, a copy must be attached. Activities must be fully described including directions, choices, timing. If the activity was selected from a text or prior experience, reference should be given.

3) Sharing: Procedures for how member individual work is to be shared/discussed with the group is given.

4 through 6) For the discussion part, a list of questions to be asked is included for each of the categories: processing, generalizing, and application. Refer to Chapter 1 for a description of these phases of the group. Your discussions will vary depending on the frame of reference you are using. It is wise to be prepared with more questions than you will need. Also keep in mind the goals of the group when choosing discussion questions. An activity is generally more effective when the clients feel it has meaning for them. Relating each session's activity back to the original goals will help keep both clients and therapist on track.

7) A verbal summary at the end of each session is important. Include for each session some points to remember for the summary.

Instructions for Preparing the Group Protocol

When you have written the entire protocol, you should type it using a computer. Each session should start a new page. When typing the protocol on the computer, use the exact headings in the order described. Capitalize the headings; use single spacing and 1-inch margins. It is not necessary to indent. Skip a line between each section or heading.

When rating sheets or worksheets are used, a copy should be attached to the outline or session to which it relates. Use the following forms to write your first draft of your Group Intervention Plan Protocol (Worksheet 11-3).

The next two chapters provide examples of group protocols. The first has a developmental focus, while the second has a cognitive behavioral focus. For each of these, the role of the leader is facilitator. However, each has a different frame of reference.

Note: James P. Klyczek was coauthor of Chapter 11 in the first and second editions. Dr. Klyczek originated the concept of the group intervention plan assignment with the six session outlines in 1985, and very kindly shared his group dynamics course materials with me. Dr. Klyczek is Assistant Professor and Clinical Coordinator in the Occupational Therapy Program, Division of Health and Human Services, D'Youville College, Buffalo, NY.

Bibliography

American Occupational Therapy Association. (2002). Occupational therapy practice framework: Domain and process. *American Journal of Occupational Therapy, 56,* 609-639.

American Psychological Association. (2001). *Publication manual of the American Psychological Association.* Washington, DC: Author.

Brownson, C. (2001). Program development for community health: Planning, implementation and evaluation strategies. In M. Scaffa (Ed.), *Occupational therapy in community based practice settings.* Philadelphia: F. A. Davis.

Worksheet 11-3
Group Intervention Plan Outline

Group title:

Author:

Frame of reference:

Purpose:

Group membership and size:

Group Intervention Plan Outline (continued)

Group goals:

1.

2.

3.

4.

5.

6.

7.

8.

Rationale, limitations, adaptations:

Outcome criteria:

Group Intervention Plan Outline (continued)

Method:

Time and place of meeting:

Supplies and cost:

References:

Group Intervention Plan Outline (continued)

Group Session Outline

Session 1 of 6

Group title:

Session title:

Format:

Supplies:

Description:

303

Group Intervention Plan Outline (continued)

Group Intervention Plan Outline (continued)

Group Session Outline

Session 2 of 6

Group title:

Session title:

Format:

Supplies:

Description:

Group Intervention Plan Outline (continued)

Group Session Outline

Session 3 of 6

Group title:

Session title:

Format:

Supplies:

Description:

Group Intervention Plan Outline (continued)

Group Intervention Plan Outline (continued)

Group Session Outline

Session 4 of 6

Group title:

Session title:

Format:

Supplies:

Description:

Group Intervention Plan Outline (continued)

Group Intervention Plan Outline (continued)

Group Session Outline

Session 5 of 6

Group title:

Session title:

Format:

Supplies:

Description:

Group Intervention Plan Outline (continued)

Group Intervention Plan Outline (continued)
Group Session Outline
Session 6 of 6

Group title:

Session title:

Format:

Supplies:

Description:

Chapter 12

A Group Laboratory Experience

The following is an example of a group protocol. It is a group designed as a laboratory experience for professional students. Ideally it is done in groups of eight students, with the instructor as the leader. It addresses some of the most common professional issues for students and serves as a context for the discussion of the principles of group dynamics described in Chapter 2. The series of six sessions is planned in a sequence that moves toward greater intimacy as the group develops. The leadership is also intended to change from directive in the beginning toward a democratic, facilitative style at the end. The group leader models therapeutic interventions with various problem behaviors and fosters the exploration of here-and-now relationships. Members have the opportunity to take on various roles and to practice group interaction skills. Process illumination should be discussed as a part of each session, with a goal of learning and personal growth.

Although this is a six-session sequence, it has been suggested by my students that three open sessions be interspersed. An open session has no planned activity, and its purpose is to discuss the process of prior sessions. After Session 3 in my group, for example, there seemed to be little time to discuss the many issues and feelings resulting from giving and receiving feedback. An open group following this session would give the members a chance to discuss their concerns and to better understand their relationship to each other. Session 4 seemed to be too structured, and several of the groups felt the need to voice their urge to rebel against the structure and/or the directive leadership style. An open session following this one would allow for the discussion of group development and the significance of their rebellion in the context of group development theories. Another interesting addition to the sequence is a leaderless group. This forces the group members to take on leadership roles and further illuminates the group process. This semester, many of the groups decided to end their group with a "termination" activity. One group brought in brunch, another had a pizza party, and another decided on a goodbye collage. With these additions, the group lab experience is expanded to 10 weekly sessions.

Group Intervention Protocol

Group title: "Developing Your Professional Self"

Author: Marilyn B. Cole, MS, OTR/L

Frame of reference: The frame of reference for this group is developmental. Students experiment with new ideas and behaviors in anticipation of the next phase of their lives, which involves taking on a professional identity. The assumption is that members are intrinsically motivated to know themselves better and to become competent professionals.

Purpose: This group is designed to help junior occupational therapy students to make the transition from a student role to a professional role. The six group activities are selected to deal with the most common areas of difficulty for students, such as being assertive, accepting feedback, and setting priorities in their lives.

Group membership and size: "Developing Your Professional Self" is designed for second semester junior occupational therapy students. Most of these students are between 20 and 22 years of age, although several are adults coming back to school. The majority are women who have lived independent of their families for at least 2 years, although there are several men and several students who commute from home. Having entered the junior year in an occupational therapy academic program, these students have all achieved and maintained a high academic average and have survived at least one semester of difficult and challenging professional coursework. All have had at least one semester of clinical Fieldwork I experiences, allowing them a taste of what it is like to work with clients (a few hours per week). In choosing to become occupational therapists, these students have set a goal and are working to achieve it. This will be a closed group of no more than eight members. The same members will be expected to attend all six sessions with no absences (Worksheet 12-1).

Group goals and rationale: The student will do the following:
1. Discuss awareness of professional self in relation to clients and peers.
2. Demonstrate ability to problem solve, behave assertively, and set goals and priorities.
3. Identify strengths and weaknesses of self and others.
4. Express feelings directly and offer respectful feedback to others.
5. Accept feedback from others and use it constructively.
6. Clearly state professional values.
7. Demonstrate ability to interact effectively with peers.
8. Identify group behaviors and group process.

Students in the junior year are learning many of the skills necessary to treat clients. However, in order to use those skills effectively, the student needs to feel comfortable in the professional role. The "Developing Your Professional Self" group is designed to promote a needed self-awareness associated with professionalism. As a professional team member, future occupational therapists will need to interact effectively, behave assertively when necessary, share in group problem solving, and learn constructively from other team members. Factors other than academic ones will influence professional effectiveness, such as warmth and empathy, flexibility and openness, ability to express feelings, and appropriate self-disclosure. The group format gives students an opportunity to explore and practice needed skills and attributes in preparation for their Fieldwork II experiences. This group design, although planned for occupational therapy students, may also be useful for students in other disciplines. Adaptations would be minimal, simply substituting for "occupational therapy," nursing, physical therapy, social work, etc. The group and interpersonal skills needed by many health professionals are quite similar.

Worksheet 12-1
Contract for Group Membership

This contract should be reviewed and signed by each member of the group before beginning the first session.

I understand I am involved in a developmental process, and therefore, it is necessary to attend all sessions to benefit fully from the process. I realize that in order for me to be an effective member, it is important that I complete all assignments and arrive on time. I agree to participate as openly, honestly, and responsibly as I am able to, realizing that I am not under any group pressure to reveal personal data that I would regret sharing with the group. I agree to speak personally and make "I" statements as objectively and specifically as I can, trying not to generalize or talk in abstractions. I realize that no personal information about any group member should ever be discussed outside of the group.

Signed: _____

Date:_____

From Cole, M. B. *Group dynamics in occupational therapy: The theoretical basis and practice application of group intervention* (3rd ed.). Thorofare, NJ: SLACK Incorporated. © 2005 SLACK Incorporated.

Outcome criteria:

1. The student will demonstrate interpersonal skills by verbal participation at least three times in each weekly session.

2. Students within the context of each session will discuss and demonstrate the skills required for self-disclosure, problem solving, giving and receiving feedback, empathizing with or confronting others, behaving assertively, and setting goals and priorities.

3. The progress of each student may be rated twice on a five-point scale, one being poor ability and five being excellent ability. The first rating should be before the first session, the second rating after the sixth session. This pre/post group rating will then show progress made by each student in each skill required. The Group Member Progress Rating chart (Worksheet 12-2) may be used to measure progress in each of these factors: self-disclosure, problem solving, giving feedback, receiving feedback, empathizing with others, confronting others, behaving assertively, setting personal goals, and understanding dynamics.

Method: Structured group activities and discussions will occur each week. The activities will be graded from a superficial and safe level to a deeper level interpersonally. The activities will also be graded so as to encourage more group interaction and less dependence on the leader as each week progresses. Group development and interpersonal learning will be encouraged, and an understanding of the process of the group will be facilitated.

Time and place of meeting: The group will meet for 1 hour each week for 6 weeks. The rooms are selected to be free of noise distraction and to preserve the confidentiality of the group. A large table and nine chairs are preferable, so that members can work on group projects. On days when only discussion takes place, chairs may be arranged in a circle without the table. For the 1-hour meeting, it is important that no one leaves or comes late, and that there are no interruptions. The door should be closed, and a sign saying "Do Not Disturb, Group in Session" should be displayed outside.

Worksheet 12-2
Group Member Progress Rating

Rating 1 (low) to 5 (high)	Session 1	Session 6 (or last)
Self-disclosure		
Problem-solving		
Giving feedback		
Receiving feedback		
Empathizing with others		
Confronting others		
Behaving assertively		
Setting personal goals		
Understanding dynamics		

From Cole, M. B. *Group dynamics in occupational therapy: The theoretical basis and practice application of group intervention* (3rd ed.). Thorofare, NJ: SLACK Incorporated. © 2005 SLACK Incorporated.

Supplies and cost

	Unit price	Total
9 sheets of white drawing paper 12 x 18 inches	donated	
16 assorted magazines	donated	
5 jars of glue	$1.50	$7.50
9 pairs of scissors	$2.50	$22.50
10 marking pens (set)	$2.50	$2.50
10 pencils (pack)	$1.50	$1.50
1 package 3- x 5-inch index cards	$1.25	$1.25
20 Xerox copies	$.10	$2.00
9 sheets typing paper	donated	
Total cost		$37.25

Rider, B., & Gramblin, C. (1987). *Activities card file*. Kalamazoo, MI: Author.

Session 1 of 6

Group title: "Developing Your Professional Self"

Session title: "Professional Self-Awareness Collage" (adapted from Rider & Gramblin, 1987)

Format:

    Warm-up—3 minutes
    Introduce group lab—2 minutes
    Instructions for activity—2 minutes
    Collage activity—20 minutes
    Sharing—10 minutes
    Discussion—20 minutes
    Summary—3 minutes

Supplies:

    9 sheets white drawing paper 12 x 18 inches
    5 jars of glue or 9 glue sticks
    9 pairs of scissors
    16 uncut magazines
    10 marking pens, assorted colors

Description:

1. Introduction:

    Warm-up—Ask each person in turn to give his or her name and something he or she likes and does not like about occupational therapy.

    Introduce group lab—Group outline will be shared with the group.

    Purpose—The purpose of this activity is to help us think about ourselves as professionals.

2. Activity:

    Give out bags and markers. "We will begin by signing our name at the top like this 'Jane Doe, OTS.'" Magazines, glue, and scissors are placed in the center of the table. "Look through the magazines and cut out pictures that represent qualities you have as a professional. We all have some characteristics that we will want to share and have others know about. These may be characteristics that will help us as professionals. Fold the drawing paper in half and paste the pictures representing these on the outside of the folder you have made. You may use both front and back covers.

    "We also have some characteristics we would rather not share. These may be a hindrance to our professional identity. Cut out pictures representing these and paste them on the inside of the folder you have made. When you are finished pasting the pictures, use markers to label each with the characteristic you intend it to represent. You have about 20 minutes to complete this task. We will discuss the collages when we are finished. This will be a good way to get to know each other better."

    Give warning when 5 minutes are left. After 5 minutes, collect all materials and place out of reach.

3. Sharing:

    Ask for a volunteer to start sharing the collages. Once started, go around the group in order, forcing no one to share more than he or she wants.

Session 1 of 6 (continued)

4. Processing:

    Questions for discussion.
    - How did you feel about doing this activity?
    - How many of us felt comfortable sharing the inside vs. the outside of the folder?

5. Generalizing:
    - How well do you know your professional self?
    - What did you learn about yourself from doing this activity?
    - What did you learn about others?
    - How difficult was it to decide which parts of yourself are "professional"?

6. Application:
    - How will an activity like this help people build a professional identity?

7. Summary:

    Points to remember are to be taken from comments of members. Some might be:
    - The "face" we show to the public is not what is really inside.
    - The outside represents what we wish to be, the inside what we fear we may be.
    - Students do not find it easy to think of themselves as professionals.
    - Some common characteristics are the wish to play a helping role and fondness and empathy for other people.

Session 2 of 6

Group title: "Developing Your Professional Self"

Session title: "Difficult Decisions"

Format:
   Warm-up—5 minutes
   Introduce activity—5 minutes
   Instructions for activity—5 minutes
   Difficult decision writing—10 minutes
   Discussion—30 minutes
   Summary—5 minutes

Supplies:
   8 3 x 5 inch index cards
   8 pencils
   Basket or box ("hat")

Description:
1. Introduction:
   Warm-up—Ask members to give names and recall one characteristic about their professional self from last session.
2. Activity:
   "Today we will discuss difficult professional decisions or problems. Each of you take an index card and a pencil and write on the card a professional problem or decision you have experienced in the past year. You may draw on Fieldwork I experiences, volunteer experiences, or situations in the classroom, as long as they concern some aspect of your chosen profession.

   "You can write about a problem you had difficulty with or had trouble making a decision about. Give necessary background and detail, but you need not identify yourself. We will be putting the cards in a hat and drawing out someone else's problem to solve. You have 10 minutes to write your problem." Give 1 minute warning.
3. Sharing:
   Collect all cards after 10 minutes and shuffle them. Put them back in "hat" and ask each member to draw one out. If someone draws his or her own, he or she has the option of putting it back and drawing another. "Now think about the problem on the card you drew and get ready to share with the group how you would solve it. Take turns sharing solutions and discuss."

   For this activity, discussion will be during the sharing rather than afterward. Members have the option of identifying their problem and asking the group for additional help.
4. Processing:
   Discussion questions:
   • What feelings are involved in making difficult decisions?
   • How did you feel hearing someone else address your problem?
   • What parts of this activity did you find difficult? Easy?
   • How does it feel to need/ask for help? Receive help?
5. Generalizing:
   • What did you learn from today's activity?
   • Who owns the problems discussed? Who should take responsibility?
   • What did you/others contribute?

Session 2 of 6 (continued)

- What is the worst/best thing you could do?
- If decision, what are pros and cons?
- Whose decision is it? Should it be?
- What additional information is needed to decide/solve?

6. Application:
   - What can we learn from each other as professionals?
   - How can we help each other as professionals?

7. Summary:

   This activity usually produces much discussion and often members own up to their own problem. They have become a group of peers working together and trusting one another. A parallel should be drawn to the ideal in practice where no one should feel afraid to ask for the help of his or her colleagues in facing a difficult problem.

Session 3 of 6

Group title: "Developing Your Professional Self"

Session title: "Giving and Receiving Feedback"

Format:
   Warm-up—5 minutes
   Introduce activity—5 minutes
   Instructions for activity—5 minutes
   Writing activity—15 minutes
   Discussion—25 minutes
   Summary—5 minutes

Supplies:
   9 sheets of paper 8 1/2 x 11 inches
   9 pens or pencils

Description:
1. Introduction:

   Warm-up—Begin by asking members to say a few words about how they are feeling today.

   Educational concepts—"Today we will be working on communication, self-awareness, and accepting feedback from others. Often the success of our professional interactions will depend on how well we understand our own feelings and express them to others. Even negative feelings can be expressed in positive terms. For example, if you are studying for a test, and your roommate is talking loudly on the phone, you might say to her: 'I know you're enjoying talking to your friend, but I'm having a hard time concentrating on my work. Would you mind calling your friend back later?'

   "Most people have an easier time giving positive feedback than negative. However, avoiding negative comments can cause all kinds of problems, especially when two people have to work together. This exercise is designed to practice giving positive and negative feedback to each other."

2. Activity:

   Pass out paper and pencils. "Fold paper in half. Put name on the outside folded half at the top. On the inside, write some ways you feel you need to grow professionally (skills needed, issues to deal with, etc.). Fold paper over so what you have written is not visible. Pass folded paper around circle. Each person writes on the outside how he or she feels the person whose name is on the paper could grow professionally. To make this chore less difficult, you may also write one thing you admire about the person. Both positive and 'change needed' comments should be expressed constructively. Even if you do not know everyone that well, do the best you can."

   Give 15 minutes for this part. After that stop, even if not finished. Each reads own paper for a few minutes.

3. Sharing:

   Members share the results with the group. If possible, each should read a few positive and growth comments to the group.

4. Processing:

   Discussion questions
   - How do you feel about the feedback you received?
   - How did you feel about giving feedback to others?
   - What problems did you encounter in doing this exercise?

Session 3 of 6 (continued)

5. Generalizing:
   - How do the comments about yourself compare with comments of others?
   - What feedback from others do you agree/disagree with?
   - What did you learn from doing this exercise?
6. Application:
   - Whom would you like feedback from in your professional role?
   - How can you use feedback in everyday life?
   - How can you become more comfortable in giving constructive feedback to others? To clients?
7. Summary:
   Ask members to summarize.

Session 4 of 6

Group title: "Developing Your Professional Self"

Session title: "Professional Values"

Format:
Warm-up—5 minutes
Introduce activity—5 minutes
Instructions for activity—5 minutes
Activity—15 minutes
Discussion—25 minutes
Summary—5 minutes

Supplies:
9 pencils
9 Values worksheets (Worksheet 12-3)

Description:
1. Introduction:
   Warm-up—Begin by summarizing last week's activity. How are people left feeling about the group? Is there any unfinished business? (Any comments, either negative or positive, should be accepted by the leader without judgment and acknowledged.)
   Educational concepts—"Knowing our professional values can help us set priorities and use our time at work and away from work more constructively. For example, if I want to balance my career with a meaningful relationship with my family, then I will be careful not to work overtime or make work-related commitments on weekends. Professional values should also guide our behavior at work. If you believe a good rapport with clients is important, you may take extra time with them to show your concern."
   Pass out Worksheet 12-3 and pencils. Follow instructions on top of sheet. Allow 15 minutes to complete. When finished, each member shares his or her responses with the group.
2. Activity:
   The discussion guidelines written on the sheet are to come up with a group consensus on values held in common. One group member can be a recorder and allow group to collaborate on what professional values they can agree on. A separate Values worksheet may be used for note taking of group values.
3. Sharing is done during the activity.
4. Processing:
   • How did the group perform without leader intervention?
   • How did you feel about doing the activity on your own?
   • How did the structure affect your interaction?
5. Generalizing is done during the activity.
6. Application:
   • How do values affect your interpersonal relationships?
   • What role do values play in your professional life?
   • How do values determine how you spend your time?
7. Summary:
   In summary, the recorder can read his or her notes back to the group and accept final revisions and/or comments.

Worksheet 12-3
Values

Directions: Complete the following sentences in your own words. Then compare your responses to those of the other members of your group in order to generate a set of commonly held values in interpersonal relations. In the discussion, you have four tasks:
1. To make yourself heard
2. To hear others accurately
3. To listen for themes
4. To collaborate on the group consensus

A professional should:

A professional should not:

A supervisor:

A student:

A colleague:

A spouse or boyfriend/girlfriend:

I want to be remembered as a person who:

Our group:

Session 5 of 6

Group title: "Developing Your Professional Self"

Session title: "Assertiveness Role Play"

Format:
Warm-up—5 minutes
Introduce activity—2 minutes
Instructions for activity—3 minutes
Activity writing—10 minutes
Sharing (role playing)—25 minutes
Discussion—10 minutes
Summary—5 minutes

Supplies:
8 3 x 5inch index cards
8 pencils

Description:
1. Introduction:
   Warm-up—Define assertive, passive, and aggressive and discuss the differences between these.
   Educational concepts—"One of the most common problems students have in making the transition to professionals is not acting assertively. Lack of assertiveness can lead to difficulty even on field-work experiences, as many of you have already discovered. For example, one student on a Fieldwork I experience overheard a discussion by staff members who were setting up a family conference in the client lounge at 2:00 p.m. This student was already scheduled to run an occupational therapy group in that room at 2:00 p.m. However, she did not say anything about it to the staff group. The student was left without a place to run group and became very frustrated. Afterward, when staff became aware of the problem, they wondered why the student did not speak up! They could have met in several other places. This situation could have been avoided if the student had behaved more assertively."

2. Activity:
   Pass out index cards and pencils. "You will now write down on the card a professional situation in which you would like to have responded more assertively but did not. You may either have been too passive or overly aggressive instead. On the front of the card, describe the situation: who, what, where, when, and whatever background information is necessary. On the back, state what your actual response was (if possible, give a quote) and state how you felt afterward."

3. Sharing:
   Each member shares the situation written on the front of the card. Then members decide as a group which situations they would like to role play. Group chooses first, second, and third choices, using group decision-making techniques to do this.
   Role play one to three situations as time allows:
   - Allow protagonist to direct role play.
   - Protagonist chooses members of group to play significant characters.
   - Protagonist sets up room, props.
   - Role play situation as it really happened first, then discuss.
   - Reverse roles and play situation using assertive behavior as discussed by the group.
   - Allow a few alter egos to present feelings and/or alternate responses.

Session 5 of 6 (continued)

4. Processing:
- How did you feel about doing the role play?
- Which characters did you identify with?
- How do you feel about being assertive? Passive? Aggressive?
- What are you feeling about the protagonist's situation?

5. Generalizing:
- What passive, assertive, and aggressive behaviors can you identify in the role play?
- What are the advantages of assertive behavior?

6. Application:
- What did you learn about being assertive professionally?
- What steps do you personally need to take to be able to behave assertively in the professional setting? As a student? As an occupational therapist?

7. Summary:
Summarize by reinforcing assertive behaviors, reviewing the role of feelings and habits, and thanking role players for their participation.

Session 6 of 6 (continued)

Group title: "Developing Your Professional Self"

Session title: "Group Evaluation"

Format:
   Warm-up—5 minutes
   Introduce activity—5 minutes
   Instructions for activity—5 minutes
   Activity—15 minutes
   Discussion/Summary of all six sessions—20 minutes
   Summary—10 minutes

Supplies:
   9 Group Evaluation worksheets (Worksheet 12-4)
   9 pencils

Description:
1. Introduction:
   Warm-up—Begin by stating that this will be the final group of the series and ask members to say how they feel about ending the group.

   Educational concepts—"An important part of the termination of groups is to review all the sessions and summarize what has been valuable. As professionals, we will all need to evaluate our client groups, so this will be good practice. Worksheet 12-4 has been designed to help you think specifically about this group and to apply some of what you have learned about group dynamics."

2. Activity:
   Give out worksheets.

   "First, you are asked to identify the roles your fellow members played in the groups, and for this you will have to name names. In our discussion, these questions will serve as the basis of giving one another feedback about our participation. Next, we will look at the events of the group. These are emotionally charged situations that often emerge unexpectedly. In the context of activities, often it is the conflicts and problems groups encounter that become the turning points from which we learn the most. You are asked to identify three such events over the last five sessions.

   "Norms are the 'ground rules' of behavior in groups. You are asked to identify the implicit or implied norms over the course of the group. The stage of development is sometimes difficult to identify in the short time this group has been meeting. We will use Schutz's stages of inclusion, control, and affection as a guide (see Chapter 2). Sometimes the characteristics of stages overlap and this can be confusing, so you are asked to justify your choice with behaviors you see or have seen in this group. Your feeling about the group may be an important clue about what stage the group has achieved.

   "Finally, you are asked to look at the group leadership. What style was used, and how has it changed over the course of the group? You have 15 minutes to complete the worksheet."

3. Sharing:
   Members share their answers to some or all of the questions on the sheet, as time allows. After each question, ask the group to discuss their answers and come to a consensus. Be sure to leave the last 15 minutes to summarize and to reflect on the past six sessions.

Worksheet 12-4
Group Evaluation

Directions: Answer the following questions about your group as it has developed from Session 1. Be sure to identify members by name.

Participation and Roles:
1. Who are the most outspoken participants?

2. Who are the least frequent participants?

3. Who talks to whom? What patterns have you observed? (Identify any subgroups that exist.)

4. Who keeps the ball rolling?

5. Who/what has blocked the group?

6. What rivalries have you observed during the group? Who has challenged the leadership?

Events: Name three interactions or situations that were high points or turning points for the group. Describe each situation briefly.
   1.

   2.

   3.

Norms:
1. What behaviors are acceptable to the group today?

2. What behaviors are not acceptable today?

3. How have norms changed from the beginning of the group?

Group Evaluation (continued)

Stage of Development:
1. What stage of development has this group achieved? Justify your answer.
   a. Inclusion
   b. Control
   c. Affection

2. How do you feel about the group right now?
   a. It means a lot to me. I'm sorry it's ending.
   b. I feel good about the other members.
   c. I feel indifferent.
   d. It feels uncomfortable. I'm glad it's ending.
   e. I strongly dislike the group.

Leadership:
1. What was the leader's style of leadership? Why?
   a. Directive
   b. Facilitator
   c. Leader as adviser

2. How has the role of the leader changed over the course of the group?

Other Process Observations:

Session 6 of 6 (continued)

4. Processing:
   - How do you feel about the group as a whole? Specific members? The leader?
   - What parts of the group experience are most memorable?
   - Which experiences did you like best/least?
   - How do you feel about your role in the group?
5. Generalizing:
   - What did you learn about yourself from being a part of this group?
6. Application:
   - What parts of this group experience can you take with you and apply to future roles both personally and professionally?
7. Summary:

   End by summarizing results and asking each person to say in his or her own words what parts of this group experience he or she values and feels good about.

Chapter 13

A Group Experience: Developing Cultural Competence

Cultural competence is essential if occupational therapists are to practice effectively in a growing multicultural society (Evans, 1992). With diverse populations on the rise across the United States, cultural competency for occupational therapy professionals cannot be viewed as a passing fad. Many professional students do not fully appreciate the meaning of culture. In its broadest sense, culture may be understood as the "sum total of a way of living, including values, beliefs, standards, linguistic expression, patterns of thinking, behavioral norms, and styles of communication that influence behaviors of a group of people and are transmitted from generation to generation" (Wells & Black, 2000, p. 279). Culture includes notions of health and illness and ways of doing everyday tasks.

Cultural competence is defined by Wells and Black (2000) as:

...the process of actively developing and practicing appropriate, relevant, and sensitive strategies and skills in interacting with culturally different people. (It involves) the capacity to respond to the needs of populations whose cultures are different from what might be called dominant or mainstream. (p. 278)

The following group protocol was designed to introduce professional students to the concept of cultural competence. Each session begins with a didactic component that reviews current thinking on the subject from a variety of sources. The group activities for each session flow from the introductory topic to promote self-awareness and allow members to learn from each other's experiences. Cultural understanding results from learning and experiencing cultural differences (Wells & Black,

2000). It is hoped that the mix of students in each group laboratory will provide enough diversity of experience for students to learn and practice strategies and skills for effectively communicating with potential clients from a variety of cultural backgrounds.

This group laboratory uses Wells and Black's Cultural Competency Model, which consists of three intrinsic components and three extrinsic components. The students' cultural perspectives consist of:

1. Attitudes
2. Perceptions
3. Behaviors

These qualities are defined by their own culture and have been passed on to them by their families or others in their culture. Cultural awareness refers to knowledge of one's own culture: what beliefs and values we hold, and how we define what is ordinary for us. Sometimes it is necessary to take ourselves away from our own everyday routines and get out of our home territory in order to recognize the cultural idiosyncrasies that make us truly unique. Therefore, the first step in developing cultural competence is to become aware of our own cultural uniqueness.

The second layer of components in the cultural competency model are extrinsic factors:

1. Self-exploration
2. Knowledge
3. Skills

These factors provide the theoretical basis for the group intervention strategies used in this group protocol. Knowledge will be imparted via short educational introductions at the beginning of each group session, while self-exploration will be encouraged through the worksheets and exercises. Students will also learn and use group interaction skills such as empathy, active listening, and open questions in learning about the cultures of other members. Cultural sensitivity assumes a certain level of cultural awareness. McGruder (2003) defines cultural sensitivity as a "readiness to explore other cultures nonjudgmentally. Contact with empowered people whose cultural, racial, ethnic, class, gender, or sexual orientation is different from one's own is the most highly valued sort of activity for increasing cultural sensitivity. The learner must be willing to leave his or her own comfort zone and enter environments in which he or she will have the experience of being the numerical minority" (p. 93). Collectively, members will develop skill in using verbal and non-verbal communication to create an atmosphere of non-judgmental acceptance in exploring the cultures of others.

The following group protocol uses the seven-step, client-centered format for group facilitation, interaction, and learning.

Group Intervention Plan Outline

Group title: "Developing Cultural Competence"

Author: Marilyn B. Cole, MS, OTR/L, FAOTA

Frame of reference: A cognitive behavioral frame of reference is chosen because it encourages students to examine their own thinking process regarding cultures of self and others. This frame of reference teaches students to use reasoning to question and dispute some of their beliefs regarding cultures different from their own.

Purpose: This group laboratory is intended to broaden the cultural perspective of students and to prepare them to practice and to live in a changing world of diverse cultures and people. The laboratory exercises will teach members to recognize their own biases and to explore cultural differences without judgment or prejudice. It will prepare students to create an atmosphere of acceptance and open-mindedness wherever they go, both professionally and socially.

Group membership and size: This group intervention was designed for professional students. Groups of eight members are ideal. An effort should be made to include a mix of persons from different cultures in each group whenever possible.

Goals and rationale: Eight specific goals are outlined for this laboratory experience. Students will:
1. Fully appreciate the meaning of culture (beyond ethnicity) in the broadest sense.
2. Develop an awareness of one's own culture.
3. Recognize and verbalize one's own attitudes and biases toward others.
4. Explore and verbalize similarities and differences among group members.
5. Demonstrate nonjudgmental acceptance.
6. Define "otherness" as it pertains to one's own culture.
7. Develop and communicate empathy with others different from one's self.
8. Demonstrate cultural awareness and sensitivity through group interactions and journal writing.

Much can be learned about culture using the members' own cultural backgrounds and experiences. Attitude change is often best accomplished through interaction with peers rather than lectures or individual assignments. During group discussions, members will be encouraged to share their beliefs through open and honest self-disclosure.

Outcome criteria: The achievement of goals can be measured through self-ratings, written answers to essay questions, and personal journals. Please refer to Worksheet 13-1 to be given as a pre/post test. In addition, members will write a journal entry (minimum two handwritten pages) immediately following each session, using guidelines as follows:
- What I learned about myself from today's session.
- What I learned about other members (give names).
- One positive aspect of the group session.
- One negative aspect of the group session.
- What are my personal barriers to nonjudgmental acceptance of others?
- What goal can I set for myself during the next session & why?
- Other issues as assigned.

Methods: The instructor begins each session by imparting educational concepts about one aspect of culture, followed by experiential learning. Sessions use structured group activities to explore various aspects of culture. The instructor then facilitates discussion of the group activity, using the seven-step format outlined in Chapter 1. During discussions, instructors will model nonjudgmental acceptance and open self-disclosure.

Worksheet 13-1

Outcome Criteria Pre/Post Test:
Developing Cultural Competence

Directions: Please answer these questions as best you can. Do not skip any questions.

1. Define culture.

2. Give an example of cultural awareness.

3. Describe your own cultural background.

4. Name five ways that members of this group are different from each other.

5. Rate your own attitude toward diversity on a scale of 1 to 10 (1 = negatively biased, 10 = positively biased) for each of the following:

___ African American
___ Homosexual male
___ Adult with cerebral palsy
___ Asian American
___ Homeless person
___ Hispanic (Mexican)
___ White American
___ Person with moderate mental retardation
___ Person imprisoned for sexual assault
___ Catholic priest
___ Muslim anti-American demonstrator
___ Female with extreme obesity

6. Give an example of how you could show empathy and sensitivity toward a client whose culture evokes negative feelings in you.

7. Write three questions you could ask to learn more about someone's culture.

Group Intervention Plan Outline (continued)

Time and place of meeting: Group meets once a week for 90 minutes. This allows ample time for both educational learning and group experiences. Either day or evening time is suitable. The room should allow for privacy and freedom from distractions. Members may sit in comfortable chairs arranged in a circle. During written exercises, members seated around one large table may be preferable.

Supplies and cost: This group is relatively inexpensive to run, using mainly copies of worksheets and pencils. Index cards (3 x 5 inches) and a roll of adhesive tape are also needed. In addition, the following are required for each member:

- Sets of 8 colored markers
- Glue sticks
- 12 x 18 inch drawing paper
- Scissors
- 2 magazines
- Bound notebooks for journal writing may also be provided
- The cost is estimated at $10 per member.

Group Session Outline (1 of 6)

Group title: "Developing Cultural Competence"

Session 1: "Your Cultural Heritage"

Format (90 minutes total):
  Introduce members—5 minutes
  Educational concepts, introduction to cultural competence—15 minutes
  Instructions for activity—5 minutes
  Worksheets—20 minutes
  Sharing—10 minutes
  Discussion—30 minutes
  Summary—5 minutes

Supplies:
- Worksheets
- Pencils with erasers for each member

Description:
1. Introduction:

  Warm-up—Ask each person to state his or her name and give national/ethnic origin.

  Educational concepts—As a beginning step in developing cultural competence, we will first explore our own cultural heritage and share some information about our families with the group. We will define the key terms for this exploration: culture, ethnicity, race, and socioeconomic status. Then we will look at a model for developing cultural competence (Wells & Black, 2000).

  Culture—In its broadest sense, culture may be understood as the "sum total of a way of living, including values, beliefs, standards, linguistic expression, patterns of thinking, behavioral norms, and styles of communication that influence behaviors of a group of people and are transmitted from generation to generation" (Wells & Black, 2002, p. 279). Culture also includes notions of health and illness and ways of doing everyday tasks. Another definition comes from Krefting and Krefting (1991, p. 102) in Crepeau, Cohn, and Boyt Schell (2003): culture is "a learned, shared experience that provides 'the individual and the group with effective mechanisms for interacting both with others and with the surrounding environment'" (p. 81).

  Ethnicity—Culture is not the same as ethnicity or race, although some people use it that way. According to Weber (1968) in Crepeau et al. (2003), ethnic groups are those which "entertain a subjective belief in their common descent because of similarities of physical type, or of customs, or both, or because of memories of colonization and migration" (p. 83).

  Race—According to McGruder (2003), both race and ethnicity are socially constructed categories, concepts agreed on in public and private discourse that can only be understood in the context of the history of their use at a specific time and place. Neither ethnicity nor race have a biological basis. Groups categorized by skin color (blacks), linguistics (Hispanics), or religion (Jews) have been shown to be more biologically diverse and heterogeneous than homogeneous. In other words, there are no common racial characteristics that can be validated statistically. Yet, as McGruder points out, the categories are psychologically and socially real. In every corner of the globe, humans are denied or given rights and privileges based on race. Therefore, psychologically, a history of privilege or oppression within an ethnic or racial group can, to a great extent, shape one's culture.

Group Session Outline (1 of 6) (continued)

Socioeconomic status—Socioeconomic status is historically based on three factors: income, place of residence, and educational level. These three factors determine our social position within a society. To a great extent, our social position influences our values, beliefs, and view of the world. Our "class" (i.e., lower, middle, or upper income level) often determines the material resources and opportunities available to us, and to our clients (Sussenburger, 2003). Persons might be upwardly mobile, in relation to their parents, or downwardly mobile, as might be the result of illness or other life events. Social status has a profound effect on a person's attitudes and beliefs and shapes culture in ways of which he or she might not be aware or cannot easily explain.

While speaking about issues of culture is socially acceptable, issues of ethnicity, race, and social status are often not acceptable topics of discussion in polite society. Therefore, one of the goals of this group is to recognize the sensitive nature of these issues and to explore our own backgrounds and attitudes, so that we will not offend our clients unintentionally by making assumptions about them based on our own cultural baggage.

We will begin this process by first developing cultural awareness (i.e., the exploration and recognition of our own cultural uniqueness).

Before we begin, are there any questions or comments members would like to share?

2. Activity:

"The worksheet you will fill out is called My Cultural Heritage. (Hand out Worksheet 13-2 and pencils). You will trace your ancestry for three generations, using a method called a genogram (McGoldrick & Gerson, 1985). On the worksheet diagram, triangles represent males, circles represent females. You will first identify yourself as either a circle (if you are female) or a triangle (if you are male) at the bottom of the diagram. Write your name in the circle or triangle. You may draw additional triangles or circles for your brothers and sisters, and write their names also. Spaces for your parents and grandparents are labeled. Follow the instructions written on the worksheet for additional information about each ancestor. Then, on the reverse side of the worksheet, write the answers to the questions outlined on the bottom of the sheet. Feel free to add information that you think is meaningful or important to share. For example, if someone's parents or grandparents are divorced, you might want to add a stepmother or stepfather or an additional set of grandparents. If any of your grandparents have died, you can add a date of death and perhaps a cause of death. You have 20 minutes to complete the worksheet. Any questions? May I have a volunteer paraphrase these instructions?"

3. Sharing:

When time is up, collect pencils. Ask for a volunteer to begin sharing. In the interest of time, members should restrict their sharing to facts that have special meaning for them. Other ways to limit sharing might be to choose the relative that had the most influence on a member's cultural identity. Questions on the back should be discussed one at a time.

4. Processing:
   - How did it feel to create the three-generation genogram?
   - What was hard for you? What was easy?
   - How did it feel to share information about your family with the group?
   - What questions do members have about each other's families or culture?

5. Generalizing:
   - What are some things members have in common?
   - What are some cultural differences?
   - What did you learn about culture from doing this activity?
   - What did you learn about each other?

My Cultural Heritage

Directions: Create a three-generation genogram using the diagram below (McGoldrick & Gerson, 1985). Write each person's name, date of birth, and primary occupation on the diagram.

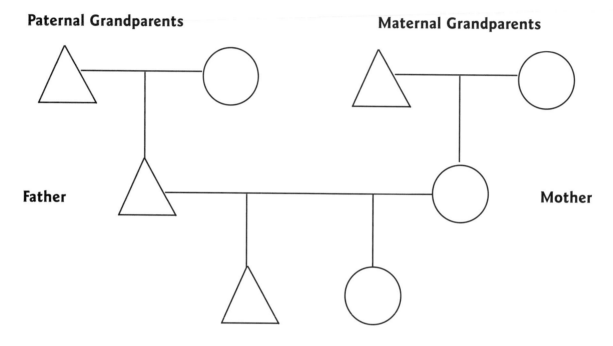

Paternal Grandparents   **Maternal Grandparents**

Father   **Mother**

You and your brothers and sisters (add circles/female or triangles/male, as needed)

List the following characteristics for parents and grandparents below: Name, place of birth, religion, special talents or abilities, and most important life achievement.

On the back of this worksheet, please answer the following questions:
- What ethnic identities do you hold?
- How are you like/unlike your parents?
- What do you believe the role of a grandparent should be?
- What values did you learn from your family about working, learning, spending money, marriage, aging, or any other significant issue?

Group Session Outline (1 of 6) (continued)

6. Application:
   - After hearing about each other's families, what do you think is unique about your own culture, that makes you different from other members?
   - What did you learn about yourself from doing this genogram?
   - How do you think your own cultural heritage affects your ability to communicate with people from cultures different from your own?
   - What are the most important values you learned from your parents/grandparents?

7. Summary:

   "May I have a volunteer to summarize our first group session?"

   Leader gives feedback to group on how well they accomplished the task.

   May give preview to next week's group topic.

   Journal entry: What cultural beliefs and values have been passed on to you from your ancestors? What is your family's socioeconomic status, and how does it affect your own beliefs and expectations of yourself?

Group Session Outline (2 of 6)

Group title: "Developing Cultural Competence"

Session title: "Gender Roles"

Format (90 minutes total):
Warm-up—5 minutes
Educational concepts—15 minutes
Worksheet—25 minutes
Discussion—40 minutes
Summary—5 minutes

Supplies:
Worksheets and pencils for each member, colored markers to share.
List of values for warm-up: Write on a sheet large enough for all members to read from a distance:
- A good love relationship
- Financial security
- Satisfying religious faith
- Freedom to do what I want
- Meaningful family life
- Success at my chosen career
- Excitement and adventure
- Power and fame

Description:
1. Introduction:

Warm-up—Each member states name and chooses one of the values on the list that has special meaning for him or her. Members tell group why the value they chose is important for them.

Educational concepts—"Cultural awareness refers to our knowledge of our own culture. What values and beliefs do we hold, and how do we define what is ordinary for us? One way to organize our thinking about what we value is to define the life roles we play. Mary Reilly used roles such as worker, housewife, student, player, and retiree to provide conceptual structure for occupational therapy's theory and practice (Jackson, 1998). Each role we play has tasks or occupations associated with it, and thus serves to define our occupational patterns or lifestyles. Furthermore, roles imply both an intrinsic and an extrinsic perspective. Roles are the parts that people play in a larger social system. One's role in a family, for example, might be a son or daughter, a spouse, a caregiver, or a breadwinner. The role carries with it not only occupational choices for the individual, but social expectations as well. The tasks of a caregiver might be to feed, clothe, or comfort a young child or an aging parent. These occupations have meaning for both the caregiver and the recipient of care. Thus, role theory takes into account the social and cultural contexts within which occupations are performed.

"Role expectations are the rules and the enabling and constraining forces defined by cultures in specific social situations. For example, what are the role expectations of a group leader?" Comments from members can be processed. "Some expectations might be to set the boundaries of time and place, to provide structure, or to allow members to have choices about the topics discussed or group activities. In fact, each of you may have different expectations of a leader. Your expectations of me will have a great deal to do with your own cultural beliefs about how a good group leader should behave. Because I understand this fact, that each of you comes to the group with a different cultural perspective, I will be careful not to judge you and not be too offended if you criticize my leadership. If this were a client group, I would need to take their cultural perspectives into account also. To do otherwise would be culturally insensitive.

Group Session Outline (2 of 6) (continued)

"Role identification occurs when a role is internalized. We see ourselves as students, workers, or family members because we see ourselves occupying these social positions and performing the occupations associated with these roles (Kielhofner, 2002).

"Role theory helps to explain a few problems with occupational performance. Role conflict occurs when a person takes on overlapping roles and finds him- or herself having to choose between meeting one role expectation or another. The mother who is called home from work to care for a sick child is an example of a role conflict. She must either ignore the sick child or leave her work undone. Role overload can occur when a person takes on more roles than he or she can handle. Some of you might know people who work night and day, yet never seem to be able to meet all of the obligations demanded by their multiple social roles.

"Roles can provide scripts that define our social interactions and behaviors. For example, our occupations, mode of dress, and style of interaction will be different when we are at work than when we are home with our families. Role confusion can occur when you and your spouse start a business together or when your boss invites you out for dinner.

"How are roles related to values or to culture? The answer to that question is different for each individual. Each of us chooses roles which are meaningful for us, or which we perceive as helping us achieve valued goals. For example, why are all of you currently in the role of a student?" May process answers from members. "Because you perceive that role as a stepping stone to achieving the status of a professional. Roles help us organize and sequence the occupations we need to perform in order to achieve a higher social status.

"To illustrate, during our warm-up, some of you chose a meaningful family life as an important value for you. What roles do you play relative to that value?" May process comments from members. "You might show your appreciation to your parents for paying for your college education by studying hard and getting good grades in your courses. That is what a good son or daughter should do, right?" Discuss.

"Our cultural background shapes our perceptions of the roles we choose and our own expectations of how those roles should be enacted."

2. Activity:

"Today, we will explore one type of role, gender roles. Beliefs about the roles of males and females have been instilled in most of us from when we were very young. The toys we are given to play with, for example, might be seen as early lessons preparing us for our roles as adults. That is the topic of today's worksheet." Pass out Worksheet 13-3 and pencils. "Please follow the instructions written on the top. You may use colored markers for your drawings. No one needs to be an artist, but please don't draw a stick figure. We will have an opportunity to explain our drawings during our discussion. You have 25 minutes to complete the worksheets."

3. Sharing:

Ask for a volunteer to start. Pictures and information in the boxes may be discussed during the first go around. Answers to essay questions should be shared one at a time, with discussion and interaction on each separate topic. Facilitator should take care to allow each member to answer each question. This could take up to half the time allotted for discussion.

4. Processing:
   - How did it feel to share your drawings?
   - Which was easier, drawing or writing?
   - What did you feel about each other's drawings and comments?
   - How do you feel you measure up to your ideal (woman or man)?

5. Generalizing:
   - What are some of the lessons learned from today's activity?
   - What are some ways that different cultures define the roles of men vs. women?

Worksheet 13-3

Gender Role

Directions: Use pencil and/or markers to draw an ideal man and ideal woman in the space provided. Then answer the essay questions below and on the back of the worksheet.

Draw an ideal man	Draw an ideal woman
Describe some characteristics of your ideal man:	Describe some characteristics of your ideal woman:
What are the roles of men in your family?	What are the roles of women in your family?
Describe a typical day for your father:	Describe a typical day for your mother:

1. How are you similar to your parent of the same gender? How are you different?
2. How have gender roles in your family affected your own roles and expectations of yourself? Who else has provided major role/gender identification for you?
3. What did your parents tell you a good girl always does? Never does?
4. What did your parents tell you a good boy always does? Never does?
5. How well have you followed your parents' advice? What happens when you do not?
6. As a child, were you treated differently because you were female/male? Give some examples.
7. What are some cultural stereotypes regarding gender role?
8. What are some actual male/female differences vs. myths?
9. Compare the status of men and women in your own culture with that of other cultures.
10. How does gender affect career choices and opportunities for power or leadership?

Group Session Outline (2 of 6) (continued)

- What occupations are required by the roles each of us holds?
- How are role expectations different according to gender in the following examples: parent, military personnel, authority figure, athlete, corporate executive?
- In addition to gender, what other roles are defined by culture? Give some examples.
- What is the relationship between culture, roles, and occupations?

6. Application
   - Why might understanding gender roles be important when working with clients?
   - Which gender is more likely to provide caregiving?
   - How do gender roles influence the occupations we enable our clients in doing?
   - How does gender affect our role as an occupational therapist?
   - What can we do to learn about our client's values and beliefs about gender?
   - What are some gender differences in the way we express emotions? Handle stress?

7. Summary

   Ask for volunteer to summarize.

   What are some new things members learned today?

   Facilitator provides feedback to members about their participation.

Group Session Outline (3 of 6)

Group title: "Developing Cultural Competence"

Session title: "Customs, Traditions, and Rituals"

Format (90 minutes total):
Warm-up—5 minutes
Educational concepts—20 minutes
Worksheet—20 minutes
Discussion—40 minutes
Summary—5 minutes

Supplies:
Worksheets and pencils, index cards for warm-up, on which the following are written:
- Introduce yourself to a potential employer.
- Introduce yourself to a new client.
- Greet your best friend from home who has come to visit for the weekend.
- Say hello to someone of the opposite sex at a singles bar.
- Greet your grandmother at her home when you arrive for Thanksgiving dinner.
- Greet your doctor at his office.
- Introduce yourself to a stranger seated next to you on an airplane or train.
- Greet your sister or brother the day after the two of you have had a heated argument.

Description:
1. Introduction:

Warm-up—Each member draws an index card. Ask members to stand and greet the person to their right, according to the role play situation on the card they have drawn.

Educational concepts—"Today we're going to explore some of the more subtle aspects of culture. As you observed in the warm-up, even the simple act of greeting one another is bound by social rules applying to different situations. These expectations are based on our culture.

"Ethnocentrism refers to the lack of understanding or appreciation of another culture. It is rooted in the belief that one's own way of life is superior. For example, someone might visit a foreign country and be offended that they do not speak English or they do not accept the American dollar (Hasselkus, 2002). Who has traveled to a foreign country? What were some of your thoughts and experiences regarding cultural differences?" Members' comments may be processed. "Even within the United States, there are differences between north and south, east and west. For example, how is a "southerner" different from a "Connecticut Yankee"? Or a Kansas farmer different from a "New Yorker"? Who is from another part of the United States?" Discuss. "Cultural sensitivity assumes a certain level of cultural awareness. The first step is to become aware that our own ways of doing things are not the only way and may not even be the best way. Perhaps there are things that other cultures do better than ours. We need to move away from the position of egocentrism and adjust our attitude about another person's culture. McGruder (2003) defines cultural sensitivity as a 'readiness to explore other cultures non-judgmentally.'"

Group Session Outline (3 of 6) (continued)

"One aspect of culture that is easily recognized and communicated is tradition. *Webster's Dictionary* (1992) defines a tradition as 'a long-established or inherited way of thinking or acting.' Traditions may be passed on to you by your families or by others of your culture. Organized religions are often said to embody traditions regarding the celebration of holidays (holy days). These religious rituals have been expanded and interpreted by many subcultures. For example, how a Christian family celebrates Christmas might have many variations depending upon which nationality or branch of Christianity one belongs to. Life events like weddings, baptisms, and funerals also differ according to the religious beliefs of one's culture.

"*Webster's Dictionary* defines a custom as 'a habitual practice; the usual way of acting in given circumstances... applied to an individual or a community... reinforced by traditions and social attitudes.' Hasselkus (2002) tells us that 'social rules for behavior in our everyday lives are part of the shared beliefs and shared webs of significance that make up our culture' (p. 47). She uses a kindergarten classroom as an example of defined social norms as to behaviors that are acceptable and not acceptable. Kindergarten children quickly learn to conform to the expectations of the teacher. What are some customs that affect your behavior in this classroom? How do we address each other? What would happen if... (add an unacceptable behavior)?

"Customs often define our choices and preferences and how we react to different contexts. For example, the foods we eat and how we eat them are defined by our culture. What do some of you consider appropriate foods for breakfast? While traveling in Europe, I noticed that the buffet breakfasts served at our hotel included many cheeses, cold cuts, and varieties of fish. In the southern United States, grits may be a common addition to a traditional breakfast. Customs can become so automatic that they can influence us in ways that we are not aware. For example, what do you say when someone sneezes? What do you say when someone accidentally bumps into you?

"Customary behaviors may be organized into routines, habits, and rituals. Hasselkus (2002) uses these three words to describe the repetitive, predictable patterns of behavior in daily life (p. 49). Habits and rituals offer stability to an otherwise chaotic existence. Clark (2000) makes a distinction between habits and routines. Habits are 'relatively automatic things a person thinks or does repeatedly,' while routines are 'higher-order habit(s) that involve sequencing and combining processes' and are related to specific outcomes. Rituals, although characterized by repetition like habits and routines, have the added feature of 'drama, symbolism, and meaning-centeredness' (Crepeau, 1995, in Hasselkus, 2002). In other words, what makes a ritual different from a habit or routine is its meaning.

"In order to begin to explore cultures different from our own, I'm going to ask you to share some of the cultural differences represented right here in this room. All of us come from somewhat different cultures. Let's explore some ways that our cultures might differ from each other by sharing some of our customs, traditions, and rituals."

2. Activity:

   Hand out Worksheet 13-4 and pencils. "You have 20 minutes to answer the questions on this worksheet. Some have choices and some do not, so please read the questions carefully. We will be sharing our answers with the group."

3. Sharing:

   Ask for a volunteer to start. Go in order around the group sharing one category at a time. Allow members to ask each other questions at the end of sharing in each category.

4. Processing:

   Questions for group discussion:

   • How did you feel about answering these questions about your culture?

   • What feelings did you have about sharing your answers?

Worksheet 13-4
Customs, Traditions, and Rituals

Directions: Please take the next 20 minutes to answer some of the questions in each category as specified. Do not skip any categories. You may continue on the back of the sheet or use additional sheets as needed.

Customs (choose 1)

- How does your family typically celebrate a favorite holiday? Choose a specific holiday and give details.
- How are birthdays celebrated in your family? Describe your most memorable birthday celebration.

Rituals (choose 1)

- Describe one daily ritual that has meaning for you. How did you get started doing this, and what are some symbolic meanings connected with this ritual?
- What task do you routinely do for/with someone else? What does this act symbolize?

Traditions (choose 1)

- What is your religion? How do you practice this religion?
- Describe the customs and rituals connected with one of the following in your culture: a wedding, a death in the family, or the birth of a child.

Subtleties

- How do you express anger, joy, grief? Give an example of each.
- How did you learn to do or say these things? Which are cultural vs. individual?

Group Session Outline (3 of 6) (continued)

- Does anyone want to ask the leader some questions? (Answer them.)
- How do you feel about other member responses to what you shared?
- What was hardest/easiest about doing the worksheet?

5. Generalizing:
   - What did you learn about culture from today's activity?
   - How would you define your own culture as compared with others in the group?
   - What do members have in common? What are some differences you observed?
   - What different cultures are represented in this group? (List them.)

6. Application:
   - How do traditions, customs, and rituals define a person's behavior?
   - How do traditions, customs, and/or rituals help persons in times of crisis?
   - What customs or traditions are liberating for you. Which are burdensome?
   - Which of your personal attitudes about these aspects of culture have changed? How?

7. Summary:

   Ask members to summarize.

   Thank members for their honesty and self-disclosures.

   Encourage members to write further thoughts in their journal entries.

   Next week: outsiders vs. insiders.

   Journal entry: What customs, traditions, and/or rituals have you experienced in your own family (holidays, special foods, etc.)? In practicing your religion (marriage, baptism, funerals, etc.)? What do you like about these traditions? What is their meaning for you? What social purpose do they serve for those of your culture?

   From today's exercise, what can you say about the cultural differences of members?

Session Outline (4 of 6)

Group title: "Developing Cultural Competence"

Session title: "Diversity Collage"

Format (90 minutes total):
    Warm-up—5 minutes
    Educational concepts—15 minutes
    Collage—30 minutes
    Discussion—35 minutes
    Summary—5 minutes

Supplies:
- Stack of assorted magazines (two per person) to share
- The following for each member:
- Scissors
- Glue stick
- 12 x 18 inch white paper
- Pencil
- Set of 8 colored markers

Description:
1. Introduction:

    Warm-up—Members seated around a large table extend one hand, palm down, toward the center of the table so that hands and arms resemble the spokes of a wheel. Middle fingers may touch in the center. Each member states name and answers the following question: "What features makes your own hand/arm distinctive and unique?" Members may consider skin, size, shape, and decorative features such as nail polish, jewelry, and clothing. A short discussion may follow in which members comment on each other's responses.

    Educational concepts—"Today's topic is diversity. The warm-up exercise highlighted only a few ways that people can be different from each other. What are some other ways that people are diverse? (List on board.) Wells and Black (2000) refer to diversity as the varied national or ethnic backgrounds of U. S. citizens and also categories of class, gender, age, ability, and sexual orientation. Health status may be added to this list of ways people differ.

    "People sometimes feel uncomfortable when they talk about issues of diversity. That may be because we have learned that we should be politically correct (PC). This term became popular around 1990 and is defined as "a set of ideas, concerns, principles, and directives that stress social non-oppressiveness, inclusiveness, and sensitivity to diverse groups of people" (Herbst, 1997, p. 183). The focus of correctness is to limit sexist, racist, or otherwise offensive language when discussing diversity issues. Language is one way that people convey elitist attitudes about nondominant groups in society.

Session Outline (4 of 6) (continued)

But there is a problem with always being politically correct. It teaches us to be color-blind. Has anyone heard this term? (May process comments from members.) We are not talking about an inability to see red and green traffic lights. Rather, it comes from the directive that we must treat everyone the same and to minimize our awareness of diversity. But is everyone the same? Of course not. That's why we've taken so much time doing exercises to make you more aware of your own culture. If we are to become culturally competent, culture cannot be invisible to us. So today, in this group, let's leave political correctness on the other side of the door. Race and skin color are not topics to avoid; they are two of many aspects of culture that we can learn to explore and appreciate. Let us acknowledge how people are different, without stereotypes or prejudice.

The context in which we hear about things like race or skin color usually involves some incidence of discrimination. Discrimination is the action resulting from stereotyping and prejudice. Prejudice is defined as "an erroneous judgment, usually negative, which is based on incomplete or faulty information. Any preconceived opinion or feeling, either favorable or unfavorable. Unreasonable feelings, opinions, or attitudes, especially of a hostile nature, directed against any group of persons" (Wells & Black, 2000, p. 283). Does prejudice apply only to race? What might be some prejudices regarding fat people, old people, crazy people, or homeless people? (May process comments from members.)

Stereotyping involves putting people into categories based on some external or perceived characteristic (e.g., "Old people can't drive" or "White men can't jump"). Categorization is the brain's natural tendency to sort out information to facilitate storage and retrieval. It is useful to categorize much of what we learn, so that we can cluster information about different topics, and remember it when we take a test or have an intelligent conversation. But when it comes to people, we should try to refrain from categorizing them too quickly. If we are to become culturally competent, we must remind ourselves that each person, whether friend, potential client, or associate, is an individual.

While prejudice and stereotyping are attitudes, discrimination is a social action. Discriminatory actions may be individual (choice of friends), community level (racial profiling by local police), or national level (better health care for those with private insurance). Most people in American society would say that discrimination is not a good thing. Yet in many ways we tolerate discrimination by looking the other way. One of our objectives for this group is to heighten our sensitivity to discriminatory acts at every level of society. The first step in reaching that sensitivity is to become aware of our own unacknowledged prejudices and stereotypes and those we have observed in our communities and in society.

2. Activity:

"Today's activity may be difficult for you if you have been taught to be politically correct. But acknowledging the prejudices and stereotypes held by many mainstream Americans is a necessary step in developing cultural sensitivity. I'm going to ask you to be honest in constructing a diversity collage from pictures you find in these magazines. You'll need to examine the social attitudes you have observed, both in others and within yourself, and to think about the stereotypes and labels that might be given to diverse groups of people." Hand out scissors, glue sticks, paper, pencils, and sets of markers; place stack of magazines in the center of the table.

"There are four steps to this task:

a. Find six pictures in these magazines of persons who are different from yourself in some way. Think about the list we made earlier about the ways in which people differ. Cut out the pictures and glue them onto the paper, leaving space to write under each one.

b. Make up a name for each picture, and write it with a marker.

Session Outline (4 of 6) (continued)

    c. List under each name, four or five adjectives, labels, or stereotypes that might be given to that person by society. Here is where I'm asking you to put aside political correctness and acknowledge the possibility of stereotypes and prejudice. What you write down does not necessarily represent your own attitudes, and we will need to agree as group that members are not to judge each other by what we write down. You may use pencil to write your list, so that you can change your mind without worry.

    d. Lastly, write three questions you might like to ask this person about their culture. Remember, not everyone is aware of their culture as we know by now you are. Be subtle in the wording of your questions, and make them reflect an open, nonjudgmental curiosity. Try to use open questions that cannot be answered by "yes" or "no."

    You have 30 minutes to complete your collage, labels, and questions."

3. Sharing:

    Ask for a volunteer to start. Members explain their collages to the group, including names and list of characteristics. In a separate go-around, each member may choose one picture for which to read their questions and discuss their reasons for asking them.

4. Processing:
  - How did it feel to do this collage?
  - What parts were hard? Easy?
  - What internal barriers did you discover when naming and labeling the pictures?
  - How did you feel about writing questions?
  - How did you perceive other members responded to your collage?
  - What was it like to share your collage with the group?
  - What feelings do you have about my asking you to do something like this?

5. Generalizing:
  - What types of diversity did the collages represent? (List.)
  - What common themes did you see?
  - What common feelings did members express about doing the collage?
  - What are some differences among the collages?
  - What parts of this exercise affected you the most?
  - What might be some reasons for doing a diversity collage?
  - What did you learn about yourself?
  - What did you learn about other members?

6. Application:
  - What does your collage reveal about you personally?
  - How has this exercise raised your awareness of your own attitudes toward diverse groups? How has it raised your awareness of the attitudes of others?
  - Which diverse groups interest you the most? Least?
  - What persons in your own life are similar to those represented in your collage?
  - What experiences have you had interacting with someone who is different from yourself?

7. Summary:

    Ask for volunteers to summarize. Thank members for their honesty. Remind members of confidentiality and not to disclose the content of the group to others outside the group. Members write their names on collages; collect collages and keep for further discussion.

    Journal entry: Discuss your feelings about today's activity. What might be some reasons for these feelings? What labels have been applied to you or someone you love? Tell about one experience you have had with someone of another culture.

Group Session Outline (5 of 6)

Group title: "Developing Cultural Competence"

Session title: "Insider vs. Outsider"

Format (90 minutes total):
   Warm-up—5 minutes
   Educational concepts—15 minutes
   Activity—20 minutes
   Sharing—5 minutes
   Discussion—40 minutes
   Summary—5 minutes

Supplies:
- Adhesive tape
- Scissors
- Index (3 x 5 inches) with the following labels written in large letters: Blame Me, Protect Me, Laugh at Me, Put Me Down, Worship Me, Ignore Me, Fear Me, Listen to Me, Call Me Stupid, Agree with Me. These labels should be kept out of sight until they are anonymously taped by the leader on members' heads.
- Clipboard with pad and pencil

Description:
1. Introduction:
   Warm-up—Members stand in tight circle, arm to arm. Members take turns being "odd man out" and from outside the circle, physically try to break in. The game ends when each member has successfully broken into the group. Briefly discuss strategies used by members to "break in" vs. "keep out."

   Educational concepts—Everyone wants or needs to be accepted. We first seek acceptance by the people around us, our family, our friends, our neighbors, our classmates. Acceptance generally means matching our own behavior to the behavior of the other members of the group to which we wish to belong. As the song says, everyone wants to be "in with the in-crowd." Sometimes being an insider is a good thing, and sometimes it isn't. What might be some reasons being an "insider" is good? What might be some reasons not to belong? (May process member comments.)

   You may be familiar with Abraham Maslow's (1968) hierarchy of needs, which are:

   a. Physiological
   b. Safety
   c. Belonging and love
   d. Self-esteem
   e. Self-actualization

   Belonging is the third greatest human need after safety and is equal in importance to love needs. According to Schutz (1958), a child's need for inclusion is initially met by his or her family. This early acceptance (or rejection) forms the basis for later behaviors with regard to inclusion or exclusion from social groups.

Group Session Outline (5 of 6) (continued)

On a societal level, Wells and Black (2000) define inclusion as the "belief that all individuals should be able to participate fully in activities of life with the same benefits and opportunities"(p. 164). This value is consistent with the philosophy and ethical principles of occupational therapy. The National Association for Multicultural Education (NAME)(2003) views the multicultural approach as "a philosophical concept built on ideals of freedom, justice, equity, and human dignity... (which are) attitudes and values necessary for a democratic society." The stated purpose of NAME is to challenge all forms of discrimination in schools and society through the promotion of democratic principles of social justice.

Why do you think we need a national association to wipe out discrimination? Who is being discriminated against in this country? (May process member comments.) Minority groups in this country might be thought of as African American, Native American, Hispanic, and others. What is the difference between a minority group and a nondominant group? (May process member comments.) What is the dominant group in the United States? Domination has to do with the unequal distribution of power. McIntosh (1998) states that "white privilege is like an invisible weightless knapsack of special provisions: assurances, tools, guides, codebooks, passports, visas, clothes, a compass, emergency gear, and blank checks" (p. 104). Wells and Black (2000) call this an "unearned privilege" that results from simply being born into a dominant group. What do you think about this statement? Is it true? (May process member comments.) How do you think white people feel about this? Wells and Black suggest that white people in positions of authority (e.g., teachers) have an obligation to promote the following goals:

- Respect human rights for all diverse peoples
- Promote the strengths and values of cultural diversity
- Accept alternate lifestyle choices for people
- Promote social justice and opportunity for all
- Attempt to equalize power among all ethnic groups

What do you think might be some special obligations for occupational therapists with regard to these goals?

2. Activity:

Imagine that you are creating the rules, regulations, policies, and procedures for an exclusive club to which only people exactly like you can belong. As a group, your goal is to make a list of 10 qualifications members must meet in order to be eligible. Does everyone understand the task? (May process questions and clarify, but don't give any specific advice.)

To add a bit more challenge, I'm going to give each of you a label, which I will tape to your forehead so the rest of the group can easily see it. You will see everyone else's label, but not your own. After the group completes its task, we will each try to guess what our label is. (Instructor randomly selects labels and tape to member's foreheads, taking care to make sure the words are visible but not seen by the member him- or herself.)

Do your best to role play what the labels say while you complete the group task. Please don't anyone take offense at what anyone says because we know that this is only pretend. So we can say whatever we like to each other during the next 20 minutes, without worrying about being polite. Agreed? Can everyone see each person's label? (May ask members to pin back hair or other obstructions or rearrange seating.) You have about 20 minutes to come up with your list of inclusionary qualifications. Here is a pad to record your list. (Place pad and pencil in center of the table, but don't say anything else. Stop the group after 20 minutes, whether or not they have completed the list.)

Group Session Outline (5 of 6) (continued)

3. Sharing:

    Before members remove their labels, ask for a volunteer to start guessing what their labels say. Allow discussion of feelings if this happens spontaneously. Each member can remove the card after he or she has guessed, even if the guess is incorrect.

4. Processing:
    - How did it feel to have a label?
    - How did you feel about treating each other according to the labels?
    - How did you like being asked to do this task?
    - What made it hard? Easy?
    - What feelings did you have toward each other as a result of role playing?
    - Who was left feeling badly? Why?
    - What do you need to say to each other to resolve these feelings?

5. Generalizing:
    - How did the labels affect the way you completed the task?
    - What do you think about the list you created?
    - Who did most of the work in creating the list?
    - How did you choose who would record the list?
    - What lessons did you learn from this experience?
    - How does this experience relate to being an outsider or an insider?
    - How does this experience relate to the concept of white privilege?

6. Application:
    - What are some social parallels with aspects of this experience?
    - What experiences in your own life are you reminded of?
    - What insights did you gain about yourself from this experience?
    - How can you apply this experience to your own life?

7. Summary:

    Ask for a volunteer to summarize.

    Thank members for their honesty and self-disclosures.

    Congratulate members on being able to put aside political correctness.

    Remind members to keep member disclosures confidential.

    Include members in reviewing important lessons learned.

    Next session will be the last.

Journal Entry

    Describe two experiences you have had in the recent past: one which made you feel like an "insider" and one that made you feel like an "outsider." Describe your thoughts about termination of the group. What unfinished issues would you like to discuss?

Group Session Outline (6 of 6)

Group title: "Developing Cultural Competence"

Session title: "Exploring Another Culture"

Format (90 minutes total):
Warm-up—5 minutes
Educational concepts—15 minutes
Worksheets—10 minutes
Sharing—20 minutes
Discussion—25 minutes
Pre/post test—10 minutes
Summary—5 minutes

Supplies:
• Worksheets
• Pencils
• Pre/post test copies for each member

Description:
1. Introduction:

Warm-up—Introduce yourself as if you were answering your telephone at your place of work. Explain where you work and who might be calling you there. In a second go-around, answer the phone as you would at home. How is this different from work, and why?

Educational concepts—People hold multiple cultural identities in the United States. This happens because each setting in which we perform occupations of daily life has its own set of norms, roles, and expectations, which are based on shared attitudes and beliefs. Some cultural environments may even have a unique language or a unique set of tools and equipment. Consider the differences in culture between a restaurant and hospital emergency room. How are the missions of these two workplaces different? What other differences come to mind? (May process member comments.) How does one's behavior change when entering these settings as a client? What other work cultures can members describe? (Discuss a few examples.)

What are some other cultures with which you are familiar? What is the culture of your college campus or educational setting? What are the roles people hold, and how are they defined? What religious groups do members belong to? (Discuss some examples, including physical setting, what occupations are involved, who organizes and structures meetings and how, what are the traditions and/or rituals, and what is their meaning?)

How do people begin to learn about an unfamiliar culture? The process involves taking the risk of leaving one's own cultural comfort zone and a willingness to become the numerical minority. Traveling to another country might be one way of doing this. What other countries have members visited? (May discuss member comments.) What cultural conflicts did you encounter while traveling? What happens if you enter an environment where you don't speak the same language? How do you feel when others can't understand you? This experience may give you some empathy for clients who do not understand your questions on an evaluation or who ask you questions that you don't understand.

Group Session Outline (6 of 6) (continued)

Empathy may be defined as "a way of seeing with the eyes of others, to appreciate their views of the world" (Egan, 2001). Rogers (1975) writes of empathy, "It means entering the private world of the other and becoming thoroughly at home in it... it means temporarily living in his or her life, moving about in it delicately without making judgments." Earlier we defined cultural sensitivity as a readiness to explore the cultures of others nonjudgmentally. Empathy is one way of developing an understanding of a person from another culture. As professionals, we may communicate empathy by identifying the feelings clients express both verbally and nonverbally. But Peloquin (2003) states that true empathy transcends procedures, calling it "not a fusion with the pain of another, but a connection with the person of another" (p. 159).

Developing empathy means taking certain risks. Rogers (1975) writes that "In some sense it means that you lay aside your self, and this can only be done by a person who is secure enough in himself that he knows he will not get lost in what may turn out to be the strange and bizarre world of the other" (p. 3). As professionals, we never know what the world may look like through the eyes of our clients. That is why we need to be aware of our own multiple cultures, whatever they may be, before attempting to explore cultures unfamiliar to us. This is another way of saying we need to be comfortable with ourselves, with who we are. Cultural awareness strengthens our own identity and sense of self and therefore, gets us ready to be open to others.

Cultural sensitivity includes the quality of empathy for individuals who are different from ourselves. A related concept from Carl Rogers (1961) is nonjudgmental acceptance; the client is accepted for the human being that he or she is, regardless of his or her feelings or behaviors. Our responses to clients need to be both respectful and genuine. These are not techniques we learn as therapists, they are attitudes we may need to work hard to develop. Because if we have not done the work of examining ourselves and recognizing our own biases, our verbal and nonverbal behaviors may communicate our prejudices to clients without our realizing it. All of the client-centered concepts discussed in Chapter 3 apply in forming therapeutic relationships with our clients, regardless of their cultural differences. According to McGruder (2003), "Looking for culture through careful observation of and interaction with others coupled with introspection of self enables the establishment of accurate empathy between practitioner and client" (p. 94).

Egan (2001) describes a way of communicating empathy by first identifying the feeling being expressed and then summarizing the situation that is perceived to have caused it. The primary accurate empathy statement essentially entails filling in the blanks in the following sentence: "You feel _____ because _____" (see Chapter 3). For example, if I'm rushing in to this meeting late and out of breath, and I tell you I've just come from a very intense meeting, how might you communicate empathy for me using this format? (May process answers from members). Perhaps you'd say "You feel distressed (tense/upset) because of something that happened in the meeting you just left." That kind of statement would tell me several things. It would tell me you didn't judge me negatively because I was late, which would be a relief. It would also tell me that you would be open to hearing about what I might be distressed or upset about. This is how an expression of empathy builds trust between you and your client. You are not only reflecting back your understanding but also your caring and concern for him or her. This opens the door for deeper, more meaningful communication.

The activity for today was designed to help us practice exploring each others' cultures in ways that show respect, genuineness, empathy, and nonjudgmental acceptance. We will role play asking questions and responding to each other, and we will examine the messages we convey about our own hidden biases or our openness and empathy with one of our peers.

Worksheet 13-5
Cultural Identities

Name at least three cultural identities you currently hold (educational, work, religious, recreational, community, family, alternate family, social activist, ethnic, etc.):

1.

2.

3.

Choose one specific identity to describe in depth:

Name of setting:

Purpose or mission:

Physical setting:

Social/occupational roles:

Norms or rules of social conduct:

Power structure (who is in charge, what is the hierarchy):

Tools and equipment, dress codes, and special vocabulary:

Rituals and traditions and their meaning:

Any other culturally meaningful factors:

From Cole, M. B. *Group dynamics in occupational therapy: The theoretical basis and practice application of group intervention* (3rd ed.). Thorofare, NJ: SLACK Incorporated. © 2005 SLACK Incorporated.

Group Session Outline (6 of 6) (continued)

2. Activity:

   Today's activity has two parts: a worksheet and a role-play exercise. First, we will describe one of several cultures with which we identify. (Pass out Worksheet 13-5 and pencils.) These will be briefly shared, and the group may decide which culture to explore as a group. One of you will then become the "client," while the other group members ask questions and/or express empathy while exploring the culture you have briefly described. You have 10 minutes to complete the worksheets.

3. Sharing:

   Ask for a volunteer to start, and each member describes one cultural identity. We will choose one cultural identity to explore as a group. Which one interests you most? (Can take several suggestions, and then take a vote).

   Members take turns asking questions to learn more about the culture of the member chosen. Allow this process to continue for about 10 minutes.

4. Processing:

   First ask person chosen to role play:
   - How did it feel to be asked all these questions?
   - Which questions made you feel most accepted?
   - Which questions were hardest to answer?

   Then ask group members:
   - Which questions might have implied judgment or bias? Why?
   - How did members feel about each other's questioning style?
   - What made this activity hard? Easy?
   - How do members feel about not being chosen to role play?

5. Generalizing:
   - What questions demonstrate genuine curiosity?
   - How does the language we use convey our attitude?
   - How did members convey empathy?
   - What nonverbal messages did you observe during the role play?
   - What level of understanding did you achieve about the chosen culture?
   - How is this culture different from your own?
   - What can you learn from doing an exercise like this?

6. Application:
   - What did you learn about your own style of asking questions?
   - What did you avoid asking? Why?
   - Which questions taught you the most about cultural sensitivity?
   - How culturally sensitive do you think you are?
   - What feedback can you give each other about respectfulness, genuineness, and nonjudgmental acceptance during the role play?
   - Why do you need to practice your skills in exploring other cultures?
   - Where in your own life can you apply this exercise?

   Pre/post test:

   Since this is the last session, we will take a short post-test. If you don't finish it in the next 10 minutes, you may have extra time after the session ends. The reason for doing it now is to become aware of what we have learned from all six sessions. This knowledge may contribute to our summarizing all six sessions. (10-minute limit.)

Group Session Outline (6 of 6) (continued)

7. Summary:

What are some lessons you have learned since this group began?

What activities were most meaningful to you? Least meaningful?

What feelings do members wish to share about our time together?

What are some ways you might apply the lessons you learned?

Thank members for their participation.

Congratulate members on their trust, self-disclosure, and openness with each other.

Final journal entry (collect journals after completed): Describe any feelings you have about ending the group. What were the most meaningful parts of this group for you? What parts didn't work so well for you? What changes would you suggest, and why?

End note: This group could be enhanced by incorporating field trips, travel, or volunteer experiences that bring members into contact with different cultures. The focus of the preceding group activities is on self-awareness and cultural awareness. Developing sensitivity is expected to be an ongoing process.

Bibliography

Clark, F. A. (2000). The concepts of habit and routine: A preliminary theoretical synthesis. *Occupational Therapy Journal of Research, 20*(Suppl.), 1235-1375

Crepeau, E., Cohn, E., & Boyt Schell, B. (2003). *Willard & Spackman's occupational therapy* (10th ed.). Philadelphia: Lippincott, Williams & Wilkins.

Egan, G. (2001). *The skilled helper: A problem management and opportunity development approach to helping.* Monterrey, CA: Wadsworth Publishing.

Evans, J. (1992). What OT's can do to eliminate racial barriers to health care access. *American Journal of Occupational Therapy, 46*(8), 679-683.

Hasselkus, B. (2002). *The meaning of everyday occupation.* Thorofare, NJ: SLACK Incorporated.

Herbst, P. H. (1997). *The color of words: An encyclopedic dictionary of ethnic bias in the United States.* Yarmouth, ME: Intercultural Press.

Jackson, J. (1998). Contemporary criticisms of role theory. *Journal of Occupational Science, 5,* 49-55.

Kielhofner, G. (2002). *A model of human occupation: Theory and application* (3rd ed.). Baltimore: Lippincott, Williams & Wilkins.

Krefting, L. (1992). Strategies for the development of occupational therapy in the third world. *American Journal of Occupational Therapy, 46*(8), 758-761.

Krefting, L., & Krefting, D. (1991). Cultural influences on performance. In C. Christiansen & C. Baum (Eds.), *Occupational therapy: Overcoming human performance deficits* (pp. 101-124). Thorofare, NJ: SLACK Incorporated.

Maslow, A. H. (1968). *Toward a psychology of being* (Rev. ed.). New York: Van Nostrand Reinhold.

McGoldrick, M., & Gerson, R. (1985). *Genograms in family assessment.* New York: W. W. Norton & Company, Inc.

McGruder, J. (2003). Culture, race, ethnicity, and other forms of human diversity. In E. Crepeau, E. Cohn, & B. Boyt Schell (Eds.), *Willard & Spackman's Occupational Therapy* (10th ed.). Philadelphia: Lippincott, Williams & Wilkins.

McIntosh, P. (1998). *White privilege and male privilege: A personal account of coming to see correspondencies through work in women's studies. Working paper No. 189.* Wellsley, MA: Wellsley College Center for Research on Women.

National Association for Multicultural Education. (2003). www.nameorg.org. Accessed November 19, 2004. Washington, DC: Author.

Peloquin, S. (2003). The therapeutic relationship: Manifestations and challenges in occupational therapy. In Crepeau, E., Cohn, E., & Boyt Schell, B. (Eds.), *Willard & Spackman's Occupational Therapy* (10th ed.). Philadelphia: Lippincott, Williams & Wilkins.

Rogers, C. (1961). *On becoming a person.* Boston: Houghton Mifflin.

Rogers, C. (1975). Empathic: An unappreciated way of being. *The Counseling Psychologist, 5*(2), 2-9.

Schutz, W. (1958). The interpersonal underworld. *Harvard Business Review, 36,* 123-135.

Sussenburger, B. (2003). Socioeconomic factors and their influence on occupational performance. In Crepeau, E., Cohn, E., & Boyt Schell, B. (Eds.), *Willard & Spackman's Occupational Therapy* (10th ed.). Philadelphia: Lippincott, Williams & Wilkins.

Weber, M. (1968). *Economy and society: An interpretive sociology.* (Originally published in 1922.) New York: Bedminster.

Webster's college dictionary. (1992). New York: Random House.

Wells, S., & Black, R. (2000). *Cultural competency for health professionals.* Bethesda, MD: American Occupational Therapy Association.

Appendix A

The Task-Oriented Group as a Context for Treatment

Gail S. Fidler, OTR

Abstract

Increasing recognition of the influence of man's social and cultural environment on behavior has extended the parameters of patient treatment. Such developments are manifested in the gradual melding of sociologic, psychoanalytic, and learning theories and the emerging focus on ego functions and adaptive skills. This paper explores concepts of the task-oriented group within this context, offering a definition and delineation of purpose for its use in occupational therapy as a remedial-learning experience for the schizophrenic patient.

Returning the hospitalized psychiatric patient to an acceptable productive role in the community and appreciably reducing the rate of recidivism is a complex problem. Such concern has led to intensive studies of both psychotherapeutic procedures and organizational structures of the mental hospital. The impact of sociologic inquiry into the mental hospital has been to add another dimension to our theoretical constructs regarding both individual feeling and behavior, and conditions under which such behavior may be altered to the benefit of the patient.

Understanding the significance of the social matrix in which the patient functions has brought more sharply into focus factors influencing ego function in addition to the intrapsychic and intrapersonal. As early as 1931, Harry Stack Sullivan[1] spoke of the importance of the social setting to the behavior of schizophrenic patients. Literature of the past fifteen years is replete with the investigations and analyses of the import of environment on patient functioning.[2-4] This focus has inevitably led to theoretical and practical attempts to relate concepts of ego psychology to social theories of the environment.[5,6] Such linkage, as well as the social scientist's interest in group phenomena, has given impetus to increased exploration of the many facets of group process and group therapy.

Group Process and Group Psychotherapy

Group psychotherapy is firmly established as a method of treatment for mental illness. It has its foundation in psychodynamic personality theories and emerged in America essentially from a psychoanalytic frame of reference stressing personality change through exploration of intrapsychic and interpersonal pathology believed to be at the root of conflicts and problems.[7-10] The group has been seen as a setting in which the individual, with the help of the therapist and through sharing with other members, could explore and work through those unconscious conflicts and problems which inhibited personality change and growth. Such a frame of reference places primary importance on unconscious phenomena and explores "here-and-now" feelings and behavior as a means to arriving at an awareness and understanding of intrapsychic conflict. The role of the therapist is to facilitate such awareness and elicit the involvement and help of members in exposing and working through personal conflicts and problems.

The social scientist's interest in groups emanated from a sociologic orientation rather than from personality theories. This frame of reference stresses the impact of society and the group on individual behavior and seeks to explain behavior based on the nature of the society in which a man lives. This ideology is exemplified by Lewin[11] who theorized that behavior was determined by the situation in which it occurred as well as by personality factors. The sociologist's beginning involvement with groups was via his interest in organizational structure, and this was reflected in an early focus on the use of the group to accomplish a task or to effect a change in management.[12] Such experimentation inevitably led to the development of theories regarding the use of such groups in teaching and learning.[13]

Theories and practice in the field of group dynamics have focused on the group as a dynamic force in facilitating learning and behavioral change. Emphasis on "the group" as the primary change-producing agent thus accentuates the importance of exploring the dynamic forces within the here-and-now group to both understand and facilitate such change. Group structure and membership roles become significant, and individual feeling and behavior is viewed only as it contributes to or deters from cohesive structure and contributory roles.

As the group therapist, the psychiatrist, and the social scientist work collaboratively in an attempt to resolve some of the complex problems of the mentally ill, these two seemingly disparate theories have moved closer together. There are increasing efforts to integrate not only practice of group psychotherapy and group dynamics but also the more apparently divergent concepts of each. One has but to survey current literature to be impressed with the ubiquity of these efforts.

Experimental Studies

In Social Psychology in Treating Mental Illness[14] Fairweather describes an experimental approach combining the psychodynamic doctrine of patient treatment with theories of social psychiatry, sociology, and the small group. This program focused around patient-led, small task-oriented groups for the chronic regressed schizophrenic. Such an approach, Dr. Fairweather points out, "called for an altered perception of the patient's role from that of a subordinate to that of a peer group member with responsibilities to himself and his group members, and away from that of a passive recipient within the limits of his abilities, despite existing psychopathology."[15] Tasks

around which these autonomous patient-led groups were organized concerned the current and future living of each member. Thus task levels ranged according to the capacity of the patient from personal care and ward responsibility to responsibility for vocational planning and placement. These groups provided the opportunity for patients to explore and develop their capacities for independent function, creating patient roles within the hospital which were more consistent with those of the outside community.

This study made an important contribution to patient programming and treatment. Although it concerned itself entirely with problems of the chronic regressed schizophrenic, there is much that would seem to be directly applicable to other patient categories and most certainly to patient groups in rehabilitation settings.

Marshall Edelson's experimental study[16] at the University of Oklahoma was concerned with "making possible the meaningful integration of both group experience and individual psychotherapy in an intensive treatment program designed to accomplish fundamental alteration in characterological disorder rather than solely rapid relief of acute secondary symptomatology and restoration of an ability to function marginally in the community." This work combines ego psychology and group dynamics in a therapeutic community as the basis for intensive psychotherapy. The focus of this study is aptly stated by Dr. Edelson in these words: "The therapeutic community (and small group) is organized to provide opportunities for the appearance of the patient's characterological difficulties or way of life as these are expressed in activities and other aspects of group living and for the confrontation of the patient and the group with these difficulties and their consequences to the life of the (hospital) community."

A third innovative experiment was Robert Morton's use of the laboratory method with psychiatric patients.[17] This study describes the design and use of the group process laboratory training program for hospitalized mental patients. The laboratory is a structured, small group experience designed to bring about change by establishing conditions whereby participants are forced to test their assumptions regarding interpersonal and group relations. Not only is the application of the laboratory experience to hospitalized psychiatric patients a creative innovation, but it is even more provocative to learn that they were autonomous, staff-leaderless, patient groups. Morton agrees with Fairweather that cohesive decision-making groups with psychotics cannot be explored if a professional leader is present. It is their contention that even the most permissive therapist-leader reinforces dependency for the psychotic to a detrimental extent. This experiment provides some useful and creative postulates regarding small group experiences for psychiatric patients and should stimulate further research and study in the adaptation of this technique in treatment and rehabilitation programs.

It is interesting to note that in follow-up studies on the Morton experiment only two findings seemed to be suggestive.[18] Training laboratory patients were employed a mean of 5.92 months during the nine month follow-up period whereas the group therapy patients were employed 4.70 months. In the Fairweather study, patients participating in the small-group program were significantly better than the control group in community adjustment with regard to areas of employment, verbal communication with others, and friendships.

These three experimental studies are examples of the way in which the small group is being used and adapted to meet treatment needs and essentially bridge the apparent gap between theories of individual psychodynamics and sociology.

The Task Group in Occupational Therapy

Development of task-oriented treatment groups approximately four years ago within the occupational therapy program at New York State Psychiatric Institute emanated from several not unrelated observations. First, the increasing conviction that as patients engaged in activities or created objects they expressed characterological difficulties and that attention to these problems as they emerged and were operant in the here-and-now seemed to be of benefit to the patient. The second observation was that a seemingly evident relationship between problems evidenced by the patient in his activity experiences and difficulties he encountered in the work-day world. Third, the nature of the occupational therapy setting which expects active involvement in doing, provides a microcosm of life-work situations that can be seen and explored as they occur rather than in retrospect. Fourth, recognition of the relationships between verbal skills and learning and our experience which indicated that learning and concomitant growth were enhanced when problems in doing

were identified and explored. Finally, our belief that the shared, small group experience is conducive to the exploration and amelioration of some problems in ego function.

Groups were organized with approximately eight members selected on the basis of their particular difficulties in doing and being productive as well as their readiness and need for a small group experience. All patients admitted to these early groups were male schizophrenics, and placement in a given group was determined by the level of ego function. Meetings were held three to four times a week for periods of one and one-half hours. Each group was responsible for choosing its own common task and arriving at a consensus regarding procedures for accomplishing that task.

Definition and Purpose

Task as it relates to such groups is defined as any activity or process directed toward creating or producing an end product or demonstrable service for the group as a whole and/or for persons outside of the group. Some examples of tasks chosen by these groups were: publishing a newspaper, cooking, building a playhouse for the children's service, gardening, organizing a patient council, play reading, and ward decoration and improvement.

The intent of the task-oriented group is to provide a shared working experience wherein the relationship between feeling, thinking, and behavior; their impact on others and on task accomplishment; and their productivity can be viewed and explored. Alternate patterns of functioning can be considered and tested within the context of the here-and-now, to the end that such learning may induce ego growth and improve function. Task accomplishment is not the purpose of the group but hopefully the means by which purpose is realized. It is seen as the catalytic agent which elicits behavior and interaction, brings into focus both functional capacities and limitations, facilitates collaboration in working through problems, and provides a concrete reality factor against which to measure learning and achievement. Furthermore, the task provides a frame of reference which helps to keep in focus what is relevant to explore and work through and what conflicts and issues belong more appropriately in other treatment settings. In such a group, issues and problems which directly effect the cohesiveness and/or task accomplishment are the appropriate agenda items.

Such groups are not unique in eliciting or diagnosing conflicts of the schizophrenic but it would seem that use of a common task within a small group setting does facilitate delineation of certain problems and their amelioration. Responsibility for selecting and accomplishing a task provides an opportunity for the group to explore problem-solving and decision-making skills, to have concrete evidence of their ability to function as well as to identify those expectations which give rise to conflict. The expectation that an activity needs to be chosen and implemented makes it necessary for the group to look at concepts regarding self and others that have impaired problem-solving skills and gives impetus to working toward their resolution.

The ability to perceive cause and effect relationships is a well-recognized problem of the schizophrenic, and learning in this area requires consistent, repeated opportunities to see and have evidence of cause and effect. The task-oriented group with its focus on the relationship between feelings, thinking, behavior, and task achievement thus creates excellent learning opportunities. Following through on a task procedure, the nature of doing or not doing, gives ample confirmation of cause and effect regarding behavior and function. When task responsibility must be shared, and when the nature of one's doing is viewed in terms of its contribution to the group, such learning is further amplified.

Reality testing through consensual validation is an essential process in every group and is of particular value to the schizophrenic. In addition to the shared reality indigenous to group structure and interaction, a clearly delineated task with standard procedures and techniques provides a shared reality from which perceptions can be tested and shared. Shared participation in an activity, the necessary interdependence, makes possible an objective, demonstrable assessment of one's capacities and limitations. One of the values of the task-oriented group is the consensual validation of the patients' capacity to grow and change as evidenced in the accomplishment of a task.

The need to work together, as well as talk together about one's doing, contributes to learning to conceptualize and verbalize more accurately and directly. Identification of problems in functioning, discussion of these as well as exploration of alternatives, combines feeling, behavior, and cognition and provides the necessary components of learning and change. The shared decision-making,

working experiences available in these groups and the opportunity to explore and work through problems that interfere with satisfactory function make integrated learning possible. If we are to teach new and better ways of functioning then we need to combine the patient's doing with his thinking and bring such relationships into awareness in order that he may integrate such learning.

Collaboration on a concrete, clearly defined task encourages more direct and clear communication and, coupled with group support, provides a safe area in which to practice such skills. In addition, experiences in working and sharing help the schizophrenic to begin to perceive and conceptualize his needs within the context of gratification potential with increasing awareness of his own potential for obtaining gratification rather that the expectation of rejection or frustration outside himself.

The task-oriented group, with its focus on function related to here-and-now tasks and doing their corresponding responsibilities, bears a closer resemblance to living in the outside community and provides learning which correlates more directly with those skills and expectations required in community adjustment.

It would seem useful at this time to make some distinction between these groups and verbal psychotherapy and delineate some values to the patient when both experiences are correlated. Within the task-oriented group setting, issues concerning feelings, perceptions, and behavior are discussed and explored only insofar as they are shared by others and impede or contribute to the problem-solving and/or activity accomplishment of the group. Personal, intrapsychic and historical determinants are not emphasized but are reserved for investigation in psychotherapy. Many personal and interpersonal perceptions and responses are elicited but not dealt with in the group. Psychotherapy provides an opportunity to explore these in depth, interrelating the unconscious, the historical, the personal, and the interpersonal to the here-and-now. Likewise, the task-oriented group provides a life-like action and doing setting in which insights gained in psychotherapy can be tested and consolidated through performance. The extent to which the task-oriented group and psychotherapy is correlated, the degree which the purpose of each and their relationship is understood by both staff and patients, may well determine the extent to which treatment potential will be realized.

Leadership

The role of staff leader or therapist is an important determinant in the group. The function of the leader is to facilitate a process and milieu which will be conducive to the kind of learning and growth to which these groups are directed. The role of the leader is to make learning possible and not to assume responsibility for the group. Fulfillment of objectives will depend in good measure on the leader's concepts of the mental patient and himself, as well as his skill in group and interpersonal processes.

Confidence in the inherent capacity of the group to be constructively self-determining, in its ability to ultimately recognize problems and reach realistic solutions to these, is a basic requirement. The foundation for such an attitude is belief in the right of the patient to be self-determining and a trust sufficient to allow exercise of freedom in exploring and testing his capacities. The group needs to be perceived as a therapeutic agent in its own right and leadership not as giving treatment but rather as the agent which helps to maximize the therapeutic and learning potential of the group.

It would seem that we tend to see patients as more fragile and thus needing more guidance and direction than seems warranted, at least on the basis of our experience. Perhaps this view of the patient is sustained by our need to be needed and important to the patient and to be recognized as having expertise. Autocratic leadership confirms for the patient his dependent position and tends to reaffirm his concept of self as inept and inadequate, while hesitant, aloof permissiveness increases his sense of vagueness, unpredictability and limitlessness. Jay W. Fidler[19] defines the nature and extent of leader activity as it pertains to working with groups of psychotics, emphasizing the importance of active interventions based on sensitivity and understanding of the schizophrenic's particular problems with reality testing and other ego functions.

Such understanding and attitude sets, however, are not the only basis of leadership skills for these groups. An intimate knowledge of and skill in problem-solving procedures is essential if the group is to be helped toward learning and developing such capacities. The extent to which problem-solving skills are an inherent part of the leader's way of thinking and functioning and his ability to make these appropriately apparent in identifying and dealing with issues will, by and large, determine the extent to which the group will be able to learn these processes and incorporate them into their functioning.

The extent and quality of the leader's receptivity to looking at himself and his relations to others, his freedom to participate in the learning and growth process, his ability to share perceptions, and his openness to exploring all aspects of his functioning in the group, will either make learning and growth possible and a less threatening expectation for members, or confirm the many doubts and distortions they bring to the experience. The leader cannot expect from his group what he is not willing or able to do himself.

Problems of the Schizophrenic

Several aspects of the task-oriented group seem to bring into focus particular problems of the schizophrenic patient. First, decision-making is particularly difficult, especially the decision regarding task choice. There seems to be little question that groups expect the staff leader to make the choice for them. Some groups have insisted that this be done while others have behaved as though this was what they both wanted and expected. Groups have discussed their anxieties and conflicts about decision-making, and these discussions suggest that problems in this area are related to dependency needs, fear of responsibility, and the ultimate unacceptability of any decision they might make. It would seem that since they conceptualize themselves as worthless and "bad", any decision they make as well as its implementation will be worthless and "bad" and reflect basic ineptness and inadequacy. It would also seem they expect authority (the parental figure) to find any decision they make unacceptable and inadequate. However, groups resent and may forcefully reject any task choice suggestion made by the leader. Ambivalence with regard to dependency, coupled with problems related to self-concept, compose one of the major conflictual areas which need to be worked through before meaningful growth can occur. Some of these findings would seem to support Fairweather's hypothesis that the dependency needs of the psychotic contraindicate staff leadership in task-oriented groups.

More recently we have been experimenting with a standard task for each beginning group in an effort to assess the extent to which decision-making problems may be altered or reduced when task choice is not an initial requirement. It is further hoped that such a procedure may lead to the development of a group diagnostic implement. However, the issue is not so much whether we deny or gratify the patient's dependency needs but rather how we can teach decision-making. It seems reasonable to conjecture that teaching such skills is a problem because of our limited understanding of the full nature of blocks to learning and thus our inability to identify and utilize techniques and procedures which facilitate learning.

Second, expectations of a shared group are frightening. It is as though fluid ego boundaries and difficulties in perceiving self as separate from others makes the closeness inherent in the small group an additional threat to identity. For some patients there is also the expectation that narcissistic needs will be frustrated and that sharing in a group will deny dependency needs. In addition, anticipation of shared doing seems to represent a threat to the schizophrenic's defenses and orientation. However, the structured, predictable aspects of the task and engagement with non-human objects increase opportunities for supportive consensual validation of observable abilities and facilitates identification of those perceptions that they share in common.

Third, great difficulty is experienced in problem-solving. Although some of the dilemmas operant in problem-solving are obviously related to dependency needs and authority relationships, difficulties which emerge in these groups suggest also that many patients have never learned even the basic procedures for identifying problems and exploring possible solutions, or have lost the ability to appropriately perceive and organize perceptions into logical concepts.

The combined thinking and doing, the cognitive perceptual skills at both the motor and verbal level inherent in the product of these groups, seem to bring clearly into focus disturbances and abilities in thinking and learning.

Fears associated with learning and related conflicts, disturbances in cognition, and resultant dysfunction become readily evident. By the same token, the structure and focus of these groups make possible a sense of competence and learning less conflictual, the task providing evidence of movement toward achievement. Furthermore, task activity furthermore creates opportunities to engage and relate in a more concrete way making it possible to be involved at a conceptual level commensurate with current capacities rather than consistently requiring a higher symbolic thinking

order. The task also facilitates gradation of learning. As we become more knowledgeable about blocks to learning and their impact on function, we should be able to articulate more meaningfully related learning experiences and use more fully the potential of the task-oriented group.

Finally, two generalized responses have been evident in these groups. There are those who find expectations of doing, the intrinsic action, learning and responsibilities, very threatening. These patients place a high premium on talking about their problems, and intellectualization is used as a way of avoiding the more hazardous and fearful doing of a task. These groups have great difficulty arriving at a choice of task, and such a decision may be prolonged for an inordinate period of time. Other patients seem driven to an excessive emphasis on the task, to a flight into activity as a means of avoiding bringing problems into awareness and working them through. Furthermore, there would seem to be a correlation between the leader's characteristic way of functioning, what he perceives as the more important "therapeutic set" and a group's sustained focus or movement toward a more equitable balance between these two responses.

One further observation would seem to be useful, and this relates to the kind of task choices made by groups. There seems to be an identifiable relationship between the task selected by a group, the level and nature of their primary emotional needs, and the conflicts surrounding those needs. Furthermore, task choice seems to reflect the group's progress or regression. Further study of this phenomenon should increase our understanding of need-gratifying processes and enhance our ability to make growth potential opportunities available to the patients.

Returning the schizophrenic patient to the community as a potentially productive, contributing member with an increased capacity to sustain such a role, is a multi-faceted, complex problem. The task-oriented group represents one of many attempts to reduce the problem. It seems that at least it provides a structure wherein dysfunction can be observed and explored. Hopefully these and other explorations will make it possible to ultimately articulate more clearly the essential factors of remedial processes. As we become increasingly able to inter-relate psychodynamic and sociologic concepts, as we enhance our knowledge of the cognitive process and its relationships to intrapsychic phenomena and overt behavior, our efforts may come closer to realizing the ultimate goal of satisfactory community living for our patients.

Acknowledgment

The author is indebted to Dr. Lothar Gidro-Frank and Dr. Eugene Friedberg for their interested support and to Miss Patricia Mayer, OTR, whose creative thinking and skillful leadership contributed so much to our learning.

References

1. Sullivan HS. Socio-psychiatric research: its implications for the schizophrenic problem and mental hygiene. *Am J Psychiat.* 1931;10.

2. Stanton AH, Schwartz MS. *The Mental Hospital.* New York: Basic Books; 1954.

3. Caudill W. *The Psychiatric Hospital as a Small Society.* Cambridge, Mass: Harvard University Press; 1958.

4. Jones M. *The Therapeutic Community: A New Treatment Method in Psychiatry.* New York: Basic Books; 1953.

5. Cummings J, Cummings E. *Ego and Milieu.* New York: Atherton Press; 1963.

6. Edelson M. *Ego Psychology, Group Dynamics and the Therapeutic Community.* New York: Grune & Stratton; 1964.

7. Slavison S. *Group Psychoanalytic Psychotherapy.* New York: International University Press; 1964.

8. Wolf A. The psychoanalysis of groups. *Am J Psychother.* 1949;3.

9. Bach G. *Intensive Group Psychotherapy.* New York: The Ronald Press; 1954.

10. Mullan H, Rosenbaum M. *Group Psychotherapy, Theory and Practice.* Glencoe Free Press; 1962.

11. Lewin K. *Dynamic Theory of Personality.* New York: McGraw Hill; 1945.

12. Schien E, Bennis W. *Personal and Organizational Change Through Group Methods.* New York: John Wiley & Sons; 1965:357-368.

13. Bradford L, Gibb J, Benne K. T. *Group Theory & Laboratory Method.* New York: John Wiley & Sons; 1964.

14. Fairweather GW. *Social Psychology in Treating Mental Illness.* New York: John Wiley & Sons; 1964.

15. Ibid, 14.

16. Ibid, 6.

17. Morton RB. The uses of the laboratory method in a psychiatric hospital. In: *Personal and Organizational Change Through Group Methods.*

18. Johnson DL, Hanson PG, Rothaus R, Morton RB, Lyle E, Moyer R. Follow up evaluation of human relation training for psychiatric patients. In: *Personal and Organizational Change Through Group Methods.*

19. Fidler JW. Group psychotherapy of psychotics. *Am J Orthopsychiat. 1965*;35(4).

The Concept and Use of Developmental Groups

Anne Cronin Mosey, PhD, OTR

Developmental groups are task-oriented groups structured in such a manner as to stimulate the various types of nonfamilial groups usually encountered in the normal development process. Five types have been identified:

1. Parallel
2. Project
3. Egocentric-cooperative
4. Cooperative
5. Mature

The concept of developmental groups was formulated in an attempt to apply recapitulation of ontogeny in the treatment of patients who are deficient in their ability to interact effectively in small groups. In dealing with this area of dysfunction, consecutive participation in the various types of developmental groups provides a framework for planned change. Group experiences are graded so as to provide opportunities for acquisition of basic group interaction skills. It is suggested that learning occurs through reinforcement of behaviors or approximation of behaviors that are necessary for successful participation in a given type of developmental group and nonreinforcement of behaviors that are inconsistent with successful participation.

A subtle change in orientation seems to be taking place among practitioners and scientists. There is movement away from the medical model, with its focus on concepts of pathology, toward an organization of thinking and effort around the concepts of growth. Scientists have shown renewed interest in exploring the development of various mature human capacities (here referred to as skills) and identifying factors that promote or cause development of these skills. Practitioners are beginning to think in terms of lags, deficits, or deviations in the normal developmental process. Classical diagnostic categories are being discarded for a more functional delineation of areas of adequate development and areas in which there is need for continued or redirected development.[1]

Treatment that emphasizes the nurturing of growth rests upon three major postulates:

1. Deviations in development can be altered.[2]
2. Subskills fundamental to mature adaptive skills must be acquired in a sequential manner.[3]
3. Mature adaptive skills can be acquired through participation in situations that simulate those interactions between individual and environment believed to be responsible for the sequential development of a given adaptive skill.[4]

It is out of this orientation, of treatment as recapitulation of ontogeny, that the concept of "developmental groups" has been formulated. It is presented principally as a heuristic device for discussing one facet of patient care.

Description of Developmental Groups

Developmental groups are clinical simulations of the various types of nonfamilial groups usually encountered in the normal developmental process.[5] These groups and their community-based counterparts are described as task-oriented and primary. Task-oriented refers to members' active engagement in the accomplishment of a definable project or task.[6] "A primary group is a face-to-face organization of individuals who cooperate for certain common ends, who share some common ideas and patterns of behavior, who have confidence in and some degree of affection for each other, and who are aware of their similarities of bonds of association."[7] The family (in its ideal form) is one example of a primary group. However, there are many nonfamilial groups that have the above listed characteristics. It is this type of group that is of concern in this paper.

Five types of developmental groups have been identified: parallel, project, egocentric-cooperative, cooperative and mature.[8] In a clinical setting, they would be described as follows:

A parallel group is made up of an aggregate of patients who are involved in individual tasks with minimal necessity for interaction. Group members may act as sources of stimulation for one another or tentatively test the effect of their behavior on others. However, task accomplishment does not require interaction. The therapist provides assistance with tasks and takes responsibility for meeting the social-emotional needs of each member.

In a project group, members are involved in common, short-term tasks that require some interaction, cooperation, and competition. The task is paramount. Mutual interaction outside the task is not expected. The therapist provides or assists the group in selecting tasks that require interaction of two or more persons for completion. He or she responds to the social-emotional needs of group members.

Egocentric-cooperative groups are characterized by group members selecting, implementing, and executing relatively long-term tasks through joint interaction. The task remains central, but satisfaction of some social-emotional needs of fellow group members is encouraged. There is emphasis on the reciprocal satisfaction that can be gained by responding to others' needs. The therapist gives support and guidance relative to the task and continues to satisfy a considerable portion of each member's emotional needs.

In a cooperative group, members are encouraged to identify and gratify each other's social-emotional needs in conjunction with task accomplishment. This type of group often includes only members of the same sex. The therapist acts primarily in the role of an advisor and may not be present at all group meetings.

A mature group is heterogeneous in composition and characterized by members taking those task and social-emotional roles that are required for adequate group functioning. Maintenance of a proper balance between productivity and personal need satisfaction is stressed. The therapist interacts as a coequal group member.

Division of developmental groups into five types is arbitrary—an attempt to provide demarcation points. It is more accurate to perceive these groups as being on a continuum. Thus, in the clinical setting, a given group may be best described as standing somewhere between two adjacent types of developmental groups.

When used in the treatment process, developmental groups are seen as agents of planned change. It is postulated that change occurs through the individual experiencing the consequence of his behavior in the group setting.[9] Developmental groups are so structured that adaptive behavior leads to a positive reinforcing stimulus while maladaptive behavior does not. A positive reinforcing stimulus is an event that causes need reduction. The need may be outer-directed as in the need for companionship, or inner-directed as in the need to be competent.[10]

Treatment of Group Interaction Skill Deficiency

The concept of developmental groups was formulated originally to delineate and describe a method of treating deficiency in group interaction skill. It grew out of the attempt to apply recapitulation of ontogeny in the treatment of patients who were deficient in their ability to interact effectively in small groups. Although developmental groups may be utilized in other areas (which will be briefly discussed later) they are seen as particularly useful in treatment of inadequate development of group interaction skill.

Group interaction skill is here considered to be an adaptive skill. It is defined, in its mature form, as the ability to participate in a variety of groups in a manner that is satisfying for oneself and for one's fellow group members. It is postulated that this skill develops sequentially, each stage in its development being marked by acquisition of behavior that is required for adequate participation in the community-based counterpart of the five types of developmental groups. It is further postulated that group interaction skill is acquired through participation in these various types of groups in conjunction with the opportunity to experience the consequences of appropriate and inappropriate behavior.[11]

It is beyond the scope of this paper to give a detailed description of evaluative methods for group interaction skill. Ideally, the therapist and patient collaborate in identifying what stages of this skill the patient has successfully integrated. Pertinent information may be acquired by observation of the patient in a group situation and discussion with the patient about his participation in groups outside the clinical setting. Evaluation also involves identifying what behavior the patient needs to acquire for successful interaction in small groups and current behavior that is interfering with successful participation.

The therapist must determine when deficiency in group interaction skill will be dealt with in the treatment process. The criterion suggested for making this judgment is treatment is initiated when the patient shows evidence of having acquired those abilities or skills that are normally learned prior to involvement in nonfamilial groups. The first step in treatment is engagement of the patient in that type of developmental group that is compatible or nearly compatible with his current capacity for meaningful group interaction.

Briefly, the treatment process consists of providing positive reinforcers for behaviors or approximation of behaviors that are necessary for successful participation in a given type of developmental group and withholding positive reinforcers for behaviors that are inconsistent with successful participation. These predetermined consequences are believed to be the central factor in bringing about change. The developmental group provides the structure; it sets and defines classes of behavior that are to be learned. Participation in a developmental group in and of itself is not conducive to planned behavioral change. Participation must be concurrent with deliberate and controlled reinforcement.

There are several methods that the therapist may use to increase the probability of the patient emitting desirable behaviors so that they can be reinforced. The method or methods selected will be determined primarily by the other adaptive skills available to the patient and his fellow group members. The most primitive method is simply to wait until the patient exhibits an approximation of the behavior he needs to acquire. This behavior is differentially reinforced as it moves in the direction of becoming an affective behavior pattern. Other initiating methods are:

1. Encouraging imitation of the therapist or other group members.

2. Suggesting specific patterns of behavior to the patient.

3. Identifying the patient's ineffectual responses and encouraging him to experiment with other forms of behavior.

4. Group discussion regarding the behavior of self and others with mutual encouragement for engaging in appropriate and effective group behavior.

5. Experimentation with various behaviors through role-playing exercises.[12]

Pragmatically, the therapist uses those initiating methods that appear to be successful.

An effort is made in all developmental groups to engage the patients in helping each other to acquire group interaction skill. Patients are encouraged to give and withhold reinforcers on the basis of the behavior exhibited by fellow group members. In order for patients to function as ancillary therapists, they must be able to comprehend what behavior is appropriate for a given type of developmental group and have sufficient self-control to give and withhold reinforcing stimuli. If it is deemed appropriate, the initial phase of treatment may be devoted to helping group members take on this ancillary therapist role.

Treatment continues to take place within the context of a specific type of developmental group until the patient has acquired the ability to function effectively in that group. He is then ready to begin learning the behavior that is necessary for competent functioning in the next, sequentially more advanced, developmental group. Depending upon the particular clinical situation and the extent to which the patient's fellow group members have progressed in an analogous manner, the patient is either placed in a new group or his original group as a whole is altered in the direction of the next type of developmental group. Treatment continues as previously outlined.

The treatment of deficiency in group interaction skill is terminated when any of the following criteria are met:

1. The patient has attained the ability to function in the type of group that is typical for his age.

2. He is able to participate in the kinds of groups that he is likely to encounter in his community environment (given its culture and the patient's preferred lifestyle).

3. The patient appears to be able to continue the development of group interaction skill outside the treatment situation.

Additional Comments

The concept of developmental groups was formulated in the attempt to apply recapitulation of ontogeny in the treatment of patients who were deficient in their ability to interact effectively in small groups. This concept may prove useful in three other areas. These areas are:

1. Treatment of deficiency in other adaptive skills.
2. Meeting mental health needs.
3. Describing the evolution of small groups.

Many of the subskills that are fundamental to the development of mature, adaptive skills are acquired through interaction in the familial group. These are usually the most basic or primitive subskills. However, more advanced subskills are often learned in the context of nonfamilial groups. The familial group may, indeed, continue to play a strongly supportive role, but interaction in nonfamilial groups is essential for adequate learning. (Treatment of those subskills that are usually developed within the family group is outside the scope of this paper.) In regard to those subskills that are partially or completely acquired through interaction in nonfamilial groups, it is suggested that they can be learned most easily through participation in a group that is structurally similar to the type of group in which the subskills are normally acquired. The concept of developmental groups could be used as a guide for selecting and forming appropriate groups. The difference between using developmental groups in the treatment of group interaction skill deficiency and deficiency in other adaptive skills is one of focus. The therapist would be primarily concerned with regulating reinforcement of behavior specific to the skill being learned as opposed to concentrating on helping the patient to learn how to function in the group. These two foci are not mutually exclusive, but it may be useful to deal with them as such to clarify treatment goals and methods.

That area of patient care here identified as meeting mental health needs refers to patient-therapist-nonhuman object interactions that are directed toward satisfying the normal human needs of the patient and maintaining his ability and desire to function.[13] The majority of mental health needs are most successfully met in a small group situation. However, needs cannot be satisfied unless there is synchronization of the individual's capacity to function in a particular group and the demands inherent in the structure of that group. In attempting to meet mental health needs, it is suggested that the therapist structure groups along a developmental continuum and that patients be encouraged to become involved in the type of group that is compatible with their group interaction skill. When a developmental group is oriented to satisfying mental health needs, the therapist is not concerned with bringing about a predetermined change in the patient's behavior. Therefore, the process of providing and withholding reinforcement is minimally important. The purpose of the group is to give pleasure, to have fun, to enjoy.

Preliminary, and somewhat superficial, observation indicates that the concept of developmental groups could be a useful tool in describing the evolution of task-oriented groups. This observation is not restricted to patient groups. As a task-oriented group moves toward becoming an effective working unit, there appear to be sequential patterns of interaction that are similar in many respects to the five types of developmental groups. Further study of this phenomenon may provide useful information for those persons who are concerned with facilitating the maturation and productivity of task-oriented groups.

The concept of developmental groups has been presented as a heuristic device. It is meant to stimulate interest and to encourage discovery. Its usefulness will be confirmed or refuted as we learn more about the human growth process, this entity that we call illness or dysfunction, and the effectiveness of treatment founded on the principles of recapitulation of ontogeny.

References

1. A. Jean Ayres, "Perceptual Motor Dysfunction in Children," paper presented at the Ohio Occupational Therapy Association Conference, 1964; John Flavell, The Developmental Psychology of Jean Piaget (New York: D. Van Nostrand Company, 1963); Anne Mosey, Occupational Therapy: Theory and Practice (printed through support of R.S.A. Training Grant No. 543-T-65 by Pothier Brothers, Medford, MA 1968); Maya Pines, "Why Some 3-Year Olds Get A's-and Some Get C's", The New York Times Magazine , July 6, 1969; Kenneth Overly, "Developmental Theory and Occupational Therapy-Considerations for Research," paper presented at the American Occupational Therapy Association Convention, Portland, Oregon, 1968; Marguerite Sechehaye, A New Psychotherapy in Schizophrenia (New York: Grune and Stratton, 1965).

2. Overly, "Developmental Theory and Occupational Therapy...."

3. Flavell, The Developmental Psychology of Jean Piaget...

4. Ayres, "Perceptual Motor Dysfunction in Children"; Mosey, Occupational Therapy....

5. Mosey, Occupational Therapy....

6. Gail Fidler, "The Task-Oriented Group as a Context for Treatment", American Journal of Occupational Therapy, 23, (1969).

7. H. English and A. English, A Comprehensive Dictionary of Psychological and Psychoanalytic Terms (New York: David McKay Co., 1958).

8. Erik Erikson, Childhood and Society (New York: W.W. Norton and Co., 1950); Anna Freud, Normality and Pathology in Childhood (New York: International University Press, 1965); T. Parsons and R. Bales, Family, Socialization and the Interaction Process (Glencoe, IL: The Free Press, 1955); J. Pearce and S. Newton, The Conditions of Human Growth (New York: Citadel Press, 1963).

9. C. Ferster and M. Perrott, Behavior Principles (New York: Appleton-Century-Crofts, 1961); Gregory Kimble, Hilgard and Margis' Conditioning and Learning (New York: Appleton-Century-Crofts, 1961); B.F. Skinner, Science and Human Behavior (New York: The Macmillan Co., 1953); A. Smith and V. Tempone, "Psychiatric Occupational Therapy Within a Learning Theory Context", American Journal of Occupational Therapy (September-October 1968); Kenneth Spence, Behavior Theory and Conditioning (New Haven, CT: Yale University Press, 1956).

10. Spence, Behavior Theory and Conditioning...

11. Parsons and Bales, Family, Socialization, and the Interaction Process; George Mead, Mind, Self and Society (Chicago, IL: University of Chicago Press, 1934); Theodore Mills, The Sociology of Small Groups (Englewood Cliffs, NJ: Prentice-Hall, 1963).

12. Fidler, "The Task-Oriented Group...."

13. G. Fidler and J. Fidler, Occupational Therapy: A Communication Process in Psychiatry (New York: The Macmillan Company, 1963).

Appendix C

Summary of Mosey's Adaptive Skills

Sensory Integration Skill: The ability to receive, select, combine, and coordinate vestibular, proprioceptive, and tactile information for functional use.

1. The ability to integrate the tactile subsystems (birth-3 months).
2. The ability to integrate primitive postural reflexes (3-9 months).
3. Maturation of mature righting and equilibrium reactions (9-12 months).
4. The ability to integrate the two sides of the body, to be aware of body parts and their relationship, and to plan gross motor movements (1-2 yr).
5. The ability to plan fine motor movements (2-3 yr).

Cognitive Skill: The ability to perceive, represent, and organize sensory information for the purpose of thinking and problem-solving.

1. The ability to use inherent behavioral patterns for environmental interaction (birth-1 month).
2. The ability to interrelate visual, manual, auditory, and oral responses (1-4 months).
3. The ability to attend to the environmental consequence of actions with interest, to represent objects in an exoceptual manner, to experience objects, to act on the bases of egocentric causality, and to seriate events in which the self is involved (4-9 months).
4. The ability to establish a goal and intentionally carry out means, to recognize the independent existence of objects, to interpret signs, to imitate new behavior to apprehend the influence of space, and to perceive other objects as partially causal (9-12 months).

5. The ability to use trial-and-error problem-solving, to use tools, to perceive variability in spatial positions, to seriate events in which the self is not involved, and to perceive the causality of other objects (12-18 months).
6. The ability to represent objects in an image manner, to make believe, to infer a cause given its effect, to act on the bases of combined spatial relations, to attribute omnipotence to others, and to perceive objects as permanent in time and place (18 months-2 yr).
7. The ability to represent objects in an endoceptual manner, to differentiate between thought and action, and to recognize the need for causal sources (2-5 yr).
8. The ability to represent objects in a denotative manner, to perceive the viewpoint of others, and to decenter (6-7 yr).
9. The ability to represent objects in a connotative manner, to use formal logic, and to work in the realm of the hypothetical (11-13 yr).

Dyadic Interaction Skill: The ability to participate in a variety of dyadic relationships.

1. The ability to enter into trusting familial relationships (8-10 months).
2. The ability to enter into association relationships (3-5 yr).
3. The ability to interact in an authority relationship (5-7 yr).
4. The ability to interact in a chum relationship (10-14 yr).
5. The ability to enter into a peer, authority relationship (15-17 yr).

6. The ability to enter into an intimate relationship (18-25 yr).

7. The ability to engage in a nurturing relationship (20-30 yr).

Group Interaction Skill: The ability to engage in a variety of primary groups.

1. The ability to participate in a parallel group (18 months-2 yr).

2. The ability to participate in a project group (2-4 yr).

3. The ability to participate in an egocentric group (9-12 yr).

4. The ability to participate in a cooperative group (9-12 yr).

5. The ability to participate in a mature group (15-18 yr).

Self-Identity Skill: The ability to perceive the self as a relatively autonomous, holistic, and acceptable person who has permanence and continuity over time.

1. The ability to perceive the self as a worthy person (9-12 months).

2. The ability to perceive the assets and limitations of the self (11-15 yr).

3. The ability to perceive the self as self-directed (20-25 yr).

4. The ability to perceive the self as a productive, contributing member of a social system (30-35 yr).

5. The ability to perceive the self as having an autonomous identity (35-50 yr).

6. The ability to perceive the aging process of oneself and ultimate death as part of the life cycle (45-60 yr).

Sexual Identity Skill: The ability to perceive one's sexual nature as good and to participate in a relatively long-term sexual relationship that is oriented to the mutual satisfaction of sexual needs.

1. The ability to accept and act on the basis of one's pregenital sexual nature (4-5 yr).

2. The ability to accept sexual maturation as a positive growth experience (12-16 yr).

3. The ability to give and receive sexual gratification (18-25 yr).

4. The ability to enter into a sustained sexual relationship characterized by the mutual satisfaction of sexual needs (20-30 yr).

5. The ability to accept the sex-related physiological changes that occur as a natural part of the aging process (40-60 yr).

Reprinted with permission from Mosey, A. (1986). *Psychosocial components of occupational therapy* (pp. 416-418). New York: Raven Press.

Excerpts From the *Occupational Therapy Practice Framework*

PERFORMANCE AREAS OF OCCUPATION				
ADL	**IADL**	**EDUCATION**	**WORK**	**LEISURE**
Bathing, showering	Care of Others (arranging, supervising care)	Formal Educational Participation	Employment Interests and Pursuits	Leisure Exploration (identifying interests, skills, opportunities)
Bowel and Bladder Participation Management (control)	Care of Pets	Informal Information Seeking/ Skill Development	Employment Seeking and Acquisition	Leisure (planning, doing, balancing)
Dressing	Child Rearing	Informal Personal Education Participation	Job Performance	
Eating	Communication Device Use		Retirement Preparation and Adjustment	**PLAY**
				Play Exploration
Feeding	Community Mobility	**SOCIAL PARTICIPATION**	Volunteer Exploration	Play Participation
Functional Mobility	Financial Management	Interactions with others/social groups	Volunteer Participation	
Personal Device Care	Health Management and Maintenance	Community (neighborhood, work, school)		
Personal Hygiene and Grooming	Home Establishment and Management	Family (roles & activities)		
Sexual Activity	Meal Preparation and Cleanup	Peer Friend (different levels of intimacy, sexual partners)		
Sleep/Rest	Safety Procedures and Emergency Responses			
Toilet Hygiene	Shopping			

PERFORMANCE SKILLS			CLIENT FACTORS	
MOTOR SKILLS	**PROCESS SKILLS**	**COMMUNICATION/ INTERACTION**	**BODY FUNCTIONS**	**BODY STRUCTURES**
<u>Posture:</u> stabilizes, aligns, positions (in task performance)	<u>Energy:</u> sustained attention and pace in task performance	<u>Physicality:</u> use of physical body when communicating	<u>Mental Functions:</u> consciousness sleep, orientation, motivation, attention/concentration, perception, reasoning and abstract thought, judgment, insight, language, calculation, emotional range and expression, sense of self (concept, esteem)	<u>Nervous System</u>
<u>Mobility:</u> walking, wheelchair, reaching/carrying objects, flexibility	<u>Knowledge:</u> use of task-related knowledge in choosing tools and materials, using goal-directed task actions, seeking needed direction	<u>Information Exchange:</u> giving and receiving information within an occupation (articulates, asserts, asks, engages, expresses, modulates, shares, speaks, sustains speech)		<u>Eye, Ear, and Related Structures</u>
<u>Coordination:</u> smooth, skilled movements in manipulating objects and performing tasks	<u>Temporal Organization:</u> initiates, sequences, continues, and completes tasks	<u>Relations:</u> maintains appropriate relationships within an occupation (collaborates, conforms, focuses, rapport, respect)	<u>Sensory Functions and Pain</u>	<u>Cardiovascular, Immunological, Respiratory Systems</u>
<u>Strength and Effort</u>	<u>Organizing Space and Objects:</u> searching and locating task-related materials, organization and sequencing use of tools, cleaning and storing appropriately		<u>Neuromusculo-skeletal and Movement-Related Functions</u>	<u>Digestive System Structures</u>
<u>Energy</u>	<u>Adaptation:</u> noting and correcting errors in task performance anticipating consequences		<u>Cardiovascular, Hematological, Immunological, and Respiratory System Function</u>	<u>Genitourinary and Reproductive Systems</u> <u>Structures Related To Movement</u> <u>Skin and Related Structures</u>

CONTEXTS		PERFORMANCE PATTERNS		
CULTURAL Customs, beliefs, activity patterns, behavior standards, expectations of society	**PHYSICAL** Objects, natural or built environments, including sensory qualities	**HABITS** Useful habits (support daily function) Impoverished habits (not well established) Dominating habits (interfere with daily functioning)	**ROUTINES** Well learned sequences, tasks performed repeatedly	**ROLES** Socially defined sets of behaviors (i.e., parent, worker, etc.)
SOCIAL Availability and expectations of significant individuals, social groups, social norms, role expectations, social routines	**PERSONAL** Age, gender, socio-economic status, education	**ACTIVITY DEMANDS**		
		Objects and their properties	Space Demands: related to physical context	Social Demands: related to cultural and social contexts
SPIRITUAL Fundamental orientation of person's life, motivation, inspiration	**TEMPORAL** Stages of life, time of year/month/day Duration of occupational performance	Sequence and Timing Required Body Structures	Required Actions	Required Body Functions
VIRTUAL E-mail, telephone, or other means of communication without physical contact				

Reprinted from American Occupational Therapy Association. (2002). Occupational therapy practice framework: Domain and process. *American Journal of Occupational Therapy, 56*, 609-639. © 2002 by the American Occupational Therapy Association, Inc. Reprinted with permission.

Group Leadership Guidelines in Six Frames of Reference

Frame of Reference	Structure	Goals	Leadership	Activities
Psychodynamic	Loosely structured, task oriented	Develop ego skills, gain insight; emotional and spiritual dimensions	Facilitative	Creative/expressive media, free choice of tasks/activities
Behavioral Cognitive	Highly structured	Specific, observable, measurable; learning skills, changing thoughts and behaviors	Directive	Educational sessions, worksheets, skill learning and practice
Allen's Cognitive Disabilities	Highly structured, groups of similar cognitive level	Ongoing evaluation, problem solving in activities of daily living, building safe environments and habits	Directive	Crafts and tasks of daily life in specific environments
Developmental	Structured around age-specific tasks and skills	Skill mastery, altering life structure, making transitions, establishing growth-facilitating environments	Directive or facilitative	Graded tasks addressing age-appropriate activities, life review
Sensorimotor	Highly structured sequence of sensorimotor activities	Stimulate development of central nervous system, adaptive functioning, normalize movement patterns, sensory integration	Directive	Movement and sensory stimulation, activities and games with minimal or graded cognitive demands

Frame of Reference	Structure	Goals	Leadership	Activities
Model of Human Occupation	Members grouped by common or expected roles, clients choose structure	Restore order in daily occupations, re-establish occupational roles, develop healthy routines, person-environment fit	Facilitator or adviser, consultant	Everyday tasks, work, play and self-care, establishing/restoring meaningful roles in families, social groups, and the community

Overview of the *International Classification of Function, Disability, and Health*, Second Edition

The purpose of the *International Classification of Function, Disability, and Health* (ICF) is to provide a common language and framework for the description of health and health-related states. The two key terms, "functioning" and "disability," are defined as follows. Functioning refers to body functions, activities, and participation. Disability refers to impairments, activity limitations, and participation restrictions. The definitions of all components of health domains and contexts enables health care workers of many disciplines (including occupational therapy) to provide a complete picture of clients with health conditions and to share useful information with others throughout the world. The classification system provides a basis for the global collection of health statistics and research and a tool for clinicians, social policy makers, and educators.

In 2001, the World Health Organization (WHO) updated its classification system to include both positive and negative aspects of health. Formerly, this global classification document focused on impairments, disabilities, and handicaps as a way to identify persons needing health care services. The updated version particularly relates to occupational therapy in its consideration of well-being and prevention in addition to the consequence of disease. Much of the language of ICF was incorporated into the *Occupational Therapy Practice Framework* (American Occupational Therapy Association [AOTA], 2002), including a broad range of activities, a hierarchy of task demands, a focus on participation, and an acknowledgment of contextual factors.

The ICF is divided into two parts, each with two components. Part 1, Functioning and Disability, includes: (1) body functions and structures and (2) activities and participation. Part 2, Contextual Factors, includes: (1) environmental and (2) personal factors. The global paradigm shift in healthcare is apparent in the ICF's inclusion of both positive and negative factors of each health or contextual factor identified. This new, holistic perspective moves beyond the medical model to the public health arena where environmental factors within the system may act as facilitators or barriers to an individual's full participation in life. The classification system lists, codes, and defines each component, and in some cases, provides a rating scale for the status of a component with percentages or ranges of severity, such as the extent of vision loss or the degree of difficulty with climbing stairs. The eight components of the ICF are as follows:

1. Body functions—Mental (learning) and physical (walking) functions of the body systems that are categorized under "client factors" in the *Occupational Therapy Practice Framework*.

2. Body structures—Include the body's anatomy (organs, limbs), also a part of "client factors."

3. Impairments—Problems with body functions or structures that are the result of some health condition and may or may not cause a disability for the client.

4. Activity—The execution of a task. The *Occupational Therapy Practice Framework* refers to this concept as "occupation."

5. Participation—"Involvement in a life situation" (p. 123), a definition that is adopted by the *Occupational Therapy Practice Framework.*

6. Activity limitations—Refers to the negative aspect of activity, formerly called occupational performance deficits in the occupational therapy literature.

7. Participation restriction—The negative aspect that is known in occupational therapy as a "barrier."

8. Environmental factors, including physical, social, and attitudinal environments, are recategorized in The Occupational Therapy Practice Framework as the seven occupational performance contexts.

Occupational therapists need to be familiar with the language and categories of ICF, in order to:

- Perform needs assessments.
- Match treatments with specific conditions.
- Document accurately for reimbursement sources.
- Substantiate the need for intervention.
- Plan for community or job market re-entry.
- Evaluate intervention outcomes.
- Advocate effectively for client needs.
- Communicate effectively with other disciplines, clients, and public policy makers.

In reviewing the ICF, it becomes apparent that there are many parallels between this document and the occupational therapy profession. Global recognition of these familiar concepts (activity demand, participation, contextual facilitators and barriers) provides an inspiration to occupational therapists everywhere to expand the role of occupational therapy and to make others aware of the broad range of skills and services we offer as a profession.

Bibliography

American Occupational Therapy Association. (2002). Occupational therapy practice framework: Domain and process. *American Journal of Occupational Therapy, 56,* 609-639.

World Health Organization. (2001). *International classification of functioning, disability, and health* (2nd ed.). Geneva, Switzerland: Author.

Index

WAIT

...There's More!

SLACK Incorporated's Professional Book Division offers a wide selection of products in the field of Occupational Therapy. We are dedicated to providing important works that educate, inform and improve the knowledge of our customers. Don't miss out on our other informative titles that will enhance your collection.